Sports Medicine

Edited by J. G. P. Williams
MA, MB, BChir, FRCS, DPhysMed

Medical Director, Farnham Park Rehabilitation Centre;
Director of Department of Rehabilitation, Mount Vernon Hospital, Northwood and
Wexham Park Hospital, Slough; and Secretary General, International Federation of
Sports Medicine

and P. N. Sperryn
MB, BS, MRCP, DPhysMed

Consultant in Rheumatology and Rehabilitation, Hillingdon Hospital and Farnham
Park Rehabilitation Centre; Honorary Medical Adviser, British Amateur Athletic
Board; and Honorary Secretary, British Association of Sport and Medicine

Foreword by The Rt. Hon. The Lord Porritt GCMG, GCVO, CBE, FRCS
President, British Association of Sport and Medicine; formerly President, Royal
College of Surgeons of England; President, British Medical Association; President,
Medical Commission of I.O.C.

Second Edition

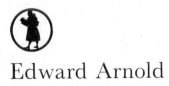

Edward Arnold

© J. G. P. Williams and P. N. Sperryn 1976

First published 1962
by Edward Arnold (Publishers) Ltd
25 Hill Street, London W1X 8LL

Second edition 1976

ISBN 0 7131 4275 8

Printed in Great Britain by Butler & Tanner Ltd
Frome and London

Contributors

James L. Kennerley Bankes, MB, FRCS, DO,
Consultant Ophthalmic Surgeon to St Mary's Hospital, London,
and the Western Ophthalmic Hospital, London.
Sub Dean for Postgraduate Studies, St Mary's Hospital
Medical School (University of London).

Hugh C. Burry, FRCP, FRACP, DPhysMed,
Wellington, New Zealand; Formerly Director, Department of
Rheumatology, Guy's Hospital, London, SE1.

Graeme D. Campbell, MB, ChB, FRCS, FRACS,
Visiting Surgeon, Waikato Hospital, Hamilton, New Zealand.

Brian Corrigan, MB, MRCP, FRACP, MRCPEd, DPhysMed,
Consultant in Rheumatic Disease,
North Shore Medical Centre,
New South Wales, Australia.

Norman Croucher,
Member of Sports Council (UK)
Member of Disabled Living Foundation Physical Recreation Panel.

Katharina Dalton, MRCGP,
Clinical Assistant, Department of Psychological Medicine,
University College Hospital, London.

Andrei Demeter, MD,
Professor of Physiology, Chief of the Department of Physiology,
Institute of Physical Education and Sports, Bucharest, Roumania.

Adrian Gagea, DiplElEng,
Professor of Physical Education,
Scientific Research Laboratory,
Institute of Physical Education and Sports, Bucharest, Roumania.

Ernst Jokl, MD,
Professor and Director, Exercise Research Laboratories,
Department of Allied Health, University of Kentucky Medical School,
Lexington, Kentucky, U.S.A.

John E. Kane, MEd, PhD,
Principal, Loughborough College of Education,
Loughborough, Leics.

D. E. Mackay, MD, DPH, Surgeon Captain, Royal Navy,
Consultant in Physiology, Royal Navy,
Staff Medical Officer, Flag Officer Sea Training.

Archibald McDougall, MB, ChB, FRCSE, FRFPS,
Consultant Orthopaedic Surgeon, The Victoria Infirmary, Glasgow.

Peter C. McIntosh, BA(Oxon), MA(B'ham)
Professor, School of Physical Education, University of Otago,
Dunedin, New Zealand.

W. R. McLoughlin, MSc,
Senior Lecturer in Physical Education,
St Mary's College, Twickenham, Middlesex.

J. A. Moncur, TD, MB, ChB, DPhysMed, DPE,
Medical Officer, Scottish School of Physical Education,
Jordanhill College, Glasgow.

W. P. Morgan, PhD,
Professor and Director, Ergopsychology Laboratory,
Department of Physical Education, University of Wisconsin, Madison, U.S.A.

David S. Muckle, MS, FRCS,
First Assistant in Traumology,
Radcliffe Infirmary, Oxford.

Dan Tunstall Pedoe, MA, MB, BChir, MRCP, DPhil,
Senior Lecturer and Honorary Consultant, St Bartholomew's Hospital;
Consultant Physician and Cardiologist, Hackney Hospital, London.

John Rayne, DPhil(Oxon), FDS, DOrth, RCS(Eng),
Consultant Oral Surgeon, Oxford Area Health Authority,
Clinical Lecturer Oral and Maxillo-Facial Surgery,
Oxford University Medical School, Oxford.

Henry Evans Robson, MB, BS, MRCS, LRCP,
General Practitioner, Loughborough, Leics.
Formerly Divisional Surgeon, St John's Ambulance.

Noel Roydhouse, VRD, MB(NZ), ChM(Otago), FRCS(Eng), FRACS,
Senior ENT Surgeon, Middlemore Hospital,
Auckland, New Zealand.

Ivan M. Sharman, PhD, CChem, FRIC,
Scientific Staff, Dunn Nutritional Laboratory, University of Cambridge,
and Medical Research Council, Cambridge.

Roy J. Shephard, MD, PhD,
Professor of Applied Physiology, Department of Preventive Medicine and Biostatistics,
Division of Community Health, Faculty of Medicine, University of Toronto, Toronto,
Canada.

Peter N. Sperryn, MB, BS, MRCP, DPhysMed,
Consultant in Rheumatology and Rehabilitation, Hillingdon Hospital, Middlesex, and
Farnham Park Rehabilitation Centre, Slough, Berks.

Harry Thomason, PhD, MSc, DLC,
Senior Lecturer (Human Performance Laboratory)
Physical Education Section, University of Salford, Lancs.

Howard C. Toyne, CBE, CStJ, MB, BS(Melb), FRCS, FRACS,
Senior Consultant Orthopaedic Surgeon, RAAF,
Melbourne, Victoria, Australia.

William Tuxworth, BA, CertEd (Birmingham),
Lecturer in Physical Education at the University of Birmingham, Birmingham.

Geoffrey Vanderfield, FRACS, FRCS,
Head of Department of Neurosurgery,
Royal Prince Alfred Hospital, Sydney, Australia.

John G. P. Williams, MA, MB, BChir, FRCSEd, DPhysMed,
Medical Director, Farnham Park Rehabilitation Centre;
Director of Department of Rehabilitation, Mount Vernon Hospital,
Northwood, Middlesex and Wexham Park Hospital, Slough, Berks.

Foreword

It is almost fifteen years since I wrote the foreword to the First Edition of this book. Those fifteen years have seen a phenomenal development in the field of 'Sports Medicine'—both in scope and general interest. This significant growth is fully reflected in this New Edition to which it is again my pleasure and privilege to write a brief foreword; a pleasure because I feel it will bring much interest and valuable information to both medical and lay readers, and a privilege because its substance bears upon a subject of increasing importance in today's mechanized and materialistic world—physical, mental and moral 'fitness'.

Of necessity it is a much bigger volume than its predecessor—as is the team of contributors which (under the able editorship of John Williams and Peter Sperryn, themselves major contributors) is now drawn from many parts of the world.

Again, as might be expected after the lapse of time between the two editions, scientific aspects of the subject bulk almost as largely as the clinical, but it maintains its basically practical approach to the general principles that must always underlie Sports Medicine.

This is well exemplified by the opening chapter—intriguingly entitled Sport in Society—which describes the historical inter-relationship of sport and health from ancient times up to today's Government controlled Sports Council. As before, one finds detailed and comprehensive descriptions of the various organs, tissues and areas of the body that may be affected by injuries and ailments—all copiously illustrated by photographs, x-rays, diagrams and graphs—and written by specialists in their particular field. But a wider vista is encompassed by consideration of such subjects as Environment, Biomechanics, Psychology, Doping, Nutrition, and First Aid—to say nothing of such interesting problems as sport for the disabled, for the young and 'not so young' and of course (essential in today's world!) for women.

Each chapter has a voluminous list of references and there is an excellent index. Indeed it is a comprehensive—I would venture to say unique—text-book, with contents of uniformly high standard and beautifully produced. It should provide interest, information and instruction to many people—not only medical men but also coaches, trainers and managers and the educated and intelligent public at large. I have no doubt it will be even more successful than its predecessor and I wish it well.

PORRITT
May 1976

Preface

The years since *Sports Medicine* was first published have seen a great expansion and development in all areas of the field. This expansion is reflected in the additional material which has had to be included in this new edition, and which has of necessity increased it in size. The development of interest in Sports Medicine throughout the English speaking world has made it appropriate to recruit a further Editor and a truly international panel of Contributors to whom we are most indebted for their invaluable contributions, without which this new edition could not have been realized.

At a time when systematic education in Sports Medicine in its widest sense is becoming accepted practice in many countries throughout the world, it is our intention here to offer a standard text covering all the relevant fields in a reasonable degree of depth. We have included extensive bibliographies both to assist our readers to follow up fields of particular interest and to indicate the wide variety of primary sources currently available.

We have based our text on the concept of Sports Medicine as an integrated multi-disciplinary field embracing the relevant areas of clinical medicine (sports traumatology, the medicine of sport and sports psychiatry) and the appropriate allied scientific disciplines (including physiology, psychology and biomechanics). In a book of this type it is clearly impossible to cover the whole subject in such a way as to satisfy every potential reader. We are ourselves aware of areas in the text which might be strengthened and developed in subsequent editions, and no doubt others will emerge from the experience of our readers.

While our text has been prepared specifically for medical practitioners, we hope that it will nevertheless prove useful to others working in or close to the field, physical educationists, physiotherapists, trainers and coaches.

We have been most fortunate in the extensive help and co-operation which we have received, not only from our contributors, but from the many others associated with the preparation of this book. We would like to express our warmest thanks to Lord Porritt, for many years a champion of Sports Medicine in the United Kingdom, not only for once again providing a Foreword to the book, but for his continuous guidance and encouragement. We would like to thank the Trustees and Council of the Winston Churchill Memorial Trust for their generosity which enabled us to study at first-hand and in depth two totally different systems of Sports Medicine during the periods of our Fellowships. We would like to thank all our friends and colleagues in the International Federation of Sports Medicine and the British Association of Sport and Medicine for their many most useful comments and suggestions for the preparation of this edition.

We have been much helped by Mr Derek Griffin, the photographer at Wexham Park Hospital, and by Mr E. D. Lacey from whom we have obtained many essential illustrations. Our various secretaries, Miss Diane Livesley, Mrs Barbara Farr, Mrs Judy Tipping and Mrs Sheila Overholt have laboured tirelessly in the production of the manuscript, and we have been singularly fortunate in the assistance given to us by Miss Barbara Koster of Edward Arnold (Publishers) Ltd. Last, but not least, we thank for their long-suffering patience our devoted wives to whom we dedicate this volume.

JW
PS

May 1976

Contents

1

Sport in society

Sport and medicine have been closely associated throughout recorded history. It is a natural relationship between client and professional adviser. As soon as sport develops out of spontaneous play into an organized activity, then practice for the competitive event takes place and the sportsman seeks systematic methods of preparation. He examines such technical and scientific information as is available about the way his body performs its athletic function and turns to the doctor as physiologist. But sport also involves injury. This may be no more serious than muscular stiffness or cramp but may on occasion be a very severe wound. The sportsman again turns to the doctor as clinician and pathologist to restore him to active competition as quickly as possible.

The interaction between sport and medicine is not all one way. Physical exercise, especially exercise taken to the limit of skill and endurance, excites the interest of the scientist and the clinician who on their own initiative feed back into sport the results of their pragmatic and scientific discoveries. The interaction between sport and medicine was particularly close in the world of the Greek city state in the fifth and fourth centuries B.C. A chance remark of Aristotle in a book on moral philosophy shows how close. He writes 'We argue about the navigation of ships more than about the training of athletes because it has been less well organized as a science.'[1] The Greeks were no fools at seafaring and the remark is highly significant. Unfortunately few of the original sources of medical advice upon sport from this period have survived. Hippocrates certainly had much to say both on clinical matters and on physiology. He appears to have been an advocate of moderation. 'Excessive and sudden filling or emptying or warming or chilling or otherwise stirring the body is dangerous.' 'Any excess is hostile to nature.'[2]

The relationship of diet to health and to athletic performance certainly was extensively studied but the chance survivals in extant literature hardly provide a coherent picture of Sports Medicine. Pausanias tells us of an Olympic victor in the long distance race of 480 B.C. who was the first to train on a meat diet. Cheese had previously been the staple source of protein. Xenophon says that athletes in training should avoid bread.[3] Later on, the moralists, headed by the playwright Euripides, condemned athletes as slaves to their jaws and victims of their bellies. But the condemnation seems to have been made on moral and social grounds rather than medical grounds.[4]

In the fifth and fourth century B.C. in Athens, Sparta and other city states, physical prowess was an ideal accepted by citizens and physical fitness was a necessity for a citizen army. Physical education of the young and physical training of the not so young were systematic and thorough. The three words used for trainers imply the use of massage, ointments and lubricants, as well as systematized exercise, and the trainers and coaches appear to have worked under some general medical direction. There were four famous athletic festivals at Olympia, Delphi, Isthmia and Nemea which attracted competitors from all over the Greek world and there were many local athletic and religious festivals such as the Panathenaic festival at Athens. There was therefore no lack of top class competition. There were wars, too, such as the disastrous one between Athens and Sparta from 431 to 404 B.C. in which athletes turned soldiers and medicine was devoted to the war wounded.

When the City of Rome extended her military empire over the whole Mediterranean world the nature of urban life changed. Cities of course increased in size. Rome in the first century A.D. had about the same number of inhabitants as Birmingham, England in the twentieth though confined in a much smaller space. Both military campaigns and athletic festivals became professionalized. The Medical profession now found itself with two groups of clients with somewhat different needs. There were on the one hand the professional performers whose livelihood depended on exploiting their physique and skill before spectators, and there were the ordinary city dwellers who were no longer called upon to fight or to work very hard—professional soldiers relieved them of the former burden and slaves of the latter. For these city dwellers keeping fit became a considerable problem.

As professional sport became more specialized so did its medical services. An attempt was made, for instance, to type athletes and relate performance to temperament and to physique. The physiology was based on the concept of opposing elements: hot and cold, wet and dry, combining in the four humours of the body; the blood, hot and wet; the bile, hot and dry; the phlegm, cold and dry; and black bile, cold and wet. Different mixtures in the body produced different temperaments: sanguine, choleric, phlegmatic or melancholic. Philostratus in the third century ruled out the melancholic from sport but recommended hard driving of the phlegmatic in training and restraint of the choleric who would try to train too quickly. The ideal performer will be the athlete of sanguine temperament. Today such a psychosomatic classification reads strangely, but 2000 years ago it was a serious attempt to systematize observations of athletic behaviour according to current concepts. Less justifiable were some discussions on diet particularly one on whether fish from swampy areas were better for the athlete than fish from the deep sea. 'Still further, the doctors brought on the flesh of swine with wondrous tales about it, directing that herds of swine down by the sea should be considered injurious on account of the sea garlic which grows in abundance along the shore and coast—the only kind of pigs they recommended eating while training were those fattened on cornel berries and acorns.'[5] Although the doctors were blamed by Philostratus for the introduction of this esoteric nonsense, there is some evidence that there was friction between coaches and trainers and the medical profession, because the latter felt that coaches were trespassing on fields which they did not understand. Galen, the most distinguished physician of the imperial era wrote a tirade against the pseudo-science of sport and the prostitution of training. Sport and medicine did not so much part company as war with each other.[6]

This friction, however, applied to professional sport only. The man in the Roman street had a way of life which involved sports medicine in a more mundane way. He had, in the first century A.D., 159 days of public holiday each year and a comparatively short working day. Much of his leisure was spent at 'The Baths'. These establishments varied in size and elaboration from modest private buildings to enormous muncipal multisport and social centres at which all manner of therapeutic and recreative exercise was taken. It was this urban way of life which stimulated Galen to write his major work on hygiene and his two shorter works on *Health—the Concern of Medicine of Gymnastics* and *Exercises with the Small Ball*. Altogether they represent a remarkable exposition of Sports Medicine. His discussion of the relationship between health medicine and gymnastics is particularly interesting. His conclusion that the art of health cannot be called either medicine or gymnastics is more than a semantic exercise. He is in fact trying to find a lasting relationship between sport and medicine within the context not of top class performance but of 'sport for all'.

The pattern of sport in our own day, dating, as it does from the stereotyping and organization of sports in the nineteenth century, has been accompanied by a corresponding growth in the contribution of medicine, both scientific and clinical, to sport. Indeed, a concern for health was itself one of the factors stimulating the development of some sports in that century. The Baths and Washhouses Act of 1846 enabled local authorities to build and manage swimming baths and many towns and boroughs took advantage of the legislation. A desire to improve the hygiene of rapidly growing Victorian towns clearly encouraged the provision of open spaces and parks for games and recreation. The main stimulus, however, came from a growing urban middle class who had initiative, leisure and resources to develop games and sports to meet their own needs. Cricket had already been organized by the aristocracy but was developed and expanded by the middle classes. Games of football, both Rugby and Association were adapted from a rural rough and tumble and refined under national codes of rules. Lawn tennis was invented for suburban gardens and club lawns. Other games and sports were similarly developed, stereotyped and organized under democratically constituted governing bodies. As leisure for wage earners increased (that is when Saturday became a half-holiday in the last quarter of the century) all sections of the population began to play and to watch these games and sports.

It would be foolish to press too far the analogy of sport in a city state of the fifth century B.C. and sport in Imperial Rome of the early centuries A.D. but there has certainly been in the present century a diminution of the need to take physical exercise in the life of ordinary men and women as there was in the urban communities of the Roman Empire. There has also been an increasing interest in sport on the part of central government in Great Britain, and in others, for political reasons. Thirdly the medical world has directed more and more attention to the relationship between sport and health in terms of both physiology and pathology.

On the diminution of casual exercise and its consequences little more need be said. One hundred years ago nearly everyone walked to work and at Christmas Mr. Pickwick and his friends took a walk of twenty-five miles to shake down one meal and prepare for another.[7] Today the use of public and private transport has had obvious physical effects on the city dwellers and also less obvious ones which are only now being scientifically discovered and assessed. Sport and physical recreation are an obvious source of exercise which is no longer obtained from going from one place to another. The relationship of sport to health therefore is increasing in importance and occupies the attention of the medical profession. At the same time the sedentary man finds that he is not fit enough to take part in the games which he enjoys and he seeks rehabilitation into sport especially after experiencing clinical symptoms which alarm him.

One of the most significant trends in the twentieth century has been the increase of interest by the central governments of nation states in sport. The interest of local government in providing facilities and opportunities is of longer standing. For 100 years, however, British Governments have been increasingly concerned at the inadequate physical fitness of young men recruited into the armed forces. The exigencies of two world wars accentuated the need for fitness. Both in the services and in civilian life the promotion of fitness and the design of systematized programmes of exercise to that end became matters of public policy. Since the 1930s, however, there has been a shift of emphasis. The desire for fitness is a powerful motivating force for exercise, but the routines of trunk and limb movements which are all that are necessary to extend the human system are not attractive and produce tedium which is self defeating. The Fitness Council set up by Act of Parliament in 1937 was a war casualty in 1939. The Central Council of Recreative Physical Training established in 1935 changed its name to the Central Council of Physical Recreation.[8]

When in 1964 the government of the day again took administrative action it was a Sports Council not a Fitness Council which emerged. At the following general election both major political parties made promises to develop sport and emphasized its contribution to the quality of life. In so far as military preparedness is still a concern of government it is now a by-product of participation in sport rather than a direct objective. Similarly the arguments of the 'thirties based upon physical training as a form of preventive medicine are no longer advanced in the crude and blatant form of that time. There is a general conviction and some meagre evidence that sport makes specific contributions to health, but sports science is not yet prepared to draw up a balance sheet. Sports medicine has in this sense advanced by taking a step backwards on to firmer ground whence it can respond with greater certainty to the claimant demands of peoples and governments to show that 'sport is good for you'. The Sports Council in 1971 produced a review of the needs of sport in the 'seventies and stated 'The economic costs of ill health, which could be attributable to lack of endurance fitness, have been studied extensively in the United States, West Germany and elsewhere, but as yet not in this country, though there is no reason to believe that our situation is very different. It is undoubtedly true that appropriate exercise could avoid hospitalization and the cost of other services in some cases as well as retaining the services of many individuals as active members of the community.'[9] There is little doubt either that expenditure by the government on sport will respond to scientific evidence of the positive connection between sport and health.

Meanwhile participation in sport by all and sundry increases. There are no sports showing a decline with the possible exception of boxing, but there are a number of sports which claim to be the fastest growing sport of the day. There are, it is true, certain groups of the population or sections of the population which are left behind. The parents of young children and particularly young mothers are underrepresented in the expansion of physical recreation, so too are those in the lower socio-economic groups. One of the functions of the Sports Council is to study the opportunities and facilities available and to ensure that no group is deprived against its wishes.[10] A sport which has developed as rapidly as any in the last twenty-five years is skiing. The expansion has taken place in mountainous countries but has not been confined to them. The same can be said of climbing, mountaineering and mountain walking. The first recorded ski competition was in 1767 in Norway, but skiing as a sport dates from the late nineteenth century.[11] Mountaineering and rock climbing as sports began a little earlier. The Alpine Club was founded in 1857. The first expedition on Welsh mountains to be recorded in the Alpine Journal took place in 1873.[12] In one hundred years the techniques of both climbing and skiing have developed to unforeseen levels, but it is the sophistication of present day equipment which would stagger the early pioneers of those sports. Sophistication, however, is not confined to one aspect; it has become a feature of all aspects, mountain rescue and emergency treatment of casualties as well as electronic timing and measuring. Both sports are fraught with danger at all levels of ability and both have high accident rates. So the mountaineer and the skier make their demands upon the doctor no less than upon the engineer and the designer of clothing. The same principle appears with less force in every sport.

There are special demands upon medical resources which emanate from sport at the highest level just because of the importance which has become attached to it. A few sports at this level manage to become commercially viable, among them Association football in Britain, baseball in the U.S.A. and ice hockey in Canada. They achieve financial success by attracting spectators. But in addition to those who pay the going price at the turnstiles are the unseen crowds of television viewers of an increasing number of sports. The Olympic Games in Munich in 1972 were visible by satellite to not less than eight-hundred million people. The advent of such a vast crowd of spectators through the mass media raises considerations not so much of profit as prestige. The Review of the work of the Sports Council 1966–9 stated 'Success in international events brings prestige and animates development of sport at all levels.'[13] The Sports Council's policy of financially supporting teams to take part in international events is supported by a research programme touching upon many aspects of sport which are directly related to policy decisions in general and success at the top in particular. The budget is small as yet, but so long as success in international sport is regarded as an important objective for national teams, all legitimate aids and scientific knowledge will be used.

The post war expansion of sport at all levels has had its repercussions upon the disabled as well as the able-bodied. Many disabled men and women have competed in different sports and by their own efforts have reached the centre court at Wimbledon or the Olympic arena. For others, success on level terms with the able-bodied is impossible. For them the British Sports Association for the Disabled and other national equivalents have opened up new horizons of prowess and achievement in local, national and international sport. Outside the realm of competitive sport a similar development has taken place. One hundred and sixty groups promoted horse riding for the disabled in 1972. Wheelchair dancing, too, has a growing number of devotees. Activities which were started as forms of therapy have become sports and recreations in their own right.

There are some who are disenchanted with sport in the modern world. Commercialization and exploitation of the young, violence in contact sports, the use of steroids and drugs in training and competition, the evasion or infringement of rules, gambling and the rigging of races, animosity in place of friendship, lionization of heroes, are all targets for criticism and condemnation. They cannot be gainsaid. Sport, although a world of unreality, cannot separate itself from the real world. It will continue to reflect as well as to shape the *mores* and values of society. It has, however, institutions of government at national and international level which for all their limitations are well established and have shown their ability to exercise restraint and to promote positive values. Changes are taking place all the time. During more than a thousand years from 776 B.C. to A.D. 393 the Olympic Games of the ancient world changed almost out of recognition. It is unlikely that the forms of sport evolved in the 1890s will suit the needs of even one hundred years later. It is much more likely that the association of sport with medicine which persisted so long in the ancient world will continue to be an important feature of the modern scene.

P.C.McI.

References

1. Aristotle. *Nichomachen Ethics*, 112, b. 5.
2. Hippocrates. Quoted by Galen. In *Sources for the History of Greek Athletics*, R. S. Robinson (1955), Cincinatti.
3. Harris, H. A. (1964) *Greek Athletes and Athletics*, London: Hutchinson.
4. Euripides. Autolycus. In Nayck *Trag. Graec. Frag.*, 282.
5. Philostratus. Gymnastics. In *Sources for the History of Greek Athletics*, R. S. Robinson (1955), Cincinatti.
6. McIntosh, P. C. (1957) *Landmarks in the History of Physical Education*, London: Routledge and Kegan Paul.
7. Dickens, C. (1972) *Pickwick Papers*. Harmondsworth: Penguin Books.
8. McIntosh, P. C. (1963) *Sport in Society*. London: Watts.
9. The Sports Council (1971) *Sport in the Seventies*. London: H.M.S.O.
10. The Sports Council (1966) *A Report*. London: Central Office of Information.
11. Lunn, A. (1952) *The Story of Ski-ing*. London: Eyre and Spottiswoode.
12. Irving, R. L. G. (1955) *A History of British Mountaineering*. London: B. T. Batsford.
13. The Sports Council (1969) *A Review 1966–69*. London: Central Council of Physical Recreation.

2

Physiological aspects of sports

In this chapter is taken a brief and somewhat intuitive look at the determinants of athletic performance. Particular stress is laid upon the traditional physiological concerns of neuromuscular performance and the associated demands of respiratory, thermal, and nutritional homeostasis. However, it is first necessary to consider briefly the interactions of physiology with psychology (Chapter 3) and constitution (Chapter 5), and it is also important in concluding the present chapter to justify the ultimate dominance of physiological limitations by reference to track records.

Psychological factors

Many observers would argue that the ultimate limit of athletic performance is set by psychological rather than physiological factors. Certainly, there is much interaction between the two. Considerations of psychology may determine whether an athlete trains to his physiological potential, and whether he realizes this potential in a specific contest. Specific factors are motivation, central inhibition, and cortical arousal.

Motivation
Under the broad heading of motivation may be listed a willingness to carry through a long and arduous training programme, a desire to excel in competition, a preparedness to sacrifice safety to speed, a determination to persist with physical effort in the face of discouragement and physical discomfort, and (particularly in the team player) a subordination of personal glory to group objectives, coupled with a preparedness to face and match the aggression of an opposing team.

Central inhibition
The physiological capabilities of the average individual are not normally seen, due to restraints imposed by impulses arising in the cerebral cortex; however, the true potential can be revealed under hypnosis, or the stress of a sudden emergency.[1] Athletes as a class undoubtedly carry themselves very close to their physiological potential, although many would claim that pressure of competition is needed to counteract their inhibitions and achieve maximum results. Inevitably, the psychological demands upon the competitor increase rapidly as the ultimate physiological limit is approached. Physiological capabilities can in this way control performance while yet remaining unrealized.

Cortical arousal
Unique environmental stimuli increase the discharge pattern of the reticular formation of the brain, with associated changes in wakefulness, vigilance, muscle

tone, cardiac frequency, and respiratory minute volume. The level of arousal is particularly critical for sports with a high skill component (such as pistol shooting and golf putting), but in some degree all activities show an inverted U-shaped relationship (Fig. 2.1) between the level of arousal and the quality of performance.

A moderate level of arousal ensures a brisk cardiac and respiratory anticipation of effort, a brief reaction time, and an adequate background of muscle tone for the development of maximum force. But the timing and extent of arousal must be appropriate to the chosen sport. Premature activation can lead to troublesome hyperventilation, sleeplessness, and general exhaustion of a contestant, while excessive arousal during performance is associated with jerky and poorly co-ordinated movements—the competitor has become 'scared stiff'.

It is normally the responsibility of the coach to manipulate the arousal of the individual or team members to an optimum level.[2] However, the physiologist

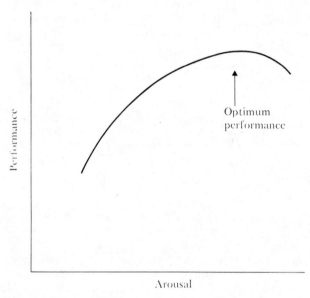

Fig. 2.1 Diagram illustrating the relationship between cortical arousal and athletic performance. The position of the optimum varies with both the personality of the competitor and the skill requirement of the event.

can sometimes assist through the development of auto-conditioning procedures. An athlete is presented with a visual display of heart rate or muscle action potentials, and he learns progressively to control these variables in the face of unpleasant and stressful stimuli.[3]

Physical factors

Body build has an important bearing upon both physiological variables and athletic performance. It has been said that for success in international competition it is necessary to choose one's parents carefully,[4] and one author has estimated that genetic factors account for 94 per cent of the variance in physiological measurements such as the maximum oxygen intake.[5] Certainly, neither physiologist nor trainer can do a great deal to modify body build.

Muscle bulk

A large muscle bulk is required in contact sports, both to provide the inertia that will dislodge an o, ponent, and also to serve as physical protection for the bones and joints of a protagonist. Some muscle-building is possible with a suitable training regime; nevertheless, the person with a mesomorphic body build (page 142) has an inherent advantage over an ectomorph.

Body mass

In some sports such as swimming and rowing, the body weight is largely supported, and an increase of total body mass is not an important consideration; indeed the Cross-channel swimmer may profit from both the buoyancy and the thermal insulation of a substantial quantity of subcutaneous fat. In other sports such as running,[6] the body weight must be raised and lowered at each pace and a heavy person is then at a substantial disadvantage. Many physiological variables such as muscle force and maximum oxygen intake are commonly expressed per unit of body weight.

Mechanics

The external work achieved for a given delivery of oxygen and a given consumption of metabolites depends upon the mechanical efficiency of the movement or activity. Efficiency is partly a question of skill, but body build also places a finite limit upon achievement. Thus *limb length* influences the transition from a ballistic to a less economic forced movement. Pace varies with length, and natural frequency with $1/\sqrt{}$ length. A long-legged person has some advantage in distance running, but in a sprint event (where mechanical inefficiency is acceptable) he may fare no better than a shorter person. A high *centre of gravity* also leads to mechanical inefficiency by increasing the postural work of maintaining body balance; it can be a serious handicap in precisely co-ordinated activities such as skating and gymnastics, but an advantage in a few sports such as basketball (where a tall body and long arms guide the ball close to its objective).

Neuromuscular performance

The quality of neuromuscular performance is determined by many different factors which may be grouped under the headings of speed, skill, flexibility, and strength.

Speed

The total time required for a sprint event includes the lag in initiating the body movement, the rate of acceleration to peak velocity, and the subsequent loss of speed as the event continues.

Reaction time

The reaction time proper depends upon the length of the neural loop between the receptor organ (eye or ear) and the responding muscles (the leg of the runner, and the hand of the pistol shooter or the table tennis player), together with delays incurred in the central processing of information. Unfortunately, the human brain can only process one unit of information at a time.[7] If underaroused, it may respond sluggishly, but if overaroused the impulse corresponding to the starter's signal may be delayed by the processing of irrelevant material. The time to completion of the movement is also modified by cumulative experience. If the required response is unfamiliar, it must be initiated through the large alpha motor fibres. However, most athletic movements have been repeated many times, and appropriate sequences of gamma loop settings[8] are now stored in the cerebellum, where they can be called into play as automatic movements. The degree

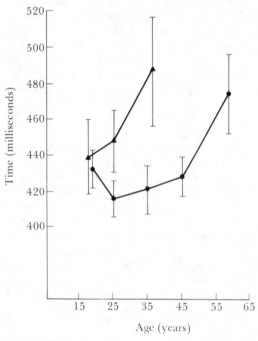

Fig. 2.2 The relationship between age and reaction time (data of the author and G. Wright for a task involving leg movement in response to a visual cue). Mean ± S.D. of results. ●——● men; ▲——▲ women.

of automaticity apparently varies with the immediately preceding thought processes;[9] if an athlete concentrates on the initiating signal ('sensory set'), a faster reaction is attained than if he concentrates upon the movement to be performed ('motor set'). Reaction times are shorter for men than for women, and normally reach a minimum between the ages of 20 and 30 (Fig. 2.2). Probably through a combination of selection and training, values are particularly small for the sprinter. The trained component, at least, seems specific to a body part, and an individual may learn to react quickly with his legs while retaining a much slower reaction rate for his arms.

Acceleration

Acceleration continues through as much as 5–6 seconds of a 9-second race. It depends upon the relationship between the inertia of the body or part, and the explosive force developed by the driving muscles. Inertia is proportional to mass. It is thus difficult for a heavily-built person to accelerate to maximum speed, and the ideal configuration for a sprinter consists of very powerful muscular legs, with little weight elsewhere in the body. The explosive force depends primarily upon the force/velocity characteristics[10] of the active muscles (Fig. 2.3). A charac-

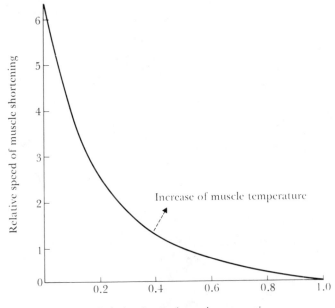

Fig. 2.3 Diagram illustrating the typical relationship between force and velocity of contraction for a skeletal muscle, with arrow to indicate the influence of intramuscular temperature upon the relationship (from *Alive, Man*, by permission of the publisher, Charles C Thomas, Springfield, Ill.).

teristic curve can be drawn for each muscle group, defining limiting combinations of force and speed of contraction at a given tissue temperature. The form of this curve is influenced by the immediate energy resources of the muscle fibres and the viscosity of the active tissues. A preliminary 'warm-up' raises intramuscular temperature, and partly for this reason[11] seems to augment sprint performance (Fig. 2.4).

The speed of movement of an individual limb is further influenced by the type of movement that is executed. If ultimate economy of energy expenditure is desired, as in distance running, then the objective is to initiate a ballistic stroke at the natural frequency of the part; the muscle fibres producing the movement show a brief burst of intense activity at the beginning of the stroke, and the antagonists are active simply in halting the stroke. In the spinter, on the other hand, economy is sacrificed to speed, and a forced oscillation at greater than the natural

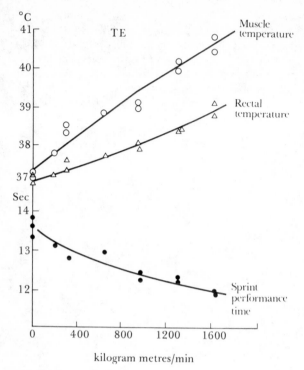

Fig. 2.4 The influence of intramuscular temperature upon the speed of sprinting, to show the effect of warm-up (data of Asmussen and Bøje,[11] by permission of the authors and publisher).

frequency is produced by continuing intense activity of the prime moving muscles. Neither ballistic nor forced oscillations are particularly accurate. In sports that require skilful movement patterns, antagonistic muscles show intermittent bursts of moderate activity that serve to slow the natural swing of the limb.[12] Additional damping is imposed by the viscous resistance of tendons, joints, and opposing skin surfaces.[13] (Fig. 2.5.)

During the final 3 seconds or so of a 9-second sprint, speed reaches a plateau and then slowly falls. A diminishing store of metabolic energy is coping with continuing resistance dependent upon air flow (proportional to the third power of wind speed[14]) and tissue viscosity,[13] friction between shoes and track,[6] and energy losses due to acceleration and deceleration of the limbs.

Skill

Some components of skill such as an unusual sensitivity of receptor organs are inherited. Thus, although the typical diver or gymnast has spent much time in skill training, he probably also commenced his career with an above average perception of body posture through the receptors of the inner ear and neck muscles. Again, a successful test-cricketer has undoubtedly done much to develop his skills, but probably started life with a peculiar receptivity to the ocular sensa-

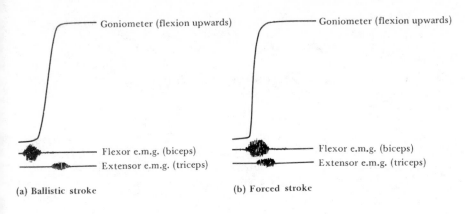

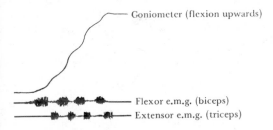

(c) Controlled stroke

Fig. 2.5 Diagrams illustrating the course of movement and the electromyographic activity of agonists and antagonists during (a) ballistic stroke, (b) forced stroke, and (c) controlled stroke.

tions of convergence and accommodation that arise as a ball approaches his bat.

Other facets of skill reflect the cumulative athletic experience of the individual, stored as movement and response patterns in the cerebral cortex and cerebellum. In the context of international competition, much depends upon very general factors. A suitable manipulation of personal arousal may be accompanied less ethically by attempts to over-arouse fellow-competitors. A proper choice of personal pace must be balanced against the less worthy objective of persuading a fellow contestant to accelerate too soon. In distance events, skill is usually associated with a diminution in the metabolic cost of a given rate of progression, but in very brief events skill may require the opposite technique—development of a forcing movement at high speed but low mechanical efficiency. In other instances, skill may be reflected in unusual feats of balance and agility, an appreciation of grace and form in movement, or an ability to place the human body, a ball, or some object with unusual precision.

Flexibility
Dynamic flexibility is essentially the inverse of viscosity, and has already been noted as a determinant of speed. In certain sports such as gymnastics, extreme static flexibility is also of importance to performance.

Strength. Strength may be sub-divided into explosive force, dynamic strength, and static strength.

Explosive force is particularly vital to the jumper, the thrower, and the sprinter. The effective power of a single violent effort depends upon all the factors discussed under 'speed', but in particular upon the force/velocity characteristics of the active muscles. The proximate basis of movement within the muscle fibres is the chemical coupling of two long chain proteins, actin and myosin,[15] using energy stored in the phosphate bond of adenosine triphosphate. The observed response depends upon the rate of chemical coupling (influenced by mineral ion concentrations), the number of actin and myosin filaments per fibre (increased by the hypertrophy of training), the number of fibres activated (often increased by learning of a task) and the leverage that can be exerted (largely determined by body build); the resultant of all these various factors is opposed by the dynamic viscosity of the part.

Table 2.1 The immediate energy resources of skeletal muscle, expressed in terms of their oxygen equivalents (data for sedentary young men based largely upon the work of Margaria and his associates[17])

Source	Power (ml/kg min)	Total store (l)	Time for exhaustion (sec)
Alactate debt	165	1·9	8
Lactate debt	68	3·1	40
Oxygen transport	45	∞	∞

Dynamic strength

If the explosive efforts are to be repeated in rapid succession (as in sprinting), the stored energy of adenosine triphosphate is replenished by the breakdown of creatine phosphate to creatine and phosphate radicals. This in effect involves dynamic strength. Performance limits are imposed on the one hand by the forces resisting acceleration and sustained movement (see speed, above), and on the other hand by the cumulative power of the two phosphagen splitting reactions and the total store of phosphagen energy within the active muscle fibres. It is convenient to equate phosphagen with the equivalent oxygen transport (Table 2.1). Di Prampero and Cerretelli[16] set the power derived from a combination of phosphagen and body oxygen stores at an average of 165 ml/kg min. In a young sprinter, figures as high as 250 ml/kg min may be encountered; this is at least four times the maximum steady rate of oxygen transport. Unfortunately, the quantity of such reserves is small (30–35 ml/kg), and the phosphagen content of active muscle can apparently be exhausted in about 8 seconds.[17] Replenishment proceeds more slowly (half-time, 22 seconds), and is dependent upon the glycolytic pathway of metabolism (Fig. 2.6). In the absence of oxygen, carbohydrate (glucose or glycogen) is broken down to pyruvate and accumulates as lactate. If maximum effort continues, this reaction is halted after about 40 seconds, probably on account of the rising tissue acidity. The oxygen power and store of this 'lactate debt' are equivalent, respectively, to some 70 ml/kg min, and 45 ml/kg. Since a well-trained athlete can disperse the accumulating acid through larger muscles and a greater total blood volume, his oxygen debt tends to be

(a) Aerobic

(b) Anaerobic

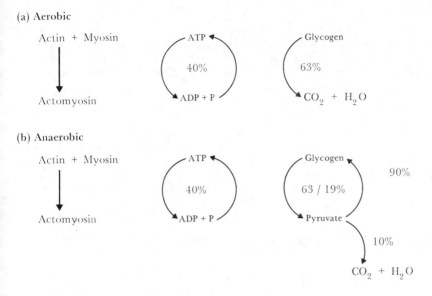

Fig. 2.6 Sketch illustrating coupling of energy-exchange reactions in skeletal muscle during aerobic and anaerobic contractions, with figures for efficiencies of several stages.

larger than that of a sedentary person; the terminal concentrations of lactate in arterial blood (about 120 mg/100 ml) are usually unexceptional, although some long distance runners may develop levels as high as 160–200 mg/100 ml (Robinson, personal communication). If oxygen is freely available, the various resources discussed to this point are progressively supplemented by a steady oxygen transport. When fully developed, this ranges from 60 ml/kg min in a typical average male athlete to 80–85 ml/kg min in an international class endurance competitor. However, the oxygen transport is not instantaneous, since both ventilation and muscle blood flow take a few seconds to reach maximum values. The speed of such adjustments can be increased by the development of conditioned reflexes that anticipate the cardiac and ventilatory requirements of exercise.

A small quantity of lactate may be metabolized to CO_2 and water by other body regions during exercise. Following effort, much lactate (Margaria suggests the high figure of 90 per cent) is reconverted to glycogen, using energy derived from the oxidation of the remainder. The reactions proceed mainly in the liver, with a half-time of 10–15 minutes. However, replenishment of intramuscular glycogen stores is a much slower process, occupying at least 24 hours.[18] In team games such as football and hockey, where repeated sprints are required, there is a progressive exhaustion of fuel for anaerobic effort, as shown by diminishing blood lactate levels in the final period of play. The endurance of many forms of vigorous muscular effort depends upon the initial glycogen content of the muscle fibres—a value susceptible to modification by diet and athletic training.

Static strength

Static strength is important in events such as weight lifting. It varies with the total number of active muscle fibres, and their individual cross-section; thus, unless a muscle is 'diluted' by fat and connective tissue, there is a rather consistent relationship between the potential force and the dimensions of a given muscle. Physiological tests measure the performance of a group of muscles, and some forms of weight training produce marked gains of measured strength without muscle hypertrophy. In such circumstances, it is probable that the contraction has been dispersed over a wider range of muscle fibres, possibly with more complete relaxation of antagonists. Central inhibition of the contraction may also have lessened, so that individual fibres can sustain a more continuous tetanic effort. The endurance of maximum static contractions is quite brief (20–30 seconds): it is unlikely that glycogen reserves are exhausted so rapidly.[19] The tolerance limit is commonly imposed by the interaction of motivation with pain and exhaustion consequent upon accumulation of acid metabolites in the active tissue; however, the fatigued muscle initially shows poor relaxation ('contracture'), and the rapid return of more normal compliance in the recovery period

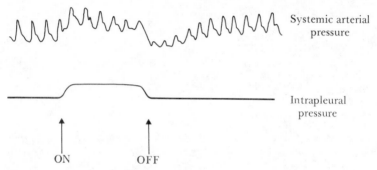

Systemic arterial pressure

Intrapleural pressure

ON   OFF

Fig. 2.7 Sketch illustrating the effect of the Valsalva manoeuvre upon the systemic blood pressure (based on an experiment of W. F. Hamilton and associates[21]).

suggests that an immediate depletion of intramuscular phosphagen stores may also be involved.[20] A further consideration is tolerance for the Valsalva manoeuvre (forced expiration against a closed glottis, used as a means of fixing the thoracic insertions of the pectoral muscles); this causes a temporary cessation of venous return, with an abrupt rise of intracerebral pressure, and a marked depression of cardiac output followed by a compensatory overshoot (Fig. 2.7).[21] In the specific context of competitive weight lifting, the apparent strength depends greatly upon the skill of the athlete. He must minimize the moment of the weights by keeping the bar close to the gravitational axis of his body, and the final elevation of the weights must be achieved by a swift 'clean and jerk' before the tolerance of maximum static effort is exhausted. The capacity to sustain repeated and prolonged but sub-maximum static contractions is important in certain sports, for example single-handed dinghy sailing. Rohmert has shown[22] that blood flow to the active muscles is impeded if they contract at more than 15 per cent of maximum force, and that flow is completely occluded at more than 70 per cent of maximum effort. In such circumstances, the contraction must be sustained by anaerobic metabolism, and because of slow resynthesis, intramuscular glycogen reserves may be exhausted by several hours of sailing.[23] Tolerance of repeated sustained static contractions can be improved by a specific strengthening of the active muscles, since they then contract at a smaller percentage of maximum voluntary force.[24]

The demands of homeostasis

If competition demands more than a minute of sustained activity, performance becomes increasingly dependent upon the demands of homeostasis—not only in the active tissues, but in the body as a whole. There must be an adequate supply of oxygen and removal of carbon dioxide, together with the achievement of thermal equilibrium and the replenishment of metabolites.

Oxygen transport
The total usable store of anaerobic energy is set at an oxygen equivalent of 75–80 ml/kg. Aerobic (oxygen dependent) metabolism thus yields about a half of the energy used in an event of one minute duration, but this proportion rises to 80 per cent with five minutes of activity, and 98 per cent with one hour of activity (Fig. 2.8). Aerobic power is commonly measured[25] as the maximum oxygen intake—the plateau of oxygen consumption reached during several minutes of progressively increasing activity on a large muscle task such as uphill treadmill running (Fig. 2.9). In theory, this provides an unequivocal expression of the ability of the cardio-respiratory system to transport oxygen from the

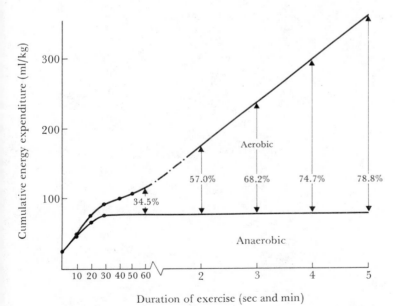

Fig. 2.8 Sketch illustrating the relationship between the proportion of aerobic work and the duration of activity (from Shephard, R. J., *J. sports Med. phys. Fitness*, **10**, 72–83, (1970) with permission).

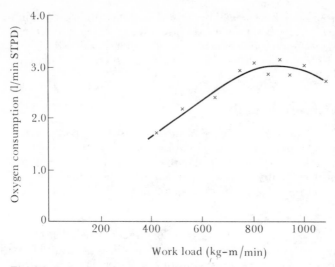

Fig. 2.9 Definition of an oxygen plateau. The athlete is required to perform a successively increasing workload (uphill treadmill running) until further increments of speed and/or slope produce no further increase of oxygen consumption (from *Alive, Man!* by permission of the publisher, Charles C Thomas, Springfield, Ill.).

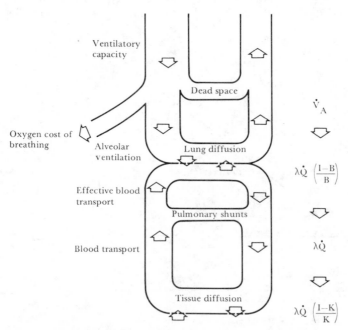

Fig. 2.10 Diagram illustrating the chain of conductances involved in the transport of oxygen from the atmosphere to the active tissues (from the author's article in the *Ontario Medical Review*, February 1968, by permission of the editor).

atmosphere to the working tissues. In practice, results vary somewhat with the test modality (treadmill, bicycle ergometer, step test, arm and shoulder ergometers), and an athlete such as a kayak paddler (who has well developed shoulder and arm muscles) may be limited by local symptoms (leg pain or weakness) rather than true central exhaustion; this is particularly likely on the bicycle ergometer, but can also occur on the treadmill.

Results are normally expressed in ml/kg min STPD, since the cost of many activities varies almost directly with body weight. However, this yields an inappropriate index of performance in endurance sports where body weight is supported (for example, rowing or swimming); attention should then be directed to absolute values (l/min STPD).

Oxygen transport may be conceived as proceeding through a chain of resistances (or more precisely conductances, the reciprocal of resistances; Fig. 2.10). These include[26, 27] ventilation (with due allowance for respiratory effort 'wasted' in both ventilation of the dead space of the airways and the oxygen cost of respiration), the interaction between the diffusing capacity of the lungs and blood transport, blood transport itself, and the interaction between blood transport and the diffusing capacity of the tissues. For the ordinary sedentary individual exercising under normal ambient conditions, by far the smallest conductance (20–30 l/min) and thus the largest resistance is presented by the blood transport term. Alveolar ventilation (60–80 l/min) also imposes some restriction upon oxygen transport, but the remaining terms are unimportant.

Ventilation

The external ventilation attained by the exercising athlete is very large, commonly averaging 160 l/min BTPS.[28] The respiratory frequency remains relatively low, often being linked with the rhythm of movement. Thus, the oarsman with a stroke of 38/min takes one breath per stroke, while the cyclist with a pedal frequency of 100 may have a breathing rate of 50/min. Many athletes show some development of both static lung volumes such as vital capacity, and dynamic lung volumes such as maximum voluntary ventilation, but it is not uncommon to find that three-quarters of both static and dynamic lung volumes are utilized in maximum activity. These are higher proportions than would be tolerated by the average sedentary person, and undoubtedly contribute to the discomfort of the contestant. Thus, in the psychological sense at least, ventilation may limit the endurance athlete. This viewpoint receives support from the importance that many coaches attach to such poorly understood phenomena as 'choking' and 'second wind'. The athlete who *chokes* may be a person who through poor pacing or excessive competition develops significant anaerobic effort at too early a point in a contest. Accumulation of lactate then gives a distressing hyperventilation better reserved for the period following a race. Alternatively, fear may provoke excessive ventilation in the absence of lactate. This is uncomfortable in itself, and the washing out of carbon dioxide from the airways may provoke a bronchospasm that augments symptoms. There is some debate as to the reality of *second wind*.[29] The present author regards it as almost the antithesis of choking. Lactate may accumulate in the early phases of a race due to tactical factors such as jockeying for position and physiological factors such as incomplete circulatory adaptation to effort. As a race continues, the pace normally steadies, systemic blood pressure rises, and muscle perfusion improves. Circulating concentrations of lactate fall, and ventilation also diminishes. At the same time, a 'warm-up' of the respiratory muscles and possibly a diminution of airway resistance reduce the sensations associated with respiration—there is what Campbell has described as an improved 'length–tension appropriateness' in the respiratory muscles.[30] Despite these sensory and psychological considerations, it is important to emphasize that blood leaving the lungs is virtually saturated with oxygen, even in maximum effort, and indeed exercise normally augments the oxygen pressure of alveolar gas.[31] Thus, there could be little gain from any further increase of ventilation. In physiological terms, external ventilation is not a significant limiting factor.

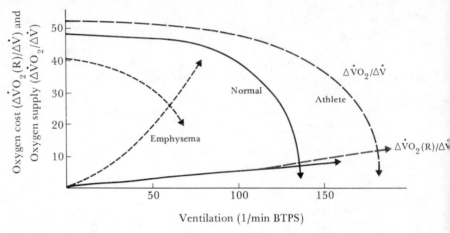

Fig. 2.11 To illustrate the critical point where a further increase in the cost of ventilation $(\triangle \dot{V}_{O_2}(R)/\triangle \dot{V}_E)$ exceeds the corresponding increase of oxygen intake $(\triangle \dot{V}_{O_2}/\triangle \dot{V}_E)$ (from *Alive, Man!* by permission of the publisher, Charles C Thomas, Springfield, Ill.).

Up to a quarter of the external ventilation is 'wasted' in the dead space. During exercise, this is attributable mainly to a 'stratified inhomogeneity', that is, an incomplete mixing of airway and alveolar gas.[32] The slow respiratory rate of the athlete allows rather more time for this mixing to occur, but there is no appreciable improvement of alveolar ventilation, since the associated prodigious tidal volume causes expansion of the airway zone in which mixing must occur.

The *work of breathing* imposes a 5–10 per cent charge upon oxygen delivery in maximum effort.[33] However, respiratory work cannot be a limiting factor unless the oxygen delivered to the circulation by additional ventilation is less than the corresponding increment of oxygen consumption in the chest muscles. Under most conditions, ventilation is nicely adjusted to ensure a maximum uptake of oxygen by pulmonary capillary blood, without surpassing the 'cross-over point' of diminishing oxygen returns (Fig. 2.11). However, the margin between normal exercise ventilation and the cross-over point is not large, and hyperventilation from anxiety or a premature accumulation of lactate could conceivably cause an athlete to pass this critical point.

Pulmonary diffusing capacity

Many athletes—particularly swimmers—have a large pulmonary diffusing capacity.[34,35] Although a part of the high reported values seems attributable to technical artefacts associated with a slow breathing rate,[36] there is little dispute that above average readings are encountered in endurance athletes, and that small increments can be induced by endurance-type training. Nevertheless, these changes are but incidental to an augmented pulmonary blood flow. Equilibration of respiratory gases between the blood stream and alveolar spaces is fairly complete even in maximum effort, and gains of pulmonary diffusing capacity can make no useful contribution to such equilibration. The only exceptions to this generalization are the athlete who must compete at moderate altitudes (Chapter 6), and the swimmer who produces a low partial pressure of oxygen in his lungs by deliberate breath-holding.

Blood transport

The blood transport of oxygen depends upon the maximum cardiac output (the product of heart rate and stroke volume), the oxygen-transporting properties of the blood, and the maximum arterio-venous oxygen difference. The effectiveness of a given cardiac output is also influenced by its relative distribution between the active muscles, skin, and viscera.

Peak *heart rates* of 250/min and more may be encountered briefly in events such as skiing, where there is a combination of stress and intense isometric exertion. However, the 'maximum' rate that can be sustained by a young man over several minutes is appreciably lower, averaging 195/min. It may be even less (about 185/min) in well-trained endurance athletes,[37] although it is difficult to be certain that the full potential of a competitor has been realized under laboratory conditions. The resting heart rate of the endurance athlete may be as low as 30/min. This reflects an alteration in the balance of vagal and sympathetic drives to the cardiac pacemaker, possibly associated with local alterations in the synthesis of transmitter substances. It has some practical importance in that it may leave the heart more vulnerable to ectopic rhythms; the Wolff–Parkinson–White syndrome is particularly dangerous to a distance competitor.

The maximum *stroke volume* depends upon body posture and the type of exercise performed. A cyclist who does not use his arms for propulsion may pool a substantial quantity of blood in the veins of the upper limbs, and in consequence he has a 20–30 ml poorer stroke volume than the runner or swimmer. A *cardiac output* of 30–35 l/min, equivalent to a stroke volume of 150–180 ml, is common in endurance athletes.[28] The large stroke volume of an athlete is achieved without marked changes of myocardial contractility—in other words, the gain of stroke output is won at the expense of not only a more complete emptying of the ventricle, but also some expansion of the end-diastolic volume.[38] It may be necessary to distinguish the enlarged cardiac shadow of the athlete from the dilated heart of disease; usually, this is possible from the form of the cardiac shadow, a consideration of the relationship between heart volume and working capacity,[39] and the size of the stroke volume observed at fluoroscopy.

The *haemoglobin* level of the blood is sometimes low in athletes, thus restricting the potential carriage of oxygen per litre of blood. Increases of circulating haptoglobins suggest that the most important cause of this problem is an enhanced destruction of red cells, either through pressure trauma (in the feet of a runner, for example), or secondary to the increased rate of blood flow. Iron loss in sweat is hardly sufficient to be implicated, but in some instances dietary fads may play a role. The carriage of oxygen per unit volume of blood depends also upon the slope of the oxygen dissociation curve between arterial and venous points; this slope can be modified somewhat by changes of diphosphoglycerate activity in response to chronic oxygen lack, but to date there has been no suggestion of a systematic modification in athletic individuals.

The *maximum arterio-venous oxygen difference* is about 160 ml/l in the endurance athlete, compared with 140 ml/l in a sedentary individual. The difference is due to a rather complete extraction of oxygen from the mixed venous blood of the sportsman. This could arise in two ways: (i) an augmentation of enzyme systems in the active muscles, and (ii) a reduction of blood flow through tissues that normally show a low oxygen extraction—particularly the skin and the kidneys. The practical role of enzyme changes is probably small. Certain types of training can increase the enzyme content of active tissues,[40, 41] but the reported changes (50–100 per cent increase) do little more than keep pace with the lengthened diffusion pathway through hypertrophied muscle. Furthermore, the oxygen content of blood draining an active muscle is low (10–12 ml/l),[42] so that the scope for further oxygen extraction by more aggressive enzyme systems is relatively small. Severe exercise normally induces a 50–70 per cent reduction of visceral blood flow,[43] and periodic reports of athletic pseudo-nephritis[44] suggest that reductions may be more drastic in the athlete than in a more sedentary individual. Nevertheless, visceral flow is never more than about 1·5 l/min, so that the possibility for a further redistribution of flow from this part of the body in vigorous exercise is slight. The potential contribution of changes in subcutaneous blood flow has apparently been overlooked by many investigators. With sustained vigorous exercise, there is an intense and generalized dilatation of skin vessels; as much as a fifth or a sixth of the cardiac output may perfuse the skin.[45] There is thus a large potential for flow redistribution. Does it occur with endurance training? There are certain parallels between endurance training and heat acclimatization, and it is likely that the well-trained athlete can accept a low skin flow since: (i) he tolerates a high core temperature, (ii) he sweats early and profusely, and (iii) convective heat loss is facilitated by rapid body movement. Nevertheless, attempts to compromise skin flow further by illegal administration of drugs is very dangerous, and may in the past have contributed to some heat deaths.

Tissue diffusion
There is currently no accurate method for measuring the 'diffusing capacity' presented by capillaries perfusing active tissues. However, indirect calculations[27] suggest the tissue diffusing capacity is several times as large as the pulmonary diffusing capacity, and for this reason no difficulty would be anticipated in the exchange of oxygen and carbon dioxide between the active tissues and the muscle vasculature. Unfortunately for theory, a difficulty does sometimes arise. A distance cyclist, for instance, may claim that his performance on hills is limited by weakness and pain in the leg muscles. The explanation apparently lies in a local obstruction of the circulation by excessively vigorous contraction of the quadriceps muscle group. However, if exercise is maintained despite this pain, systemic

blood pressure tends to increase to the point where local vascular occlusion can be overcome. Since there is no suggestion that the capilliary bed itself is at fault, it can be argued that we are here dealing with but one more manifestation of a cardiac limitation—failure to develop an immediate and adequate rise of blood pressure.

Carbon dioxide homeostasis

Thus far we have ignored problems of CO_2 homeostasis. Normal tissue function may be disturbed by excessively high or low partial pressures of carbon dioxide. Accumulation of CO_2 is unusual. The ventilatory conductance is as for oxygen, but owing to the shape of the CO_2 dissociation curve, blood transport is at least five times as effective as for oxygen.[26] The total pressure gradient from the active muscles to ambient air is thus about half that for oxygen. The main practical circumstances where a build-up of CO_2 can limit performance is in scuba and industrial diving. Swimming is a rather inefficient mode of progression, and the scuba diver is thus faced by: (i) a high rate of CO_2 production, (ii) a decrease of maximum voluntary ventilation (due to the increased density of respired gas, expiratory collapse of the airway, and external resistance imposed by the scuba set), (iii) added external dead space, and (iv) rapidly exhausted and somewhat inefficient CO_2-absorbing canisters. At altitude, the opposite problem of excessive CO_2 elimination may be encountered, with problems of intermittent ventilation and mountain sickness; repeated bouts of maximum effort in the first few days may make the athlete vulnerable at a rather lower altitude than a more sedentary person.[46]

Thermal homeostasis

The mechanical efficiency of performance is poor, even in an athlete. Theoretically (Fig. 2.6), it is around 13 per cent for anaerobic work, and 25 per cent for aerobic performance, and a high proportion of the chemical energy used by the athlete must thus be dissipated as heat. In runners, surprisingly high efficiency values (up to 40 per cent) are sometimes encountered; the expectations of thermodynamics are apparently exceeded because a part of the energy of descent is absorbed by the stretching of elastic tissue, providing a store that can be used in making the next stride.[47]

Intramuscular temperature increases rapidly during the first five minutes of activity. The general body temperature continues to rise for at least 15 minutes, but if effort continues a plateau is reached.[48] This reflects in part the increase of thermal gradient associated with the rising core temperature, in part the onset of copious sweating, and in part a progressive increase of subcutaneous blood flow. With sustained effort, equilibrium is largely dependent upon evaporation of sweat (Fig. 2.12). The endurance athlete can tolerate very high core temperatures; values of 40–41 °C have been recorded from marathon runners even under temperate conditions.

The immediate effect of a rise in local muscle temperature is to improve physical performance[11] through a reduction of muscle viscosity and a dilatation of intramuscular blood vessels. However, the rising core temperature increases oxygen utilization in inactive tissues (the so-called Q_{10} effect), and even if cardiac output can be maintained, an increasing proportion of the available blood flow

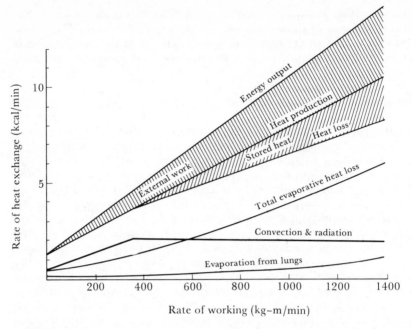

Fig. 2.12 Sketch illustrating routes of heat loss during physical activity (based on data of Nielsen, from *Alive, Man!* by permission of the publisher Charles C Thomas, Springfield, Ill.).

becomes diverted to the widely patent skin vessels, leaving a smaller potential perfusion of the active muscles.

With sustained activity in the heat, there is a progressive reduction of central blood volume and thus cardiac stroke volume. In the first few minutes of activity there is an enhanced formation of tissue fluid, and the capacity of the peripheral veins also rises coincident with the increase of core temperature;[49] in a hot dry climate there may also be an increased water loss in respired gas. As sweating develops, this contributes largely to the fall of blood volume; under adverse conditions, secretion may amount to two or more litres per hour.

If the environment is extremely hot and humid, or heat loss is impeded by attractive but impermeable team garments, cardiac output may fall to the point where the cerebral circulation can no longer be maintained. Heat collapse has occurred. If cutaneous and renal flow also fail, fatal hyperpyrexia may supervene. Cumulative loss of mineral ions over several days of competition can also lead to cramps, muscle weakness and neurasthenia.

Nutritional homeostasis

The fuel required varies with the intensity and duration of activity, but in the vigorous effort typical of the athlete a high proportion of energy is initially derived from carbohydrate. The proximate source is glycogen, stored within the muscle cell. This normally amounts to 1·5 g/100 g of wet muscle,[18] or (assuming 20 kg of active muscle), some 1200 kcal (5·2 MJ) of energy in all. If carbohydrate is providing 75 per cent of the needed energy, then fuel is available for 80 minutes of activity at an expenditure of 20 kcal (0·08 MJ)/min. Blood sugar (total 6 g = 24 kcal (0·10 MJ)) is a negligible energy resource for physical work, but there is a further labile reserve of glycogen in the liver (total 100 g = 400 kcal (1·69 MJ)); this can be mobilized at a rate of about 1 g/min.

Unfortunately, fat cannot serve as a substrate under anaerobic conditions and once glycogen reserves are exhausted, it becomes difficult for a contestant to tackle hills and other obstacles that call for anaerobic effort; the sole possibilities are the already depleted blood sugar and the breakdown of protein. Hultman[18] has shown experimentally that a cyclist can exhaust muscle glycogen in 80–90 min; perhaps becaue it is a different and somewhat less intense type of activity, the glycogen of the marathon runner is eked out over a much longer period (Costill, personal communication).

The total reserves of energy stored as fat are, from the athletic viewpoint, almost infinite. A normally nourished male contestant may have 10–15 per cent of his body weight, 10 kg or more, in the form of adipose tissue. This is equivalent to some 70 000 kcal (294 MJ) of energy, or (assuming expenditure at a rate of 10 kcal (0·04 MJ)/min) 7000 hours' supply. Unfortunately, most of this fat is at some distance from the active muscles. Intramuscular lipids are soon exhausted, and subsequent usage is set by the rate of mobilization from depot fat and/or transport across the muscle cell membrane. Accurate statistics have yet to be obtained, but maximum transport is probably 1–2 g/min (7–14 kcal (0·03–0·06 MJ)/min), being somewhat higher for endurance than for sprint athletes.

A muscular postscript

Many athletes and their coaches have an inherent respect for muscular strength, even in endurance events.[50] This is reflected in training manuals and in the statements of international class competitors that they use their strength to 'smash' opponents. Movements may certainly be poorly co-ordinated towards the end of an endurance event, and coaches wonder whether this loss of co-ordination could be avoided if the chest and arm muscles were stronger. They are also perplexed by the promising endurance athlete who apparently reaches a plateau of development at an aerobic power of perhaps 65 ml/kg min, despite rigorous cardio-respiratory training: could the chances of such an individual be improved by an increase of muscular strength?

The physiologist can immediately suggest several areas where strength is of practical value to the endurance competitor. In sports such as cycling, performance is commonly limited by occlusion of blood vessels in the active muscles. Experimental proof includes: (i) the peripheral nature of symptoms during maximum effort,[25] (ii) the accumulation of blood lactate at a relatively low percentage of maximum oxygen consumption,[51] and (iii) an inverse relationship between quadriceps strength and the extent of lactate accumulation.[24]

The importance of avoiding lactate accumulation until the final spirit has already been stressed. An athlete with local muscle weakness may indeed be 'smashed' by becoming prematurely breathless, and if the active muscles are strengthened, he can operate closer to his aerobic power before significant lactate accumulates. Costill[52] has recently drawn attention to the practice of the marathon runner, who habitually operates just below his lactate threshold (70–80 per cent of aerobic power for a distance runner).

A reduced accumulation of lactate can in turn alter the 'perceived stress'[53] at any given level of exertion, thereby improving motivation; if the end-point of an athlete's effort is extreme breathlessness, weakness, or muscular pain, then a selective gain of strength in the most active muscles is very likely to improve performance. Strength may also speed long-term recovery by minimizing the micro-traumata secondary to local weakness and lack of oxygen.

Deterioration of skill in the latter stages of a race may reflect either muscular or central fatigue. Muscle fatigue is due in part to poor perfusion, and to the extent that a strong muscle is easier to perfuse than a weak one, the strengthening of shoulder, back and arm muscles could conceivably minimize the loss of skill as exhaustion is approached. However, the usually associated symptoms—particularly the ashen-grey pallor and cerebral confusion—suggest that the staggering and poorly co-ordinated gait, so wasteful in terms of energy expenditure, should be attributed mainly to a reduced blood flow through the posture-regulating centres of the brain.

Certain disadvantages of undue muscularity must be stressed to balance the picture. Although it has been claimed that weight lifters maintain normal flexibility, some increase of viscous resistance to movement may be anticipated with bulky musculature, and problems can arise from a physical apposition of hypertrophied fleshy tissues. Muscle hypertrophy also increases the body mass to be raised, lowered, accelerated and decelerated, and since strength training does little to develop the heart, aerobic power per unit of body weight is often low in the muscular athlete. Most forms of muscle building are highly specific, and the pattern of any training programme must closely mimic the muscle usage of the intended sport if bulk is not to accumulate in the wrong region of the body.

For many purposes, it may be useful to concentrate on skill training that increases strength without bulk (see above). Specific hypertrophy of leg muscles may help the cyclist who must compete in hilly country, or the distance runner who wishes to indulge the sport of 'smashing' his opponents by sudden bursts of speed. But indiscriminate hypertrophy of muscle seems likely to impair performance, particularly in true endurance contests—track events of 3000 metres and up, and comparable durations of cycling, swimming, skiing, and skating.

Relation to track records

It is finally of interest to test how well physiological theory fits the observed performance of the athlete in international class competition. Lloyd[54] has completed an elegant analysis of this type for track times over the range of 50 metres to marathon races. He points out that the relationship between the contested distance X (in metres) and the record time t (seconds) for a given distance has the form:

$$\log_{10} X = 1 \cdot 00 + 0 \cdot 9 \log t.$$

However, the physiological theories discussed above apparently relate the energy of the runner (E) to a store (S) and an income (R) per unit time. Thus, the energy available for a race of t seconds duration should be described by the linear relationship

$$E = S + Rt.$$

Furthermore, the power of the runner P is equal to the rate of energy usage $[(S/t) + R]$, and the running speed V is a function of power such that

$$P = A + B(V)^n$$

where A and B are constants, and n is an exponent. Assuming for simplicity that $n = 1$, we obtain on rearrangement

$$B(V) = S/t + (R - A).$$

Further, the distance travelled $(X) = Vt$, so that we may write

$$B(X) = S + (R - A)t.$$

In other words, physiological theory might seem to demand a linear rather than a logarithmic relationship between distance and time. The paradox is explained by the broad span over which data have been plotted; given a more limited range, it is indeed possible to show a linear relationship. Lloyd has distinguished six performance zones (Fig. 2.13). The first covers distances from 50 to 200 m; here, the performance is determined by anaerobic capacity and power. Times for 50-metre distances are a little longer than predicted from the linear relationship, due to energy used in accelerating the body mass, while times for 200 metres are also a little protracted due to progressive exhaustion of phosphagen stores. The second zone covers distances from 400 to 1500 metres. Here are covered an anaerobic energy store and an aerobic income, and by making reasonable assumptions about the oxygen cost of running, the line is described by an intercept (store) of 4·6 litres, and a slope (oxygen intake) of 5·1 l/min; there thus seems

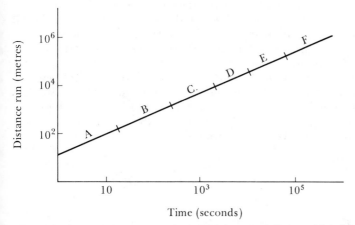

Fig. 2.13 The relationship between record times and distance (sketch based on an analysis by Brian B. Lloyd, from *Alive, Man!* by permission of the publisher, Charles C Thomas, Springfield, Ill.). Note that although the relationship is logarithmic, it may be divided into 6 zones (A–F) over which an approximately linear relationship can be seen.

a reasonable accord between record times and their supposed physiological basis. In the third zone (1500 to 9000 metres), there is a small decrease of slope (about 6 per cent); again this readily fits physiological theory, since at this stage the effective cardiac output and thus maximum oxygen intake are being reduced by a diversion of blood to the skin and venous reservoirs. In the fourth zone (30 to 120 minutes) the claims of heat increase, and there is a further diminution of slope. In the fifth zone (2–5 hours) the relationship has an intercept equivalent to only 0·87 kcal (0·003 MJ), and a slope equivalent to 14·1 kcal/min (0·06 MJ/min), or 3·3 litres of oxygen per minute; these are substantially below the anticipated oxygen debt and maximum oxygen intake of an athlete. Putting 1 g of glycogen equal to 3·8 kcal (0·016 MJ) of energy, the intercept could be related to a glycogen store of 230 g, a not unrealistic figure for the total glycogen content of the active muscles, while the slope of 14·1 kcal/min (0·06 MJ/min) would correspond quite well with predictions of fat mobilization. The final zone (times over five hours) has a very shallow slope; here, the speed is determined more by pauses for refreshment, massage and sleep than by transport processes.

The measurement of distance and the timing of athletic events are more precise than the usual laboratory physiological test, and it is thus significant that physiological concepts are sustained by examining the achievements of the world's best performers. However, a second question has greater practical importance for the sports physician, coach and trainer. How valid are physiological concepts as a basis for predicting the outcome of a race? The largest volume of information on this point relates to the maximum oxygen intake and its derivatives. Cooper[55] found a correlation coefficient of 0·90 between the aerobic power (ml/kg min), and the distance middle-aged men could run in twelve minutes; in other words, more than 80 per cent of the variation in track performance was described by this single variable. However, in women (presumably because of poor motivation), the coefficient of correlation was much poorer ($r=0·7$). In athletes, the problem is difficult because there is little difference of speed between the best and the worst performers. Ishiko[56] compared the 5000 m times of Japanese athletes with aerobic power per unit body weight, and found a correlation coefficient of 0·67. Rather similar correlations have been found between predictions of maximum oxygen intake and the performance of Scandinavian cross-country skiers.[57] In closely matched endurance competitors, the differences of maximum oxygen intake thus account for only 40 per cent of the observed differences of performance, leaving 60 per cent to other factors such as motivation, tolerance of oxygen debt, skill, and strength. In short, the current generation of physiologists can explain why an athlete performs well, but the man with the stop watch still has an advantage in predicting which of a group of athletes will win a contest.

R.J.S.

References

1. Steinhaus, A. H. (1963) Some factors modifying the expression of human strength. In *Toward and Understanding of Health and Physical Education*. Los Angeles: Brown.
2. Cratty, B. J. (1971) Activation and athletic endeavor. In *International Symposium on the Art and Science of Coaching*, ed. Percival, L., Toronto: Fitness Institute.

3. Brener, J. and Kleinman, R. A. (1970) Learned control of decreases in systolic blood pressure. *Nature*, **226**, 1063.
4. Åstrand, P-O. (1967) Commentary. Proceedings of International Symposium on Physical Activity and Cardiovascular Health. *Canad. med. Ass. J.*, **96**, 730.
5. Klissouras, V. (1971) Heritability of adaptive variation. *J. appl. Physiol.*, **31**, 338.
6. Margaria, R. (1971) Current concepts of walking and running. In *Frontiers of Fitness*, ed. Shephard, R. J., Springfield, Ill.: Charles C Thomas.
7. Poulton, E. C. (1970) *Environment and Human Efficiency*. Springfield, Ill.: Charles C Thomas.
8. Granit, R. (1966) *Muscle Afferents and Motor Control*. New York: John Wiley & Sons, Inc.
9. Henry, F. M. and Rogers, D. E. (1960) Increased response latency for complicated movements and a 'memory drum' theory of neuromotor reactions. *Res. Q. Am. Ass. Hlth phys. Educ.*, **31**, 448.
10. Hill, A. V. (1964) The effect of load on the heat of shortening muscle. *Proc. R. Soc.* B, **159**, 297.
11. Asmussen, E. and Bøje, O. (1945) Body temperature and capacity for work. *Acta physiol. scand.*, **10**, 1.
12. Hubbard, A. W. (1960) Homokinetics: muscular function in human movement. In *Science and Medicine of Exercise and Sports*, ed. Johnson, W. R., New York: Harper.
13. (a) de Vries, H. (1966) *Physiology of Exercise for Physical Education and Athletics*, Dubuque, Iowa: Brown.
    (b) de Vries, H. (1971) Flexibility, an overlooked but vital factor in sports conditioning. In *International Symposium on the Art and Science of Coaching*, ed. Percival, L., Toronto: Fitness Institute.
14. Pugh, L. G. C. E. (1967) Athletes at altitude. *J. Physiol.*, **192**, 619.
15. Huxley H. E. (1965) The mechanism of muscular contraction. *Scient. Am.*, **213**, 18.
16. di Prampero, P. E. and Cerretelli, P. (1968) Maximal muscular power (aerobic and anaerobic) in African natives. *Ergonomics*, **12**, 51.
17. di Prampero, P. E. (1971) Anaerobic capacity and power. In *Frontiers of Fitness*, ed. Shephard, R. J., Springfield, Ill.: Charles C Thomas.
18. Hultman, E. (1971) Muscle glycogen stores and prolonged exercise. In *Frontiers of Fitness*, ed. Shephard, R. J., Springfield, Ill.: Charles C Thomas.
19. Shephard, R. J. (1972) *Alive, Man!* Springfield, Ill.: Charles C Thomas.
20. Edwards, R. H. T., Hill, D. K. and Jones, D. A. (1975) Effect of fatigue on the time course of relaxation from isometric contractions of skeletal muscle in man. *J. Physiol.*, **251**, 287.
21. Hamilton, W. F., Woodbury, R. A. and Harper, H. T. (1944) Arterial, cerebrospinal and venous pressures in man during cough and strain. *Am. J. Physiol.*, **141**, 42.
22. Rohmert, W. (1960) Ermitlung von Erholungspausen für statische Arbeit des Menschen. *Int. Z. angew. Physiol.*, **18**, 123.
23. Thomas, V. (1971) Some effects of glucose syrup upon extended sub-maximal sports performance. *Brit. J. sports Med.*, **5**, 212.
24. Kay, C. and Shephard, R. J. (1969) On muscle strength and the threshold of anaerobic work. *Int. Z. angew. Physiol.*, **27**, 311.
25. Shephard, R. J., Allen, C., Benade, A. J. S., Davies, C. T. M., di Prampero, P. E., Hedman, R., Merriman, J. E., Myhre, K. and Simmons, R. (1968) The maximum oxygen intake—an international reference standard of cardio-respiratory fitness. *Bull. Wld Hlth Org.*, **38**, 757.
26. Shephard, R. J. (1971) The oxygen conductance equation. In *Frontiers of Fitness*, ed. Shephard, R. J., Springfield, Ill.: Charles C Thomas.

27. Shephard, R. J. (1969) *Endurance Fitness*. Toronto: University of Toronto Press.
28. Saltin, B. and Åstrand, P-O. (1967) Maximal oxygen uptake in athletes. *J. appl. Physiol.*, **23**, 353.
29. Lefcoe, N. M. and Yuhasz, M. S. (1971) The 'second-wind' phenomenon in constant load exercise. *J. sports Med. phys. Fitness*, **11**, 135.
30. Howell, J. B. L. and Campbell, E. J. M. (1966) *Breathlessness*. Oxford: Blackwell.
31. Åstrand, P-O., Cuddy, T. E., Saltin, B. and Stenberg J. (1964) Cardiac output during sub-maximal and maximal work. *J. appl. Physiol.*, **19**, 268.
32. Shephard, R. J. and Bar-Or, O. (1970) Alveolar ventilation in near-maximum exercise. Data on pre-adolescent children and young adults. *Med. Sci. Sports*, **2**, 83.
33. Shephard, R. J. (1966) The oxygen cost of breathing during vigorous exercise. *Q. Jl exp. Physiol.*, **51**, 336.
34. Newman, A. F., Smalley, B. F. and Thomson, M. L. (1962) Effects of exercise, body and lung size on CO diffusion in athletes and non-athletes. *J. appl. Physiol.*, **17**, 649.
35. Mostyn, E. M., Helle, S., Gee, J. B. L., Bentivoglio, L. G. and Bates, D. V. (1963) Pulmonary diffusing capacity of athletes. *J. appl. Physiol.*, **18**, 687.
36. Shephard, R. J. and Anderson, T. W. (1968) Training, work, and increase of pulmonary diffusing capacity. In *Muskelarbeit und Muskeltraining*, ed. Rohmert, W., Stuttgart: Gentner Verlag.
37. Roskamm, H. and Reindell, H. (1972) The heart and circulation of the superior athlete. In *Training—Scientific Basis and Application*, ed. Taylor, A. W. Springfield, Ill.: Charles C Thomas.
38. Roskamm, H. (1973) Limits and Age Dependency in the adaptation of the Heart to physical stress. In *Sport in the Modern World*, Berlin: Springer Verlag.
39. Holmgren, A. (1967) Vaso-regulatory asthenia. Proceedings of International Symposium on Physical Activity and Cardiovascular Health. *Canad. med. Ass. J.*, **96**, 853.
40. Gollnick, P. D. (1971) Cellular adaptations to exercise. In *Frontiers of Fitness*, ed. Shephard, R. J., Springfield, Ill.: Charles C Thomas.
41. Holloszy, J. (1967) Effects of exercise on mitochondrial oxygen uptake and respiratory enzyme activity in skeletal muscle. *J. biol. Chem.*, **242**, 2278.
42. Stainsby, W. N. (1966) Some critical oxygen tensions and their significance. In *Proceedings of International Symposium on Cardiovascular and Respiratory Effects of Hypoxia*, ed. Hatcher, T. D. and Jennings, D. B., Basel: Karger.
43. Rowell, L. B. (1971) Visceral blood flow and metabolism during exercise. In *Frontiers of Fitness*, ed. Shephard, R. J., Springfield, Ill.: Charles C Thomas.
44. Kachadorian, W. A., Johnson, R. E., Buffington, R. E., Lawler, L., Sarbin, J. J. and Woodall, T. (1970) The regularity of 'athletic pseudonephritis' after heavy exercise. *Med. Sci. Sports*, **2**, 142.
45. Shephard, R. J. (1968) The heart and circulation under stress of Olympic conditions. *J. Am. med. Ass.*, **205**, 150.
46. Jokl, E. (1968) Indisposition after running. In *Exercise and Altitude*, ed. Jokl, E. and Jokl, P., Basel: Karger.
47. Cavagna, G. A. (1970) Elastic bounce of the body. *J. appl. Physiol.*, **29**, 279.
48. Saltin, B. and Hermansen, L. (1966) Esophageal, rectal, and muscle temperatures during exercise. *J. appl. Physiol.*, **21**, 1767.
49. Henry J. P. (1951) The significance of the loss of blood volume into the limbs during pressure breathing. *J. aviat. Med.*, **22**, 31.
50. Shephard, R. J. (1971) Values and limitations of muscular strength in achieving endurance fitness. In: *International Symposium on the Art and Science of Coaching*, ed. Percival, L., Toronto: Fitness Institute.

51. Shephard, R. J., Allen, C., Benade, A. J. S., Davies, C. T. M., di Prampero, P. E., Hedman, R., Merriman, J. E., Myhre, K. and Simmons, R. (1968) Standardization of sub-maximal exercise tests. *Bull. Wld Hlth Org.*, **38,** 765.
52. Costill, D. L., Branam, G., Eddy, D. and Sparks, K. (1971) Determinants of marathon running success. *Int. Z. angew. Physiol.*, **29,** 249.
53. Borg, G. (1971) The perception of physical performance. In *Frontiers of Fitness*, ed. Shephard, R. J., Springfield, Ill.: Charles C Thomas.
54. Lloyd, B. B. (1966) The energetics of running: an analysis of world records. *Advancement Sci.*, **22,** 515.
55. Cooper, K. H. (1968) *Aerobics*. New York: Evans.
56. Ishiko, T. (1967) Aerobic capacity and external criteria of performance. Proceedings of International Symposium on Physical Activity and Cardiovascular Health. *Canad. med. Ass. J.*, **96,** 746.
57. Dahlstrom, H. (1964) Reliability and validity of some fitness tests. In *International Research in Sport and Physical Education*, ed. Jokl, E. and Simon, E., Springfield, Ill.: Charles C Thomas.

3

Psychological aspects of sport

This section* presents a series of concepts which hopefully can be employed in
the daily work of sports medicine physicians, coaches, trainers, and physical educationalists. These concepts are derived from research conducted over the past
eight years involving rather diverse samples, including young-age group athletes,
university level athletes, and world class performers. In addition the roll of physical fitness in the development and maintenance of mental health has been evaluated in normal middle-aged male and female subjects, as well as emotionally
disturbed children and adult psychiatric patients.

Concept 1. Athletes from various sub-groups differ in a variety of
psychological states and traits

This particular point has been demonstrated in numerous studies over the past
two decades, including detailed reviews in recent chapters by Kroll,[1] and Morgan,[2] as well as earlier reviews by Cooper,[3] and Cofer and Johnson.[4] However,
it has also been noted that even though athletic sub-groups have characteristic
profiles (e.g. wrestlers are extroverted and marathon runners are introverted),
highly successful athletes from given sub-groups may not fit the group stereotype.
Indeed, Morgan and Costill[5] found that one of the most successful U.S. runners
in the history of the Boston Marathon possessed the psychological profile which
characterizes the world class wrestler.[6]

Implication
Athletes from various sub-groups, as well as athletes within a given sub-group
possess different personality structures. Therefore, they presumably have different psychic needs and should be handled in a personalized fashion. Application
of psychological methods to groups will likely be just as ineffective as the group
prescription of medication; that is, personalized needs must be taken into
account. A further implication is that those persons responsible for the athlete's
care and treatment must be thoroughly acquainted with the athlete's personal
history. In addition any decision about treatment must be based upon input from
as many sources (e.g. coach, trainer, physician, perhaps team-mates, and the
athlete himself) as possible. This point was reinforced during the 7th SEAP
Games on the occasion of Nor Azhar Hamid's record shattering high jump performance of 2·12 m (6 ft 11½ in). In responding to his failure to break the 7 ft

* Based in part on a paper entitled 'Selected Psychological Considerations' by William
P. Morgan and published in the *Research Quarterly* (1974) **45,** 374. This material is
reproduced here with permission of the American Association for Health, Physical Education and Recreation.

barrier, Nor stated 'My target was a Gold for Singapore and this I achieved—seven feet was only a dream.'[7]

While one might be tempted to classify Nor's reply as rationalization, it might also be proposed that it reflects sound goal-setting judgement on his part. That is, he left the SEAP Games with a gold medal around his neck; the pride of his countrymen; the respect of his fellow athletes as well as his athletic contemporaries throughout the world: and, equally as important, his 'dream' of a seven-foot jump remained. Of course, had he jumped seven feet in the 7th SEAP Games, he would have been forced to strive for greater heights in the forthcoming Asian Games. The danger inherent in such a feat would have been the possibility of his peaking too early in preparation for Montreal. It will be recalled that Pat Matzdorf of the University of Wisconsin set the World Record of 7 ft 4 in (2·24 m) in the high jump during 1972, but he was unable even to qualify for the U.S. Olympic Team later that year. Clinical impressions, as well as conversations with coaches, team physicians, trainers, and athletes reveals that Nor and Matzdorf possess comparable personality structures. Readers interested in the matter of goal-setting and self-imposed limits in athletics should refer to the 'fear of success phobia' described by Ogilvie and Tutko.[8] Conversations with the team physician, physical therapist, and dentist who treated Nor the day of, and the day following his record performance, revealed a complex psychobiologic mosaic centering around the experience of pain. While professional confidences would be violated were the details disclosed, it is fair and reasonable to simply say that Nor's performance was associated with a significant psychic component.

Conclusion

It is absolutely imperative that all persons concerned with the athlete be made aware of the need to manage athletes on a highly individual basis. Put another way—'you must know your athlete(s)'. Also decisions concerning training intensity and duration, as well as goal-setting should be based upon *objective* input from the coach, trainer, team physician, and consultants such as exercise physiologists, sport psychologists, or psychiatrists, where possible.

Concept 2. High-level performers in athletics are characterized by psychological profiles which distinguish them from lower-level performers

This particular viewpoint is not supported by all exercise scientists working in the area of personality. Also, this matter has been reviewed in detail by Morgan[2] in a recently edited volume, and it is sufficient simply to state here that the failure to find psychological differences between athletes of differing ability levels to a great extent reflects problems of methodology.

It will be noted in Fig. 3.1 that wrestlers participating in the 1966 World Championships were found to be characterized by extroversion and stability when taken as a single composite.[6] However, when the Canadian, South African, and U.S. wrestlers were examined separately a different picture emerged; that is, the South African contingent scored significantly higher on the neuroticism-stability dimension. This may well have been a cultural factor, however, and one must be extremely sensitive to cultural differences when employing

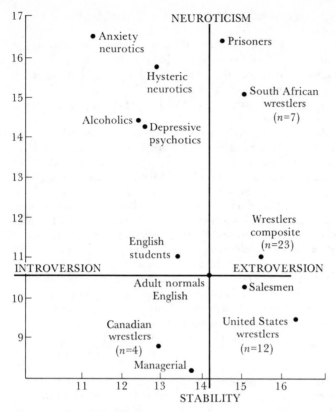

Fig. 3.1 Extroversion–introversion and neuroticism–stability in English-speaking wrestlers participating in the 1966 World Games. (Reprinted with permission from the *Journal of Sports Medicine and Physical Fitness*, 1968, **8**, 212–16.)

psychometric devices. At any rate, this investigation supported the viewpoint that high-level competitors are extroverted and stable. Furthermore, it seems fair to state that stability is a pre-requisite for high-level performance. Also, it was found in this study of high-level wrestlers that extroversion was significantly correlated with success in the 1966 World Tournament. More recently it has been demonstrated that extroversion is not a requirement for success in all sports. For example, Morgan and Costill[5] have reported that marathon runners score low on extroversion—that is, they tend towards introversion. This finding is illustrated in Fig. 3.2 which depicts marathon runners as introverts and wrestlers as extroverts. Nevertheless, it will be noted that both of these athletic sub-groups are characterized by stability.

Reinforcement of Concept 1 seems appropriate here in the consideration of group averages and profiles. While it is safe to generalize and state that world-class marathon runners are introverted and world-class wrestlers are extroverted, one must not lose sight of the importance of individuality. For example, one of the best marathon runners have evaluated is an extrovert, and conversely, one of the best wrestlers was found to be an introvert. Extroversion is correlated

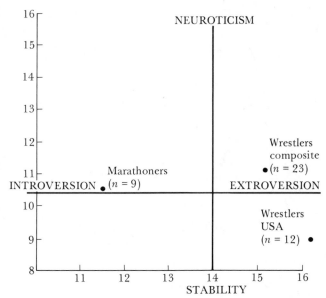

Fig. 3.2 Extroversion–introversion and neuroticism–stability in marathon runners and world-class wrestlers. (Reprinted with permission from the *Research Quarterly*, 1974, **45,** 374–90.)

with a variety of factors which are important in the athletic domain. For example, Ryan and Kovacic,[9] and Ryan and Foster[10] have found that contact athletes have higher pain tolerance than non-contact athletes, who in turn have higher pain tolerance than non-athletes. Further, pain tolerance, an important factor in many sports, is high in the extrovert and low in the introvert. Also, contact athletes score high on extroversion, whereas non-contact athletes score low on this factor. Eysenck and Eysenck[11] provide a thorough discussion of extroversion–introversion and neuroticism–stability, as well as a method of measuring these two psychological traits.

The 1972 Olympic Freestyle Wrestling Team was by far the most outstanding team ever fielded by the U.S., winning a total of 6 Olympic Medals; that is, six of the ten participants won medals. It was possible to test these ten Olympians, as well as the thirty athletes who were eliminated in the final trials. Psychological testing of the forty aspirants for the U.S. Olympic Wrestling Team was performed prior to the final selection process which consisted of round-robin wrestle-offs in each division. The results of this investigation[12] are presented in Fig. 3.3. It will be noticed that the Olympians scored lower on tension, depression, fatigue (psychic), confusion, and higher on psychic vigour. However, only the differences in tension, vigour and confusion are regarded as significant. This particular study will be discussed in more detail below. The important point is that the Olympians and unsuccessful athletes differed on a number of psychological variables.

Throughout all of this research one question has remained unanswered. Are the differences between: (i) athletic sub-groups, (ii) high- and low-level performers, and (iii) athletes and non-athletes the result of athletic participation or did these differences exist from the outset? Put another way, are the differences

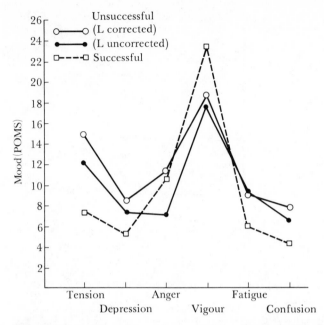

Fig. 3.3 Profile of mood states for successful and unsuccessful candidates for the 1972 U.S. Olympic wrestling team. (Reprinted with permission from the *Research Quarterly*, 1974, **45,** 374–90.)

due to heredity or environment? This is an important question since it bears on the matter of selection and prediction. It has previously been proposed that these differences can be largely attributed to genetic factors.[2,13] Space does not permit an exhaustive discussion of this topic, but it should be stated that this viewpoint is based upon theoretical considerations to a greater extent than empirical evidence. One pioneering study has been performed by Lukehart[14] who tested a group of 12- and 13-year-old boys prior to their decision to become members of an organized sport team. Those boys who elected to join the team (American football) were significantly more extroverted than those who elected not to participate (non-athletes). Both groups were retested following the first year of competition and the differences were found to be the same—the season of football did not modify the personality structures of these young men. Yanada and Hirata[15] offer additional support for the genetic or gravitation model. They found that athletes who dropped out of their sports clubs at the University of Tokyo were more depressed, neurotic, and hypomanic than those who remained. Hence, selective mortality (fall out) also supports the genetic argument.

Implication
Since athletes of differing ability levels are characterized by different psychological profiles it would seem appropriate to pursue at least two avenues in attempting to counsel and advise athletes regarding sport adoption, as well as in developing national teams. Firstly, attempts can be made through screening to identify athletes with desired profiles, and secondly, behaviour modification might be

attempted where appropriate. Of course, care must be taken that the self-fulfilling prophesy is not permitted to operate in the first instance, and it should be emphasized that no attempt at behaviour modification should be attempted by persons without the appropriate training in clinical psychology or psychiatry. Furthermore, any decision regarding selection or attempts at behaviour modification should be derived on the basis of input from the athlete, coach, trainer, team physician and consultants where appropriate.

Conclusion

Successful athletes tend to be extroverted and the exceptions to this generalization are the long distance and marathon runners who tend towards introversion. Outstanding athletes possess stable personalities in terms of the neuroticism–stability dimension, and it is unlikely that unstable athletes can perform at a high level on a consistent basis. In terms of behavioural states, the successful athlete tends to be less anxious, depressed, confused, and he possesses more psychic vigour than the unsuccessful athlete.

Concept 3. Attempts to elevate anxiety ('Psych-up') and reduce tension states should be used cautiously and on a personalized basis

While coaches frequently employ 'pep talks' as a means of energizing their teams, there is little or no evidence to suggest that such practices are of any value in the competitive situation. However, there is considerable evidence from research studies of anxiety states in relation to motor behaviour of both a simple and complex nature. Martens[16] has reviewed this literature in detail, and it seems that the evidence is equivocal; that is, there is evidence which suggests that anxiety plays a role in performance of motor skills, but there is an equal amount of evidence suggesting it does not.

Actually, this issue is not unique to sport. It has represented a continuing controversy in psychology for many years. Essentially two theoretical views have been advanced. The first is the Drive Theory which holds that increases in drive level are thought to be associated with increments in performance in a linear fashion. (Here drive level can be translated to mean anxiety.) Hence, as anxiety increases the theory would predict increases in performance. The second theoretical position, which tends to conform more consistently with everyday experiences, is the inverted-U concept or Yerkes–Dodson Law. This position holds that increases in anxiety will be followed by increments in performance up to a given point, following which further increases in anxiety will result in performance decrements. While it is difficult to state with certainty to which of these viewpoints coaches generally subscribe, it is fairly clear that a large proportion of coaches employ a variety of techniques ('pep talks', punishment, threats, etc.) in their attempt to increase tension states ('Psych-Up') in their athletes. A thorough review of this matter by Martens reveals that neither the drive theory nor the inverted-U concept is supported by an impressive body of evidence.

It should be pointed out that exercise *per se* has the effect of reducing state anxiety. Therefore any benefit to be accrued from elevating pre-competitive anxiety states would presumably be short lived since subsequent physical activity would reduce anxiety. This viewpoint is consonant with the common observation

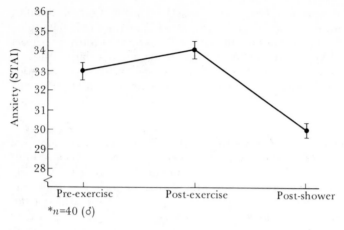

Fig. 3.4 Influence of vigorous physical activity on adult males–1. (Reprinted with permission from the *Research Quarterly*, 1974, **45**, 374–90.)

that pre-competitive tension in the form of nervousness, stomach upset, excretory frequency, dry oral mucosa, etc. passes almost immediately upon the initiation of competition. However it should be remembered that any activity is capable of reducing anxiety. This point is illustrated in Fig. 3.4. It will be noted that anxiety increased slightly following exercise in these 40 adult males.[17] However, a reduction in state anxiety was observed following 30 minutes of recovery which also included a shower. Hence, the shower following exercise may have played a role in the associated anxiety decrement. However, this possibility was not substantiated in a subsequent investigation involving 15 adult males who completed psychological inventories immediately before, immediately following,

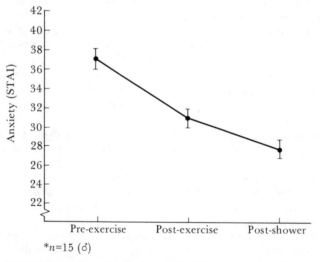

Fig. 3.5 Influence of vigorous physical activity on adult males–2. (Reprinted with permission from the *Research Quarterly*, 1974, **45**, 374–90.)

and 30 minutes following vigorous physical activity. It will be noted in Fig. 3.5 that this group experienced significant decrements in anxiety immediately following exercise, as well as after the shower. These findings have been reproduced in a series of investigations, and it is now fairly certain that vigorous exercise *per se* will reduce state anxiety in high-anxious, as well as normal adult males and females.[17]

Of course, there are many factors which might regulate pre-competitive anxiety states. For example the practice of 'making the weight' which is so common in certain athletes, especially wrestlers, has been found to decrease state anxiety. This is illustrated in Fig. 3.6 where it will be seen that a 4 per cent loss of body weight can provoke a significant decrement in anxiety.[6]

In another study designed to evaluate the state of anxiety of college wrestlers prior to both difficult and easy matches, it was found that significant *decrements*

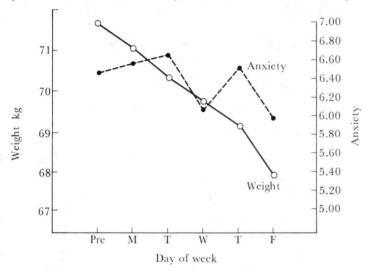

Fig. 3.6 Influence of rapid weight loss on state of anxiety. (Reprinted with permission from *Medicine and Science in Sports*, 1970, **2**, 24–27.)

in anxiety took place one hour pre-competitively as contrasted with control levels.[18] Also, the state of anxiety of the opposing team was also assessed prior to the difficult match and they were found to possess a similar level of anxiety. These findings are portrayed in Fig. 3.7. In other words, the anxiety or drive state of the winners did not differ from that of the losers when assessed precompetitively.

In a somewhat related investigation Langer[19] assessed the anxiety of a college football team approximately three hours prior to each of ten football games, as well as during the pre-season. Langer also employed coaches' ratings of performance for each game. He found that a shift in anxiety from a low score to a 'more moderate game score' was essential to good performance. It is also important to note that Langer found large fluctuations in pre-game anxiety to be detrimental to performance. In other words, the better football players were able to 'work themselves up' to a consistent level for each competition. In view of the

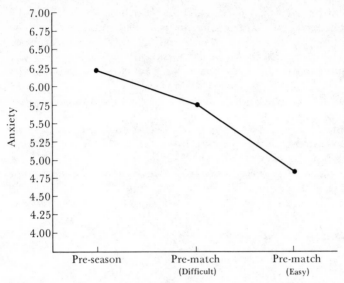

Fig. 3.7 State anxiety prior to easy and difficult competition in college wrestlers. (Reprinted with permission from the *Research Quarterly*, 1974, **45,** 374–390.)

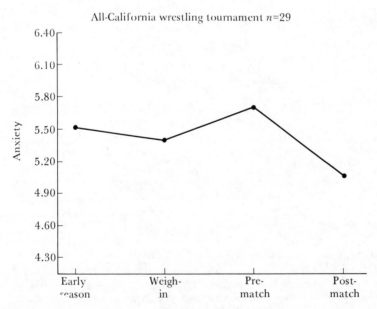

Fig. 3.8 Alterations in state anxiety during a wrestling tournament. (Reprinted with permission from *Medicine and Science in Sports*, 1974, **6,** 58–61.)

fact that team success did not co-vary with anxiety, the notion of being 'up' or 'down' for a given game was not borne out.

More recently, Morgan and Hammer[20] evaluated state anxiety of wrestlers from four different colleges (i) at the beginning of the season, and (ii) four hours before, (iii) one hour before, and (iv) immediately following competition in a state tournament. The findings are illustrated in Fig. 3.8. It will be noted that anxiety was not altered between the early season and weigh-in period (four hours prior to competition) which took place some two months later. Hence, two months of training and dual competition apparently did not alter state anxiety of these athletes. It will be noted, however, that anxiety increased significantly one hour pre-competitively which is in disagreement with the earlier findings presented in Fig. 3.7. Of course, the former represented dual competition during the regular season whereas the latter was associated with round-robin competition in a state tournament. Such conditions are obviously different in a variety of ways. It will be noted in Fig. 3.8 that a significant reduction in anxiety took place post-competitively. It should also be emphasized that the data points in Fig. 3.8 represent the average for the four teams. The data were expressed in this fashion because the four teams *did not differ at any point!* That is, the preseason, pre-tournament, and post-tournament anxiety levels of the first, second, third, and fourth place teams did not differ. Hence, anxiety did not apparently play a role in success or failure, a finding which was noted in an earlier study. Furthermore, if the data are grouped according to high- and low-anxious athletes, disregarding team affiliation, the same trend emerges; that is anxiety does not appear to be a critical factor.

Referring back to Fig. 3.3 which illustrates the profiles of Olympic wrestlers and wrestlers who failed to make the team, it will be noted that the successful wrestlers scored lower on the tension–anxiety variable pre-competitively than the unsuccessful wrestlers. Also, both groups scored below the population mean under these pre-competitive conditions. This finding suggests that, if anything, success is dependent upon low-anxiety states.

Implication
Attempting to increase performance levels by altering pre-competition anxiety states seems to be a questionable practice.

Conclusion
Anxiety levels of winning and losing teams do not seem to differ either before or following competition. Also, physical activity *per se* has the influence of reducing anxiety, and therefore, successful attempts to elevate anxiety pre-competitively would presumably be reversed very rapidly once vigorous physical activity was initiated.

Concept 4. Mental health plays an important role in athletic success, and it is quite likely that 'emotional first aid' following competition is just as important as physical first aid

Coaches have historically been concerned with the psychological preparation of their athletes for competition. This has frequently taken the form of pep talks and various other techniques thought to possess motivational value. The previous section raises the question of whether such techniques are of any value whatsoever, and existing evidence implies that the answer is no. On the other hand, a neglected, and probably far more important consideration, is the athlete's post-competitive psychological state. While coaches have historically attempted to get their teams 'up' for competition, there is little published evidence which suggests they attempt to bring them 'down'. On the other hand, there is some evidence which suggests that, win or lose, athletes return to normal psychological levels post-competitively (see Fig. 3.8). At any rate, it is reasonably clear that strains, sprains and fractures are treated immediately or shortly following their occurrence, whereas months may pass before any attention is given to serious psychological problems. Furthermore, certain psychological ailments of athletes are never even detected, much less treated. As with the case of physical injuries, preventive measures and early detection procedures should be employed. It is especially important that team physicians, coaches and trainers 'sensitize' themselves to the potential existence of psychological problems. Dismissing any athlete's problem as a 'head problem' does not solve anything. It should also be noted that 'emotional first aid' should not be limited to the athlete who experiences obvious failure. Indeed, the mediocre athlete who suddenly is catapulted into the spotlight following a record-setting performance, is probably in need of more scrutiny than the occasional failure. In this context the papers by Carmen, Zerman and Blaine,[21] Little,[22] and Pierce[23] appear to be of particular value.

Implication
Athletes should not be left to their own psychological resources following either successful or unsuccessful competition. The coach should talk with his athletes following competition, with an aim towards ego strengthening in the case of traumatic failure, as well as counsel and 'insulation' following record-setting performances. The athlete is not left to crawl off and nurse his physical wounds, and he should not be expected completely to manage his psychological trauma either. Indeed, he is probably less likely to possess the resources to perform the latter.

Conclusion
Coaches should pay careful attention to the post-competitive psychological condition of their athletes. It is in addition reasonable to state that psychological stability is a pre-requisite for success in the high-level sportsman. Successful athletes who are *truly* neurotic are the exception rather than the rule.

Concept 5. There is frequently a lack of congruence between the athlete's conscious and unconscious motives

It is not uncommon for an athlete to set a record and subsequently be unable to reproduce his performance or even come close to it. This sometimes occurs despite the fact that the athlete verbalizes his willingness to 'do anything' in order to achieve his previous level of performance. However, there is frequently a lack of congruence between the athlete's conscious verbalization and his unconscious motivation. This particular point of view is illustrated in a recent hypnoanalytic case.[24]

The athlete was a 21-year-old college distance runner. He had previously established a school and conference record in the 3-mile run, but he was unable to match this performance, nor could he even come close. Indeed, he was frequently not even capable of completing races he started. The athlete's coach interpreted his failure as reflecting a 'lack of desire' and willingness to 'put out'. The athlete on the other hand felt the coach was not offering him the necessary instruction to regain his previous performance high. At any rate, the runner was willing 'to do anything' to perform well once more. He was examined by the team physician and found to be perfectly healthy. There was no medical explanation for his poor performance. He was next examined by an exercise physiologist and found to have a maximal $\dot{V}o_2$ of 70 ml/kg of body weight which compares favourably with the aerobic power of distance and marathon runners described by Morgan and Costill.[5] The runner's previous record performance in the 3-mile run was calculated to have taken place at about 96 per cent of his maximal aerobic power. While others have noted that runners can work at such a per cent of maximum in similar races, such a performance across a 3-mile course is obviously demanding to say the least. The runner's psychological profile suggested normality in all respects. However, he possessed the characteristics of the world-class wrestler to a greater extent than the distance runner; that is, he was extroverted rather than introverted, and he scored high on hypnotizability. Subsequent sessions revealed that he was capable of entering a deep trance during which he could age-regress to earlier periods.

Under deep hypnosis the athlete was age-regressed to the day of his championship performance and requested to describe the entire race. He was able to visualize this event quite clearly, and after a very short period of time he began to experience 'pain in the side' as well as respiratory discomfort. He explained that he could not continue the race because of the intense pain (he had been running at about 96 per cent of his maximum aerobic capacity). Just as he began to terminate the race a group of his team-mates appeared and exhorted him to 'kick'. He explained that he could not let his team-mates down, and therefore, he was able to continue, with the effect that the pain was no longer noticeable. However, it returned later in the race, and he again decided to quit only to experience a double-visual hallucination on the horizon. It consisted of two television sets. He was depicted on one set as if the race were being televised (it was not), and his parents appeared on the other monitor. They in turn were thought to be viewing him run on an additional television set. He was unable to carry out his plan to stop because of these 'complications' and within a short period of time he felt as though he was in a vacuum. He could not feel any wind resistance, nor could he sense his feet hitting the ground. He described the conclusion of the race in which his chest hit the tape as being a very 'weird' experience.

The runner elected to have a post-hypnotic recall for all of these events in the waking state. When asked if he cared to continue with 'insight training' he replied that he would prefer to give the matter some additional thought. He subsequently elected not to continue with the 'insight training' (hypnoanalysis), and presumably he had gained the necessary insight he lacked earlier. His running did not improve, but his understanding of his inability to reproduce his previous record apparently did. That is, the record race was extremely painful, and he had apparently repressed this experience from his conscious. However, this repressed perceptual experience was 'replayed' during hypnosis with the effect that he elected not to continue delving into the matter. Of course, it would have been quite simple to construct 'cognitive strategies' during hypnosis with an aim towards dissociation of pain during running competition in the waking state. However, since the athlete did not wish to pursue such avenues 'the case was closed'.

Implication
A significant discrepancy may exist between the athlete's stated desires and his 'actual' (unconscious) attitude(s) towards record-setting performance.

Conclusion
The coach and physician should look beyond the athlete's past performances and current conscious verbalizations. The essence of 'failure' is best understood within a psychobiological framework which relies upon such specialties as sports medicine, exercise physiology, and sport psychology.

W.P.M.

Personality and performance in sport

Accounting for individual differences in learning and performance is the constant operational problem of the teacher. Physical educationists and coaches are certainly as aware and as sensitive as others to variations in individual's aptitude, abilities, aspirations, and general motivation, but they appear to be especially fascinated by the possibility that, in the last analysis, differences in skill and athletic performance may be attributable to variations in personality structure. One explanation offered by the physical educationists is that the environments in which gross physical abilities are displayed (e.g. in games and sports) constitute an ideal setting for the development of such socially desirable personality characteristics as confidence, sociability, self-reliance, co-operativeness, and general personal adjustment. The relationship between personality and athletic ability is also strongly supported by those who coach and advise champion athletes. These coaches, usually quite sophisticated in their understanding of the physical factors accounting for the large proportion of the variance in athletic performance, seek additional insights for the selection and training of athletes, and the prediction of their competitive behaviour from personality data. Such expectations derive from the writings and research reports of, for example, Cofer and Johnson,[4] and Ogilvie and Tutko.[8] Cofer and Johnson have suggested that in personality, athletes are a 'special breed', and that in the final assessment personality is the vital factor in the discriminating process which singles out the champion from those who appear to have similar physical gifts. Ogilvie and Tutko claim to have identified personality dimensions which are essential to competitive success, and have indicated some common personality problems of athletic 'under-achievers'. In a much wider context, it can also be said that physical educationists have become increasingly attracted to the possibilities of explaining observed individual differences in the learning and performance of a wide range of skills which constitute the curriculum of physical education and recreation, in terms of personality dispositions such as perceptual style, selective attention, risk-taking propensity, achievement motivation, and persuasibility.

The amount of published research concerning the proposed link between personality and demonstrated physical ability is not extensive, but is increasing, no doubt due to the improved validity of the measures available. A number of broad-based investigations (e.g., Fleishman,[25] Ismail and Gruber,[26] and Cratty[27]) have begun to give increasing clarity and dependability to the understanding of the factors involved in gross physical ability. At the same time personality assessment has become theoretically sounder and better standardized, even though Adelson felt impelled to open his review of personality studies in the 1969 edition of Annual Review of Psychology with the sentence, 'The field of personality these days is marked by abundance, diffusiveness and diversity.' The Cattell 16 PF inventory and Eysenck's E.P.I. are currently the favoured tools for personality studies in this area, and at least this has the advantage of making possible comparisons between the findings of different investigations. Reviewers are, however, still confounded by the variety of systems used for classifying subjects, by the different analytical methods employed, and in general by the absence of either formulated hypotheses or theoretical frameworks. Nevertheless, a number of detailed reviews of the empiric research are available (e.g. Warburton and Kane,[28] Ogilvie,[29] Husman,[30] Hendry,[31] and Harris[32]) though the studies included tend to be limited to relatively simple personality descriptions of selected groups of athletes. Even so, the reviewers find difficulty in coming to unequivocal or generalized conclusions, although it is more usual for male athletes to be described in terms of extroverted and stable tendencies (such as high dominance, social aggression, leadership, toughmindedness and emotional control) and for women athletes to be described as relatively anxious extroverts. It must be said immediately, however, that there are many exceptions to these general descriptions. This is hardly surprising since the nature of the sport or physical activity, and the subject's level of participation are two intervening variables affecting the relationship between personality and performance. If, for the sake of argument at this point, it is accepted that certain personality traits are found to be linked with outstanding goalkeeping or goal scoring ability in soccer, it would be most surprising to find that all the same traits were linked with high-level performances in javelin throwing, cross-country running or rifle shooting.

However, when the activity and level of participation are held constant, interesting consistencies in personality profiles have been reported, and evidence presented in support of the existence of certain sports 'types'. For example, Ogilvie[29] argues for a 'racing driver type' on the basis of very similar 16 PF profiles of the outstanding drivers in his research. Kroll suggested[1] that competitive wrestlers may also constitute a personality type when he could show no discriminant space between the profiles of three groups of these athletes. Kane[33] came to the same conclusion with respect to gifted soccer players when the profiles of his three groups of subjects (described as professionals, young professionals and amateur internationals) could not be separated by discriminant function analysis. Williams[34] similarly found good class women fencers from different teams to display no major profile difference, while Kane[33] had earlier demonstrated that British women Olympic swimmers and track athletes had almost identical personality profiles, and argued that this finding might well indicate a very narrow selection of women for high-level competitive athletics attributable to either the constraints of societal expectation or to the special female

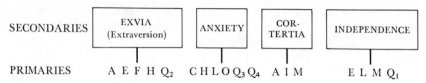

Fig. 3.9 Personality structure.[43]

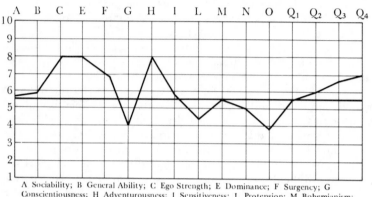

A Sociability; B General Ability; C Ego Strength; E Dominance; F Surgency; G Conscientiousness; H Adventurousness; J Sensitiveness; L Protension; M Bohemianism; N Shrewdness; O Insecurity; Q_1 Radicalism; Q_2 Self-Sufficiency; Q_3 Will-Power and Q_4 Tenseness.

Fig. 3.10 Champion athletes.[35]

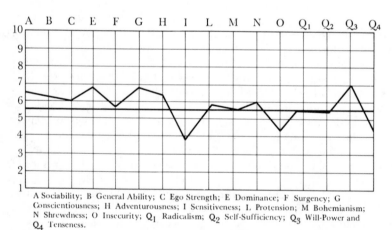

A Sociability; B General Ability; C Ego Strength; E Dominance; F Surgency; G Conscientiousness; H Adventurousness; I Sensitiveness; L Protension; M Bohemianism; N Shrewdness; O Insecurity; Q_1 Radicalism; Q_2 Self-Sufficiency; Q_3 Will-Power and Q_4 Tenseness.

Fig. 3.11 International rugby.[36]

requirement of very particular personality supports for successful competitive involvement.

To clarify the argument developed thus far, it may be helpul to introduce a few illustrations. Fig. 3.9 outlines the personality traits and the major higher order structure according to Cattell. Fig. 3.10 represents Heusner's[35] 16 PF profile of Olympic champions, and demonstrates the almost classic stable extroversion of

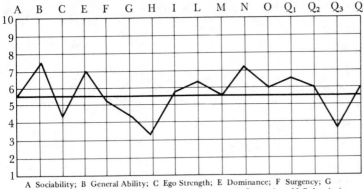

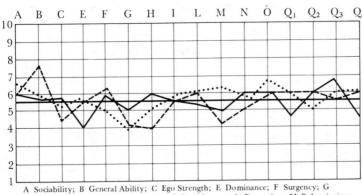

A Sociability; B General Ability; C Ego Strength; E Dominance; F Surgency; G
Conscientiousness; H Adventurousness; I Sensitiveness; L Protension; M Bohemianism;
N Shrewdness; O Insecurity; Q_1 Radicalism; Q_2 Self-Sufficiency; Q_3 Will-Power and
Q_4 Tenseness.

Fig. 3.12 British swimmers.

these men. It is worth noting that subsequent studies have never shown such
clear-cut profile description. Fig. 3.11 is a profile of British rugby players of international class[36] which also supports the stable extroversion description of athletes,
but by contrast Fig. 3.12 illustrates a profile of anxious introversion based on
the personality scores of 126 British swimmers. Figs. 3.13 and 3.14 represent the
similarity of profiles found among samples of soccer players and women athletes,
giving rise to the notion of personality 'types'.

It must be admitted, however, that a review of the research literature reveals
great confusion and contradictions due not only to the diversity of criterion groups
and methods employed, but essentially to a lack of any sort of theoretical framework or insight into the way in which personality dimensions may account for
differential performance. Eysenck[37] has constantly drawn attention to the importance, for instance, of parameter values and the mechanics of the measures used

A Sociability; B General Ability; C Ego Strength; E Dominance; F Surgency; G
Conscientiousness; H Adventurousness; I Sensitiveness; L Protension; M Bohemianism;
N Shrewdness; O Insecurity; Q_1 Radicalism; Q_2 Self-Sufficiency; Q_3 Will-Power and
Q_4 Tenseness.

Fig. 3.13 Soccer: professionals, amateurs, apprentices.

48   *Psychological aspects of sport*

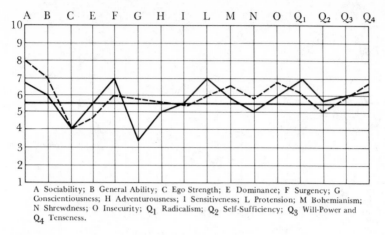

A Sociability; B General Ability; C Ego Strength; E Dominance; F Surgency; G Conscientiousness; H Adventurousness; I Sensitiveness; L Protension; M Bohemianism; N Shrewdness; O Insecurity; Q_1 Radicalism; Q_2 Self-Sufficiency; Q_3 Will-Power and Q_4 Tenseness.

Fig. 3.14 Women swimmers and track.

in experimental psychology. He refers, in particular, to the proposed link between extroversion and conditionability and explains the contradictory findings of researches as being a direct reflection of the parameter values used; weak unconditioned stimulus values favouring quick conditioning of introverts relative to extroverts, while strong unconditioned stimulus values have the opposite effect. Careful attention to the niceties of both personality theory and other parameter values is therefore needed in order to clarify the nature of such experimental relationships. In the area of research into the relationship of personality to athletic performance, no such sensitive account has so far been taken of these theoretical niceties. There would seem to be still a limitation to relatively inductive approaches aimed at personality description of criterion groups. If the results are unclear it is not surprising since such gross approaches suffer from well known experimental and methodological limitations such as the reliance on mean scores, the use of non-situationally specific inventories and the lack of fine control of subjects, either on athletic performance or on personality grounds.

More obviously it would seem to be unreasonable to expect that personality should constitute an equally important factor in different athletic activities. Physiological understanding is sophisticated enough to know that success in different sports depends on fitness factors (such as strength, cardiovascular endurance and flexibility) to a greater or lesser extent. Sprinters are not noted for their cardiovascular fitness, nor cross-country runners for their strength. Moreover, it is recognized that different sports appear to need different admixtures of skills and fitness. Consider in this connection the skill and fitness demands of bowling, cross-country running, tennis playing and weight-lifting. Is it not reasonable then to suspect that personality factors may have a different weighting in the successful performance of various athletic events; being highly important for some, of small importance in others, and of no importance at all in the remainder? If this is so then it is hardly surprising that researchers find different relationships between personality dimensions and ability in different athletic sports.

Moreover, conjecture on the nature of the personality/physical ability relation-ship from the framework of Eysenck's theoretical and empirical evidence might be better based on hypothesizing links between his E and N scales and athletic activities (such as tennis and soccer) in which the perceptual processes (in particu-lar, vigilance and selective attention, kinesthetic awareness and recall) are emphasized or where conditioning (especially to stress) may be critical.

On the other hand it is difficult to find theoretical models for hypothesizing the personality dimensions that might be important to success in, say, javelin throwing, sprinting, forward play in rugby, or even swimming.

Even within a particular athletic sport when personality differences between gifted athletes and others are found, or between these athletes and the general population norms, speculation arises as to the inferences which may be drawn. Are the personality characteristics found to be considered as pre-requisites for success, or are they to be taken as the result of long term involvement in the sporting activity? Kroll[1] has plausibly outlined four ways in which personality correlates of athletic ability may have meaning, and ventures to suggest that most research has been limited to the first of these possible interpretations. First, it may be that a set of personality factors exists which prompts individuals to become involved in a particular activity or sport. Those who possess these personality qualities in the appropriate combinations are then seen as capable of persisting long enough to become successful. According to this explanation, novices and veterans will possess similar personality patterns, the only possible difference being in the extent to which they are present. A second possibility is that there is no specific 'entry' pattern. Then, either by modification of personality over time, or by rejection of inappropriate patterns, only those developing a suitable personality pattern continue to retain their interest and progress satisfactorily. In this case, novices would exhibit different personality patterns, but veterans would possess a similar one. Educationally the therapeutic implications are obvious in this kind of model. A third explanation points to the possibility of there being a similar pattern for novices and veterans existing at entry to the physical activity or sport, but participation or selective rejection results in dissimi-lar patterns for veterans. A fourth possibility is that both novices and veterans possess dissimilar and non-discriminant patterns, and that significant research findings are purely artefacts.

Further cross-sectional comparisons of groups of athletes at different levels of achievement within a particular sport would certainly be helpful to test the validity of Kroll's postulates. In this connection the use of discriminant function analysis, which seems to have become fashionable recently with sports researchers, would seem to have great advantages for comparing multi-dimensional profiles, since it can take into account the variability over entire profiles and hence reflect total personality differences more accurately than bivariate techniques. Kroll has himself demonstrated the possibilities of the dis-criminant function approach in a personality study of winning and losing football teams, in which he found a function which significantly differentiated between the teams in personality terms.

Of even more significance in testing Kroll's models would be well controlled longitudinal studies of athletes involved in training and competitive performance. Very few such studies have so far been reported, and even then the experimental periods have been rather short. However, three recent investigations using adult athletes are in accord in finding no personality change attributable to athletic involvement over periods of three and four years. Werner and Gottheil[38] traced 16 PF profiles for West Point cadets involved in general athletics; Rushall[39] had as subjects high-level swimmers, footballers, and track and field athletes under regular training; and Kane[33] compared the personality profiles of men and women physical education students at the beginning and at the end of their four-year course of training. However, in Kane's study it was clearly demonstrated that both men and women students involved in physical education (and therefore presumably in athletics and sports) differ in personality from the general body of students. If these personality differences are in any way attributable to the 'athletic environment' then presumably the cause and effect reaction takes place before maturity. Support for this interpretation is given by Tattersfield's[40] findings for boys involved in an extensive training programme for 'age-group' swimmers. Boys aged 10 years had their personality profiles carefully documented over a period of four years. In this case highly significant changes were shown to have taken place over the experimental period. The changes were towards greater extroversion, more stability and greater dependence. From an educational standpoint it might be considered that the first and second of these personality changes were desirable, but the third one—towards greater dependency—probably not. More pertinently, however, the point might be made, on the basis of these few longitudinal studies, that personality changes due to athletic involvement are unlikely to be demonstrated among adults, since presumably their personality structures are well established and less susceptible to alteration. However the effecting of change in the developing and more plastic personality of the young, through athletic training and participation, is apparently possible.

Correlational approaches

So far this section has dealt only with the problems of squeezing useful information from the descriptive surveys of athletes that constitute the largest amount of evidence available in this area. It is somewhat surprising to find that almost no substantial correlational studies have been undertaken in an effort to tease out the nature of the personality/physical performance relationship. If and where a relationship exists it would seem that appropriate correlational procedures could best demonstrate the circumstances under which it is maximized, and this in turn could give rise to a better understanding of the nature of the relationship.

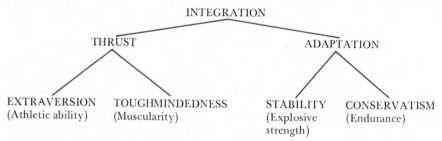

Fig. 3.15 Personality—athletic ability—hierarchical factor structure.

One attempt to consider the values of correlational strategies has been reported[33] and gives hopeful indications for further work of this sort that would clarify relationships under different parameter values. In these correlational studies two domains—personality and gross physical performance—were each assessed by sixteen variables among men and women physical education students. Figure 3.15 summarizes the factor structure and emphasizes that the largest second order factor links extroversion with general athletic ability (e.g. speed, strength and power). A series of multivariate analyses demonstrated, as expected, the increasing value of correlation coefficients from bivariate techniques through multiple regression to canonical analysis (see Kane).[33] In summary the findings were:—

(1) Among women, stability is significantly linked with the appropriately weighted physical performance domain. Approximately 15 per cent of the variance in stability is accounted for by the physical measures.

(2) Among men, extroversion is significantly linked with the physical performance vector. Approximately 16 per cent of variance in extroversion is accounted for by the physical measures.

(3) An index of sports participation is significantly linked with the multiple personality vector (which accounts for about 20 per cent of the variance) among both men and women. The most important contributing personality variables were found to be Q_2 (group dependence), E (dominance), and Q_4 (low ergic tension).

(4) The canonical correlations between the two domains for both men and women were both significant and emphasized a relationship between extroversion and athletic ability.

Apart from other implications that may possibly be developed from these correlational studies, the findings give clear corroboration to the notion that personality and physical performance are related, and that the relationship seems to depend essentially on the link between extroversion and general athletic ability.

Possible explanations and implications

Even at the descriptive level it has been pointed out that the research has produced equivocal results, and although some of the problems militating against a clear interpretation have been outlined, the fact remains that so far the research programmes have lacked rigour and perseverance. This is due essentially to the lack of any guiding theoretical framework, and possibly to the lack of suitable instruments for assessing behaviour in the specific athletic environment. What the physical education teacher and coach require from research in this area are helpful and reasonably reliable suggestions which will enable them to deal most effectively with individual differences in personal dispositions in learning and performance. At present, purely on the evidence available, this is clearly a difficult task unless an attempt is made to re-interpret existing evidence within established theoretical frameworks.

It cannot have been missed in what has gone before that such interpretations as have been offered were mostly set out in terms of the two major personality complexes proposed by Eysenck. Although Cattell's 16 PF tests have been widely used, interpretations from scores on his primary factors have not helped very much, and only derived second order factor scores (for extroversion and anxiety) which are more or less equivalent to the Eysenckian dimensions have proved useful. Eysenck's personality theory defines two broad personality scales E (extroversion–introversion) and N (neuroticism) which give a description of the phenotype, but do not in themselves represent any theory of causation. He has continued to emphasize, however, that underlying causal substrates of personality may be at the genotypic level and has continued to refine a theory linking overt personality and behaviour with causal biological sources. He proposes five levels which elaborate the genotypic links with the descriptive phenotype. The first level relates to genotypic differences between organisms and emphasizes the constitutional control of excitation and inhibition. The second level reflects differences in psychophysiological measures of genotypic variables (EEG, EMG, etc.), while at the third level environmental influences are represented as affecting behaviour, which is measured by experimental tests of conditioning, vigilance, etc. The fourth level refers to habitual personal behaviour patterns as represented by the major personality traits, which in turn give rise to types of socially relevant behaviour (neurosis, crime, accident-proneness, drug taking, etc.) at the fifth level. Most personality research has, of course, been concerned with the development and use of major personality dimensions at Eysenck's fourth level, but the earlier antecedent causative stages, and the consequent social behaviour are vital to Eysenck's theory.

Behavioural causation is, therefore, directly traceable (according to Eysenck) to idiosyncratic neural organization: neuroticism is explained as the lability or excitability of the autonomic nervous system, mediated by the hypothalamus, while extroversion–introversion is seen as reflecting the strength of the excitatory and inhibitory functions of the central (cortical) nervous system. Originally Eysenck proposed two separate but interrelated neutral circuits to explain his two main personality dimensions. The first, with which extroversion–introversion is identified, involves a system of recticular and cortical loops; the second, associated with neuroticism, is identified with the hypothalamus. Claridge[41] therefore suggested two related sources of personality arousal, i.e. sensory–recticular arousal and autonomic (hypothalamic) arousal. A great deal of recent research in personality causation has centred on arousal mechanisms, and it would seem that there is a possibility of rapprochment here between the rather different approaches of Russian and Western psychologists to the explanations and effects of arousal in man. Soviet psychophysiology has for a long time centred on the theory of the basic properties of the nervous system elaborated in its initial form by Pavlov, and developed and applied to man by Teplov[42] and his colleagues. The most recent postulates identify the properties of the highly organized nervous system as:

(1) Strength of the nervous system with regard to its endurance in the face of prolonged excitation.
(2) Strength of the nervous system to endure prolonged inhibitory stimuli which is thought to be reflected in its dynamism.
(3) Mobility of the nervous processes reflected in speed of transformation of stimuli.
(4) Lability of the nervous system characterized as the speed of initiating and terminating nervous processes.

It is suggested by Teplov[42] that the Russian psychologists' notion 'equilibrium of the nervous system' must now be taken to refer to the balance of excitatory and inhibitory processes for each of these properties separately considered. He also indicates that extensive research has only been carried out on the first of these suggested properties—strength of the nervous system. A number of researchers in the East and West have recently noted that the property called 'strength of the nervous system' may be equivalent to, or at least equated with, the higher order personality dimensions. Cattell[43] in fact used the title 'strength of the nervous system' to describe his proposed main third order factor, which combines his second order factors exvia (extroversion), and cortertia (cortical alertness). Gray[44] in discussing the issue concluded, '... there appears to be sufficient evidence for it to be worth devoting serious attention to the hypothesis that the dimensions of strength of the nervous system, and introversion–extroversion, are identical, both being based on arousal.' Moreover, Morton[45] suggests that higher levels of arousal appear to be characteristic of *both* neuroticism (high drive level) and introversion. Claridge[41] had earlier made the same point in elaborating Eysenck's theory into an equivalent arousal model which gave more emphasis to the excitatory processes than to inhibitory processes emphasized by Eysenck. His studies of the excitation–inhibition balance in perceptual and perceptual-motor tasks allowed Claridge to conclude that both extroversion and neuroticism contribute to arousal. He further suggested that one may consider two functionally related arousal mechanisms; the first he identified as a 'tonic arousal system' which is concerned with maintaining the individual's gross level of arousal, and the second is suggested as the 'arousal modulating system' which controls the level at which the tonic arousal system functions, and also integrates the stimulus input by appropriate facilitation or suppression. In other words, arousal might be considered operationally as comprising two components: (a) *chronic arousal* representing a relatively stable personality trait, and (b) *arousability* describing a variable reactivity factor concerned with the individual's lability to arousal-producing situations and with arousal modulation.

For the present purposes, therefore, the argument being offered is that the link between personality and performance may best be explained through the mechanisms of arousal and particularly through a consideration of the way in which stimuli are mediated and modulated through the arousal system.

The way in which an individual's situationally specific arousal level is related to performance has been well documented, and in general seems to be best expressed by an inverted U-shaped curve[46,47] in which performances improve with arousal from a low level up to an optimum, after which performance deteriorates with further increases in arousal.

Welford[48] has developed this point by suggesting that poorer performances might be expected from stable extroverts, whom it may be assumed are lower in both (chronic) arousal and arousability, and cites Furneaux's studies of student examinations which seem to be in line with this generalization, though extroverts tend to perform better than introverts when the environmental circumstances increase or sustain their arousal level (as with noise and at later times in the day when presumably the extrovert has had time to be aroused). The relationship does, however, rather depend as well on a number of factors (e.g. the difficulty of the task, ability, incentive value, previous experience, susceptibility to punishment) which together add up to perceived stress giving rise to a situationally specific and idiosyncratic level of arousal. Moreover, in the context of gross motor and athletic type performance, where endurance may be important, some evidence exists to link stability rather than anxiety with efficiency, in that trait anxiety (or high N) has been consistently associated with high scores on physiological measures such as cardiac and cardiovascular response. Endurance athletes tend to capitalize on their low physiological activation.

In general, therefore, if personality may be adequately and satisfactorily interpreted as arousal, it would seem to be a useful step towards understanding the personality/performance relationship. Enough has been said already, however, to indicate that a rigorous explanation would need to go a lot further. Even the attractive inverted U hypothesis for linking arousal with performance does not take one very far in terms of prediction, since on the one hand for a given performance (except the optimal) there will be two possible values for arousal, and on the other it has been shown that incentives differentially affect the relationship for introverts and extroverts.[47] This arousal/performance model is, however, of some help in considering competitive behaviour in sport. It has been strongly argued that anxiety is the most important factor affecting competitive performance.[19] Anxiety, which is a composite of relatively stable traits and situationally specific states, may be regarded as a strong drive to both autonomic and possibly cortical arousal. The net arousal level in a given stressful situation may well depend mostly on the athlete's chronic level, and ability to control anxiety. The coach's problem would seem therefore to be in manipulating, as far as possible, the athlete's anxiety-based arousal with a view to bringing him into the competition at a level which will give rise to optimal performance. Some success in such a daunting task has been reported by sports psychologists, e.g. Ogilvie.[29]

If anxiety (or neuroticism) appears to be the most important constituent of athletic *performance*, then it might appear that the other major personality dimension, introversion/extroversion may be of greater significance for athletic *training*. The essentially physical training that athletes undergo is intended to increase performance potentials by regular and systematic submission to strenuous programmes aimed at physiological adaptation and contextual skill development. The extent to which an athlete submits and perseveres with these demanding, repetitive, and often dull programmes, and therefore the benefit he gains in performance potential, is likely to be associated with his standing on the introversion/extroversion continuum. It seems not unreasonable to expect, for instance, that the more extroverted athletes, compared with the more introverted, would persevere longer where pain is involved, would react more positively to incentives, would need more variation in training stimuli, would condition more slowly to risky and dangerous situations, would react more positively to public criticism, would train better in group situations, would more quickly develop reactive inhibition especially in massed practice circumstances, and would be less consistent in training effort and results. Additionally, Eysenck and his colleagues have demonstrated the way in which extroverts and introverts systematically differ in the learning and performance of a number of fine and gross skills. In all, such a catalogue of the behavioural patterns of introverts and extroverts must constitute a very useful basis on which coaches may plan schedules to maximize the training effect on their athletes.

There seems no doubt that the wide spectrum of activities covered by such terms as 'sports' and 'athletics' make for almost insuperable difficulties in developing a general theoretical explanation of the proposed association between personality and sports performance. Some type of sports taxonomy is needed before speculations can be taken much further. It would seem in fact that personality profiles, which have been reported as describing the behavioural dispositions of participants in a particular sport, may be reflecting aspects of social selectivity rather than behavioural ones. If, however, sights are narrowed to those sporting and athletic pursuits which throw a heavy burden on the perceptual processes, it is possible to draw not only on the theoretical and experimental findings of experimental psychology in general (and the work of Eysenck in particular) but also on the work of those researchers concerned with explaining behaviour through perceptual styles of selecting and processing information. It would seem that within the confines of perceptual-motor performance, the relevance of Eysenck's personality theory and supportive evidence could be assessed, especially with respect to vigilance and selective attention. Not only would his postulates regarding his N and E scales and their interaction seem to be useful for these purposes, but this recently formed P (psychoticism) scale deserves close consideration. Additionally, the work of, for example, Witkin, Petrie, and Lacey offers other similar explanations of individual differences. Witkin's concept[49] of psychological differentiation is based on modes of perceiving, summarized in the continuum field dependence–field independence, and attention has been drawn by a number of workers[50] to the possible links between Poulton's classification of skills into 'open skills' (in which the reading of the environmental display is vital) and 'closed skills' (in which there is relative independence of environmental stimuli). Petrie has suggested[51] that in their perceptual processing, individuals may be said to be at a point of a bipolar dimension, describing at the extremes augumenters and reducers of perceptual input. Clearly Petrie may well be identifying a process not greatly dissimilar from Eysenck's E. Lacey's similar proposal[52] was based on the differential patterns of fluctuation in autonomic arousal levels which he claims to have observed consistently. He consequently described people as stabiles or labiles. Stabiles apparently show an even, quiet, unchanging autonomic functioning, while labiles demonstrate greater variability involving spontaneous bursts of physiological activity. In terms of related behaviour it is hypothesized that labiles would be impulsive in motor activity; would, for instance, find difficulty in withholding incorrect responses; and would tend to be more susceptible to external stimuli. Whiting has additionally suggested[53] that in fast ball games, differences in perceptual sampling strategies, and inferences drawn from them, may be different for extroverts and introverts.

Even so one should not expect too much from laboratory findings, and their direct applicability to the specific situation in sport. Variability attributable to personality factors in the laboratory may be accounted for by other factors in the real game or sports situation, particularly by ability and previous experience, which give rise to associated anticipatory behaviour. The way in which sports and games strategies and performance are reflective of an individual's ability, and his experience, are not well understood. Not all those with high N or high arousability are failures in competitive sport. The drive associated with these dispositions can clearly be of great benefit so long as the individual can learn to persevere and control them for productive purposes.

Summary
It is here attempted to interpret and account for reported evidence of, and associations between, personality measures and performance in sport. Some support is presented from descriptive studies for personality 'types' participating at high level in certain sports. In general, however, the findings from descriptive studies are equivocal and difficult to tie to a theoretical or causative framework without categorizing sporting activity according to some behavioural taxonomy. Nevertheless, Eysenckian theory seems to be useful even at this stage for attempting explanations for a personality/performance association in sport. This is argued as being best explained by arousal and arousability mediated by factors such as ability and experience.

J.E.K.

References

1. Kroll, W. (1970) Personality assessment of athletes. In *Psychology of Motor Learning*. ed. Smith, L. E., Chicago: Athletic Institute.
2. Morgan, W. P. (1972) In *The Psychomotor Domain*, ed. Singer, R. N., Philadelphia: Lea and Febiger.
3. Cooper, L. (1969) Athletics, activity and personality: A review of the literature. *Res. Q. Am. Ass. Hlth phys. Educ.*, **40,** 17.
4. Cofer, C. N. and Johnson, W. R. (1960) In *Science and Medicine of Exercise and Sports*, ed. Johnson, W. R., New York: Harper and Row.
5. Morgan, W. P. and Costill, D. L. (1972) Psychological characteristics of the marathon runner. *J. Sports Medicine & Phys. Fitness*, **12,** 42.
6. Morgan, W. P. (1968) Personality characteristics of wrestlers participating in the world championships. *J. Sports Medicine & Phys. Fitness*, **8,** 212.
7. Ziegelaar, R. (1973) Golden Nor delights the fans. *The Straights Times*, 3rd September, p. 24.
8. Ogilvie, B. C. and Tutko, T. A. (1966) *Problem Athletes and How to Handle Them*. London: Pelham.
9. Ryan, E. D. and Kovacic, C. R. (1966) Pain tolerance and athletic participation. *Percept. Mot. Skills*, **23,** 383.
10. Ryan, E. D. and Foster, R. L. (1967) Athletic participation and perceptual augmentation and reduction. *J. Personality Soc. Psychol.*, **6,** 472.
11. Eysenck, H. J. and Eysenck, S. B. G. (1962) *Manual for the Eysenck Personality Inventory*. San Diego: Educational and Industrial Testing Service.
12. Nagle, F. J., Morgan, W. P., Hellickson, R. O., Serfass, R. C. and Alexander, J. F. (1975) Spotting success traits in Olympic contenders. *Physician and Sports Medicine*, **3,** 31.
13. Morgan, W. P. (1974) In *Sports Medicine*, ed. Ryan, A. J. and Allman, F. L., New York: Academic Press.
14. Lukehart, R. (1969) The effect of a season of interscholastic football on the personality of junior high school males. *Abstr. Am. Ass. Hlth, Phys. Educ. Recreation*, **5,** 122.
15. Yanada, H. and Hirata, H. (1970) Personality traits of students who dropped out of their athletic clubs. *Proc. Coll. Phys. Educ.* University of Tokyo, *No. 5*.
16. Martens, R. (1973) In *Ergogenic Aids and Muscular Performance*, ed. Morgan, W. P., New York: Academic Press.

17. Morgan, W. P. (1973) Influence of acute physical activity on state anxiety. *Proc. Nat. Coll. Phys. Educ. Ass.*, **76**, 113.
18. Morgan, W. P. (1970) Prematch anxiety in a group of college wrestlers. *Int. J. Sports Psychol.*, **1**, 7.
19. Langer, P. (1966) Varsity football performance. *Percept. Mot. Skills*, **23**, 1191.
20. Morgan, W. P. and Hammer, W. M. (1974) Influence of competitive wrestling upon state anxiety. *Med. Sci. Sports*, **6**, 58.
21. Carmen, L. R., Zerman, J. L. and Blaine, G. B. Jr., (1968) Use of the Harvard psychiatric service by athletes and nonathletes. *Ment. Hyg.*, **52**, 134.
22. Little, J. C. (1969) The athlete's neurosis—a deprivation crisis. *Acta Psychiat. Scand.*, **45**, 187.
23. Pierce, R. A. (1969) Athletes in psychotherapy: How many, how come? *J. Am. Coll. Hlth Ass.*, **17**, 244.
24. Morgan, W. P., Nagle, F. J. and Ryan, A. J. (1972) Psychobiologic interpretation of 'failure' in sport. Paper read before American College of Sports Medicine, Philadelphia.
25. Fleishman, E. A. and Rich, S. (1963) Role of kinesthetic and spatial-visual abilities in perceptual motor learning. *J. Exp. Psych.*, **66**, 6.
26. Ismail, A. H. and Gruber, J. (1967) *Motor Aptitude and Intellectual Performance*. Ohio: Merril.
27. Cratty, B. J. (1967) *Movement Behaviour and Motor Learning*. Philadelphia: Lea and Febiger.
28. Warburton, F. and Kane, J. E. (1967) Personality related to sport and physical ability. In *Readings in Physical Education*, ed. Kane, J. E., London: Physical Education Association.
29. Ogilvie, B. C. (1968) Psychological consistencies within the personality of high-level competitors. *J. Am. Med. Ass.*, **205**, 780.
30. Husman, B. (1969) Sport and personality dynamics. *Proc. NCPEAM*, University of Minnesota.
31. Hendry, L. (1970) A comparative analysis of students characteristics. *M. Ed. Thesis*, Leicester University.
32. Harris, D. V. (1973) *A Somatopsychic Rationale for Physical Education and Sport*. Philadelphia: Lea and Febiger.
33. Kane, J. E. (1970) Personality and physical abilities. In *Contemporary Psychology in Sport*, ed. Kenyon, G. S., Chicago: Athletic Institute.
34. Williams, J. M., Hoepner, B. J. and Moody, D. L. (1970) Personality traits of champion female fencers. *Res. Q. Am. Ass. Hlth Phys. Educ.*, **41**, 446.
35. Heusner, W. (1952) Personality traits of champion and former champion athletes. *M. A. Thesis*, University of Illinois.
36. Sinclair, E. (1968) Personality and Rugby football. *M. A. Thesis*, University of Leeds.
37. Eysenck, H. J. (1972) Human typology, higher nervous activity and factor analysis. In *Biological Bases of Individual Behaviour* ed. Nebylitsyn, V. D. and Gray, J. A., London: Academic Press.
38. Werner, A. C. and Gottheil, E. (1966) Personality development and participation in college athletics. *Res. Q. Am. Ass. Hlth Phys. Educ.*, **37**, 1.
39. Rushall, B. (1970) An evaluation of personality and physical performance. In *Contemporary Psychology in Sport*, ed. Kenyon, G. S., Chicago: Athletic Institute.
40. Tattersfield, C. R. (1971) Competitive Sport and Personality Development, *Ph. D. Thesis*, University of Durham, 428.
41. Claridge, G. (1967) *Personality and Arousal*. London: Pergamon Press.
42. Teplov, B. M. (1972) The problem of types of human higher nervous activity and method of determining them. In *Biological Bases of Individual Behaviour*, ed. Nebylitsyn, V. D. and Gray, J. A., London: Academic Press.

43. Cattell, R. B., Eber, W. and Tatsuoka, M. (1970) *Handbook for the 16PF*. Illinois: IPAT.
44. Gray, J. A. (1967) Strength of the nervous system: introversion–extroversion, conditionability and arousal. *Beh. Res. Therapy*, **5**, 151.
45. Morton, M. L. (1972) The theory of individual differences in neo-behaviourism and in the typology of higher nervous activity. In *Biological Bases of Individual Behaviour*, ed. Nebylitsyn, V. D. and Gray, J. A., London: Academic Press.
46. Duffy, E. (1962) *Activation and Behaviour*. New York: John Wiley and Sons.
47. Corcoran, D. W. J. (1972) Studies of individual differences at the Applied Psychology Unit. In *Biological Bases of Individual Behaviour*, ed. Nebylitsyn, V. D. and Gray, J. A., London: Academic Press.
48. Welford, A. T. (1968) *Fundamentals of Skill*. London: Methuen.
49. Witkin, H. A. (1962) *Psychological Differentiation*. New York: John Wiley and Sons.
50. Poulton, E. (1957) On prediction in skilled movement. *Psychol. Bull.*, **54**, 467.
51. Petrie, A. (1960) Some psychological aspects of pain and relief of suffering. *Ann. N.Y. Acad. Sci.*, **86**, 13.
52. Lacey, J. I. (1959) Psychophysiological approaches to the evaluation of psychotherapeutic process and outcome. In *Research in Psychotherapy*, ed. Rubinstein, E., Washington: National Publishing Co.
53. Whiting, H. T. A. and Hutt, J. W. R. (1972) The effects of personality and ability on speed of decision regarding the directional aspects of ball flight. *J. Mot. Behav.*, **4**, 2.

4

Training

The days are long gone when natural endowment alone was enough to secure success in sport. In activities where performance is most directly and objectively measurable, such as athletics and competitive swimming, training for physical conditioning has been assumed an essential pre-requisite from the earliest days of serious competition. More recently, however, not only has training spread to most games and sports, but the level of participation at which players are expected to indulge in serious, time-consuming programmes of physical conditioning is becoming lower. A glance at fitness programmes proposed for aspiring club players in the *Squash Player* magazine illustrates this well;[1] these describe schedules including heavy weight training, interval running and pressure training. Thus even an activity which is itself a 'fitness' game, and used for that purpose by other games players, has its own fitness training. Relative to their physical capacity, many successful women players train just as hard as men.

The sheer volume of time and effort put into training nowadays is remarkable; 10 000 m runners may put in over two hundred miles a week of running, and swimmers may spend in excess of five hours a day in the pool. That this raises important ethical considerations is beyond doubt. The discussion of them is, however, beyond the scope of this chapter. Suffice it to say that it raises the most serious questions when one considers such intensive training for young adolescent swimmers and athletes with their comparative immaturity, vulnerability to dominance by coaches and parents, and the inappropriateness of obsessional behaviour, such as intensive training demands, to a period of growth, development and education that would seem to require the greatest flexibility.

'Training' and 'practice' are different concepts in the world of sport. 'Training' is used to mean the improving or maintaining of physical capacity, for example the use of systematized exercises to increase strength, endurance, and so on. 'Practice' refers to the repetition of techniques used in the sport concerned so that they may become more effectively executed. Thus a tennis player might practise his forehand, hoping that its timing and accuracy will be improved, and also that correct execution of the stroke will become a more habitual response, leaving the mind clear for tactical considerations. Broadly speaking then, 'training' involves taking the physical capacity factor out of the context of the sport and doing exercises to improve it, while 'practice' merely involves taking the technique, or the skill as it is often called, out of the context of the whole game or event so that it may be improved through repetition. Activities vary in the degree of emphasis placed on each. In some, such as golf and tennis, by far the major amount of time is devoted to practice, only a few individuals feeling it necessary or desirable to train 'out of context'. In men's team games a considerable amount of time is spent on physical conditioning, but the major part of preparation for skilled activities, such as racket and team games, tends to be a mixture of training and practice of which 'pressure training' is typical. The idea of this is for techniques to be practised repeatedly under simulated game conditions, speed and endurance being taxed by the pressure of set opposition or time limits for the completion of the manœuvre. Whilst this would appear to be a most logical form of preparation, it should be appreciated that if the techniques so practised are not already competently executed, deterioration of skill rather than improvement may result.[2]

Despite the near universality of training in competitive sport, it is important to realize that training can only at best embellish performance; a racehorse cannot be made out of a shirehorse, nor the reverse. Training can only build on a substantial foundation of appropriate genetic endowment.[3]

The physiological rationale of training

It would be wrong to suppose that training is an exact science, or even a consistently rational application of physiological knowledge concerning the limiting factors of performance. While much training method is sound physiological common sense, much of it is based on hunches, trial and error, traditional beliefs, and the current practices of eminent, successful athletes. Fads and vogues follow one another in rapid succession; nothing is too wayout to try if it might, just might give that vital, microscopic edge over a rival. If the new Olympic 10 000 m champion trained by running backwards and eating live frogs, both the method and the diet would be seriously considered and probably adopted by some aspiring athletes. Of course, many of the methods devised and instigated by great runners and their coaches *are* sound, and with time there is a gradual overall rationalization of approach based on effective experience.

One major obstacle to the evaluation of training methods is the enormous difficulty in devising satisfactory experimental conditions. In any form of training, motivation is such an important factor, that, without it, the same order of results just does not occur. It is virtually impossible to obtain a control group with similar motivation to that of the experimental group. The only sort of motivation that makes sense in this context is positive motivation, and no highly motivated athlete will submit to a form of training about which he is uncertain, let alone deny himself training altogether; the practicality of double-blind trials is even more remote. Another problem is that the approach of the exercise physiologist tends to be to put physical work capacity factors into somewhat watertight compartments, for example, strength, aerobic capacity, anaerobic capacity, and so on (Fig. 4.1). This, if applied too directly, can lead to a form of training which does not relate effectively to performance. For example, the isolation of muscular strength as a factor in performance was brought to an extreme degree, for valid purposes of study, by Müller.[4] His discoveries relating to the nature of strength and the optimum stimulus and frequency for training, caused a furore in the sporting world. Isometric schemes of training were devised and used; numerous investigations were carried out testing isometric against isotonic methods, and eventually it was realized that increases in isometric strength did not necessarily benefit dynamic performance. Müller's work had had the important effect of underlining the complexity of factors involved in what previously most had con-

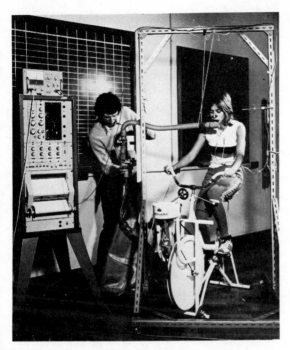

Fig. 4.1 Physiological testing in the laboratory: the middle-distance runner shown here is having her heart rate and oxygen consumption monitored at a number of known workloads on the bicycle ergometer using E.C.G., Douglas Bag, and gas analysis. (Photo: S. K. Joshi.)

sidered to be activities relying for their successful performance on pure strength. In this respect Whitney[5] gives a fascinating account of the multiple factors affecting the strength of lifting action in man.

This compartmentalization of factors may bring with it a further over-simplification. For example, ability to run a marathon is primarily dependent upon a very high oxygen uptake capacity—not just a high maximum but, more importantly, the ability to sustain for over two hours a very high sub-maximal level (of the order of 85 per cent of maximum). However, the ability to win a particular race against a particular opponent may depend on the one competitor's superior capacity to sustain sporadic pace variations, that is incurring a number of states of oxygen debt during the race; or again, it may be a hot day and specific acclimatization may determine the outcome. However, exercise physiologists are progressively analysing the variables relating to performance, showing which are trainable and which are not, although many may nurse a private hope that the picture will never be entirely clear. The day when the prediction of potential and the design of training become a matter for the collection and computerization of data, will also be the day that competitive athletics dies.

What then are the trainable variables? Åstrand lists them comprehensively in his *Textbook of Work Physiology*.[6] For a broad categorization of trainable components of performance, Munrow's classification[7] is most useful, and indeed is now common currency in the physical education world. He is careful to point out that most activities require a blend of these components and that the components themselves merge, strength being a factor in local muscular endurance for example. He classifies the components as follows:

(1) Strength.
(2) Endurance, sub-divided into
    (a) local muscular endurance;
    (b) circulo-respiratory endurance;
    (c) expedition type endurance.
(3) Mobility.
(4) Skill.

The last, skill, is in a category of its own, the most specific and least transferable of all the qualities above. It is the end product of practice, not of training and therefore comes outside the scope of this chapter. However, it is important that skill should always be borne in mind when considering a sportsman's best use of the time available to him for preparation. It would be absurd to spend more time on training than practice if glaring deficiencies in technique were apparent, and limited time were available.

Of great interest is the third category of endurance, 'expedition type' endurance. Within this can be included and examined all the very important and specialized aspects of fitness: some highly specific such as acclimatization to altitude; some general such as tolerance of discomfort, development of judgement of the degree of exhaustion attained and how much energy remains, and the conscious marshalling of resources for the supreme effort. It often seems that a top-class performer is something more than the sum of his parts.

The fundamental principle of all training stems from the fact that the healthy human body thrives on use, provided of course that adequate nutrition and energy supplies are available. Not only does it thrive on use, but adaptation occurs to maintain a functional reserve capacity above the habitual demand placed on organs and systems. Different estimates exist concerning the margin of reserve capacity above the habitual demand. In a relatively sedentary person, both habitual demand and maximum capacity are low, the reserve capacity being relatively large, however. Hettinger claims[8] that the habitual strength demands are of the order of 25–30 per cent of maximum. For the sportsman, however, making continual near-maximal demands on his strength or endurance, the margin of reserve capacity over habitual demand is small. The response to the stimulus of an increase in habitual demand is an attempt by the adaptive processes to develop a functional reserve above this new habitual demand. This used commonly to be called 'overload' but now the term 'progressive resistance' is more generally used. This principle is most obviously demonstrated in strength training.

Strength and strength training

Early work formalized by Delorme[9] for rehabilitation exercises, demonstrated that muscles required to contract against increasing loads or resistances became progressively stronger. This increase in strength is generally accepted to be accompanied by hypertrophy. However, no great precision has been achieved in attributing a standard amount of available contractile force to a unit area of

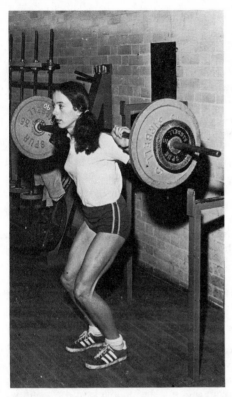

Fig. 4.2 Weight training: an outstanding young cross-country runner lifting substantial weights with confidence and good style giving the lie in so doing to the common fear among women that such activity brings gross overdevelopment. (Photo: S. K. Joshi.)

muscle cross-section. This has led to some suggestion that hypertrophy is not the inevitable consequence of all strength increases.

Classical weight training still forms the basis of most strength training (Fig. 4.2). It is so well known that perhaps it is only necessary to point out that it differs from the sport of weight-lifting. The latter consists of highly skilled, pre-scribed lifts performed competitively, the objective being to lift the heaviest weight, employing the strongest involved muscle groups at the point of greatest mechanical advantage, in a subtly efficient summation of forces. Weight training consists of devising exercises which require muscle to exert greater forces. Often positions of poor mechanical advantage are exploited to place heavy resistance on large muscle groups, or to develop strength throughout the range of move-ment. Weight training has the disadvantage of unidirectional resistance, i.e. in always combating gravity. However, the use of pulleys, ingeniously developed in physiotherapy, can overcome this disadvantage; so also can the use of rubber strands or springs. Conforming to Hooke's Law, resistance increases in propor-tion to stretch, a property which can be most usefully exploited to counteract increasing mechanical advantage, enabling 'overload' to be sustained through a large range of movement. Such devices, however, are not easily calibrated, and one of the main appeals of weight training is the exact knowledge of poundage achieved. Detailed regimens are specialized matters. Every coach, and almost every sportsman, has his own theories concerning how many repetitions should be performed of each exercise, how many sets of repetitions, what the relationship is between many or few repetitions and hypertrophy, and what type of weight training is best for 'power'. Answers to these questions are complex.[10] Astrand, however, concludes, after an extensive examination, that Delorme's original guidelines are still valid, in that low repetition–high resistance exercises produce power, high repetition–low resistance exercises produce endurance. The question of power, however, is particularly interesting. Since 'power' is defined in mechanical terms as 'the rate of doing work', it has traditionally been assumed that to enable muscles to contract faster against a given resistance, for example body weight, it is necessary merely to make them stronger. Early work by Chui[11] and others showed vertical jump scores to be increased by programmes of heavy weight training. McCloy[12] claims that the only trainable variable in speed of muscle contraction is muscle strength, and the other variable, viscosity of tissue, is unalterable. Recent developments, however, including the recognition that slow and fast muscle fibres may respond quite specifically to training, and some questioning of the relationship between strength gained by weight training and improvement in performance, have affirmed the validity of jumpers, sprinters and others performing fast training movements with relatively light weights for the development of power. 'Jump-squats' are an example of such exercises. This raises again the whole issue of taking physical components out of context of the activity for training. It is possible to discern circular trends in the history of training. Once, training was by doing, synonymous with practice, it then became progressively taken out of context. 'Isometrics' was the *reductio ad absurdum* of this. The trend now is to seek to put the strengthening action back into a context

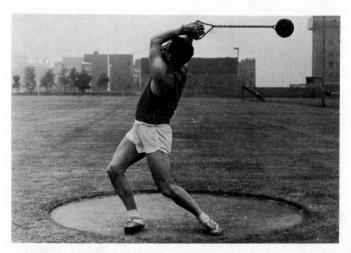

Fig. 4.3 A world-class hammer thrower trains with a 28 lb (12·6 kg) hammer (12 lb (5·4 kg) more than the weight he will use in competition). This example of overload raises the question of whether the complex pattern of skilled technique is disrupted by such a practice. (Photo: S. K. Joshi.)

simulating the movement of the technique for which one is training, or even to practise the technique itself with increased resistance such as heavier equipment. Two examples of the latter are illustrated here (Figs. 4.3 and 4.4).

Müller's work, already referred to, made a valuable contribution to the understanding of the nature of strength. The Sporting World, however, responded somewhat extremely to the staggering initial claims that one isometric contraction, 40 per cent of maximum per day, held for a few seconds, would bring

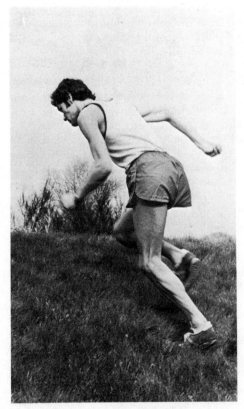

Fig. 4.4 The cross-country runner seeks overload above the normal stress by storming up steep grass banks. This particular runner had undergone a decompression and strip of the left Achilles Tendon (see chapter 25) some ten weeks previously. (Photo: S. K. Joshi.)

about the maximum possible increase in muscular strength. Although this claim was subsequently modified as a result of further work, the idea had been conveyed that all the sweat and endeavour of the weight room could be replaced with a few minutes sub-maximal effort, posturing with protagonists and antagonists locked in mild opposition (the 'dynamic tension' of Charles Atlas). Isometric exercises became very much in vogue, though, with a mixture of common sense and anxiety not to relinquish a proven method, most athletes continued to include a substantial amount of isotonic work in their routines.*

Following Müller's work came a number of comparative studies of isotonic and isometric methods, of which three examples are listed.[10, 13, 14] All suffered from the problem referred to earlier, i.e. that of setting up valid training experiments. The technical difficulties of measuring isotonic strength also meant that either isometric measurements were used to assess the effects of both regimes, or the poundages achieved in isotonic regimes were compared with dynamometer measures of isometric strength, neither being a very satisfactory method. Müller and other workers somewhat modified his early claims for isometric training,[15] mainly to the effect that a certain duration of contraction was necessary, 60 per cent of the maximum duration, and that for people in the upper echelons of fitness a higher frequency than once per day would be more effective. Most published work showed isotonic training to be the more effective and Gardner[16] showed the training effect of isometrics to be confined to a range of movement 20 degrees either side of the angle at which the training contraction was performed.

Two other pieces of work stand out for their contribution to the understanding of the complexity of strength, although in a way they ask more questions than they give answers. First of all, Ikai and Steinhaus[17] demonstrated the overriding importance of motivation in strength performance. Using various artificial motivators, such as a shot fired at the moment of the attempt, amphetamines, intravenous injections of alcohol, and hypnosis, they obtained significant improvement in strength scores of the order of 7–12 per cent for most artificial motivators and *of 26 per cent for hypnosis*. Shephard in Chapter 2 refers to the importance of the effect of central inhibition on performance. The effect of increasing motivation, coupled with a reassuring accumulation of experience, clearly reduces inhibitory restraints, and could be one factor which accounts for increases in effective strength without hypertrophy. Secondly, a most ingenious and perceptive piece of work by Rasch and Morehouse[18] reveals the importance of familiarity of movement and position to the voluntary production of maximum contractions. Strength increases produced by an isotonic exercise programme 'disappeared' when the subjects were tested in an unfamiliar position or by an unfamiliar test, even though the angle of pull of the muscles involved was rigorously standardized. Substantial increases in strength of contralateral but unexercised limbs were also recorded. One of Rasch and Morehouse's conclusions is that 'learning' is responsible for a large part of apparent strength increases. These findings merit closer attention and investigation.

Recently, attempts have been made to resolve the problems of measuring strength in action and at the same time to produce apparatus which allows the application of an infinitely variable progressive resistance. One of these devices is the 'mini-gym' (Fig. 4.5). The term 'isokinetic' has been coined to describe

*N.B. 'Isometric', meaning equal in length, and 'isotonic', meaning equal in tone, are the terms conventionally used to describe contraction or muscular activity which occurs without and with shortening of the muscle respectively. Both are to some extent misnomers: the former involving a certain degree of initial shortening due to stretching of tendons; the latter, equal in tone, describing a state not normally occurring during the movement because of changing resistance and mechanical advantage. These terms are often replaced by 'static' and 'dynamic'.

the sort of muscular contraction it allows. From the term it will be apparent that the speed of movement theoretically remains the same after initial acceleration. The device automatically increases resistance in response to the subject's attempts to move the limb faster. More refined, research specification, isokinetic dynamometers have a variable speed control and produce a graphic representation of muscular force exerted throughout the movement.

It would be wrong to leave the topic of weight training without a word of caution. Many types of lifts produce enormous stresses on highly vulnerable structures; for example, during a dead lift of 200 lb (90 kg) by a 170 lb (76·5 kg)

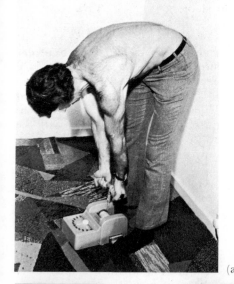

(a)

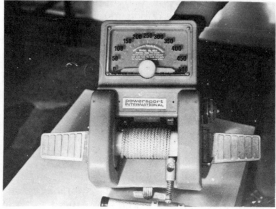

(b)

Fig. 4.5 (a) The 'MINI-GYM' in use. (b) Close-up of the apparatus. (Photo: S. K. Joshi.)

man, Morris and his co-workers[19] have calculated that the force on the lumbosacral disc is of the order of 2000 lb (900 kg), while during the deep-squat, severe
stresses on inappropriate tissues and structures are often inevitable if a lift is to
be performed to conform to the strict definitions of competitive weight-lifting.
They constitute a hazard of the sport, but there is no need whatsoever for the
weight-trainer, who merely wishes to strengthen muscles, to subject himself to
the same hazard, perhaps risking injury which may keep him out of his sport
for a very long time or even permanently. Plenty of viable alternatives exist to
the squat for strengthening leg extensors; for example, a leg press machine, where
the weight-trainer lies on his back and pushes weights up on a sliding framework
with his feet, or the Klein bench.[20] Even the half-squat is greatly preferable for
safety. The point of no return is less likely to be reached, and the position of
the spine and pelvic girdle are much more stable.

Endurance training

This is a more complex component. Strength is a factor in local muscular
endurance, such as that required by the sprint canoeist, for example, or by a
tennis player who needs to serve and smash repeatedly for five hard sets. It makes
sense, therefore, to use weight training for this factor, or some sort of over-loaded
repeated exercise in the context of the activity, provided that sufficient repetitions
are possible. Too heavy a load will defeat the object and may interfere with the
technique for the activity. Increased endurance will result from muscle hypertrophy, increased vasculature, augmented myoglobin, and increased glycogen
stores.

The importance of strength to performance normally associated with a high
circulo-respiratory capacity has already been referred to. A very substantial
analysis is made in Chapter 2 of the many determinants of this, longer term, whole
body endurance. When contemplating preparation for an activity or event of
this nature, it is important to consider the total situation of the event. The relative
importance of strength, aerobic capacity, and anaerobic capacity must be understood in terms of (a) the event itself, (b) the individual's relative sufficiency or
weakness with regard to the requirements of the event, and (c) particular circumstances such as venue, or type and likely tactics of opponent which may modify
such requirements. Wilt[21] analyses the percentage of time spent in developing
these three components by athletic training for track events of different distance.
These range from the marathon with 5 per cent of the time devoted to speed,
90 per cent to aerobic capacity, and 5 per cent to anaerobic capacity, through
the mile, (20 per cent speed, 25 per cent aerobic, and 55 per cent anaerobic)
to the 100 m sprint with 95 per cent speed, 2 per cent aerobic capacity, and 3
per cent anaerobic capacity. To be sure that such effects were occurring with
such precise distribution is another matter!

The Åstrands' studies of intermittent work[6, 31] are very illuminating indeed in
demonstrating the energy resources predominating in different types of physical
exercise. In particular, they identify the threshold of duration and intensity of
work at which alactacid supplementation of excess oxygen requirement over
maximum rate of steady-state supply is exhausted, and supplanted by true
anaerobic metabolism. They show that the pattern of effort and rest intervals for
a given amount of work in a given time critically determines whether or not

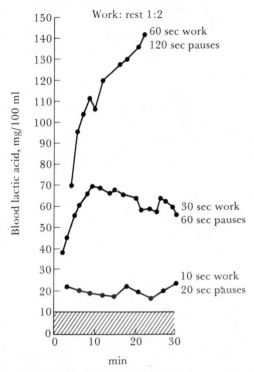

Production 25 200 kpm in 30 min

Fig. 4.6 The blood lactic acid concentration in a total work production of 25 200 kpm in 30 minutes. The work is accomplished with a load of 2520 kpm/min, the work periods being 10, 30, and 60 seconds, and the corresponding rest periods 20, 60, and 120 seconds respectively. (From Åstrand and Rodahl[6] by permission of the publishers.)

lactate levels rise (Fig. 4.6). As excess lactate is one of the major determinants of fatigue, it is clearly important tactically in a distance race to confine spurts creating energy demands above one's steady-state maximum to those which can be met by alactacid (myoglobin) resources, and to hope that one's opponents are forced to exceed theirs! The principal contribution of the intermittent work studies, however, is to produce a rationale for the design of 'interval training'.

Interval training
This has for some years been the principal training method for most runners. Doherty[22] attributes the method to the work of several pioneer coaches in Germany and Finland in the 1920s and 1930s. It comprises a system of repeated efforts in which a set distance is run on a track at a timed pace a certain number of times with a standardized recovery interval between efforts. Permutations of length, time, number of runs and duration of recovery interval are as manifold and individual as weight training schedules. Progression is made by shortening the time for the runs, increasing the number of runs, and decreasing the rest intervals. Obviously, shorter, faster runs will tend towards increasing strength

and anaerobic power, and longer runs will develop aerobic capacity, the length of the recovery interval often determining the extent of anaerobic demand. More recently, and for many years in swimming, in the controlled interval training method, pulse rate has been used rather than time to determine the length of the recovery interval, and to control the pace of the efforts. The heart-rate criteria for this practice stem from work by Karvonen,[23] who observed that 'the heart rate during training has to be more than 60 per cent of the available range from rest to the maximum attainable by running, or above approximately 140 beats per minute, in order to produce a decrease of the working heart rate.' Thus if the swimmer's heart rate at the end of an effort swim were less than 140 beats per minute he would be required to swim faster in the next effort. Rest intervals terminate when the heart rate has fallen to a pre-arranged level. If it is to be carried out strictly, such a system needs a skilled administrator for each athlete or swimmer in training.

Not every athlete has an inexhaustible appetite for such dourly prescribed forms of training. The monotony of repetition, the featureless regularity of the track and the cold precision of the stop watch can, if unrelieved, make training degenerate from stimulus to drudgery, reinforcing expectation of inadequate performance. Training needs elements of freshness and variety. More important still is the need for training which allows the athlete to exercise his own will and judgement during the effort, to respond to how he feels and to the terrain—essentially, to *enjoy* his running and exult in his fitness. *Fartlek*, or 'speed-play', is a system of training, or more commonly an ingredient of training, in which the athlete runs over varying terrain, preferably natural and beautiful (traditionally pine forests), and responds to the challenges presented by the terrain by jogging, sprinting, pacing, and striding, at will or to some prescribed framework. Clearly the athlete must be motivated to set himself challenges; he must feel eager to sprint up hillsides, coast down long inclines, to keep the pressure *on himself*, rather than rely on his coach or the watch. So, as Doherty points out, the freedom and naturalness which are such valuable assets in Fartlek require a high level of self-discipline. The embracing of such a form of training as described by one authority, quoted in Doherty,[22] gives some insight into the pressures on the track athlete. 'Fartlek was perhaps the most alluring discovery since the beginning of the century in the realm of training. A window was opened on the forest and at the same time an idea of training emerged which one would classify as "happy". Fartlek with its walks, its runs at slow pace through the woods, its short sprints, was able to revolutionize the training of the track world....' What an extraordinary state of affairs, when the pleasure of running in natural surroundings has to be rediscovered, not by sedentary man, but by athletes themselves! This type of work forms a substantial part of the training of endurance athletes, particularly during the winter season. From the purely clinical point of view it has the great advantage of reducing the number of injuries attributable to training on hard surfaces, but may produce more sprains because of uneven terrain.

Circuit training

A further form of training which trains both general endurance and local muscular endurance in particular, but also may be designed to increase strength, is circuit training, designed by Morgan and Adamson[24] in 1952 in response to their findings that schoolchildren developed more fitness during the holidays than while undergoing school physical education programmes. It is very widely used now for all sorts of training requirements; being particularly popular and appropriate for team games and suiting the indoor 'club training night' situation admirably (producing a fine thirst)! It consists of a series of exercises done in sequence, the permutation and variety of which are infinite; but typically a circuit may comprise 'step-ups', often with a loaded pack, 'pull-ups', 'press-ups', 'shuttle runs', abdominal exercises such as sit-ups, perhaps some simple, safe weight exercises such as 'curls', and a carefully designed exercise for strengthening dorsal muscles. This basic battery of exercises will be supplemented by exercises which will meet the specific requirements of the activity being trained for. There are 8–10 exercises in all. At the first session the individual is tested on each exercise for his maximum number of repetitions, either to exhaustion or within a given time. This score is divided by three to determine the training rate for each exercise. The participant then, at each subsequent session, performs three circuits of all the exercises at the training rate, as fast as possible. His time to complete three circuits will progressively diminish. An adjustment can then be made to his training rate, either by re-testing the maximum or, arbitrarily, by the addition of repetitions to each exercise. Often this procedure of testing and re-testing individuals is simplified by setting up three grades of load on each exercise, or more simply still, three grades of circuit. However, the circuit is not then so closely tailor-made to the requirements of the individual. One of the important advantages of this form of training is its sociable and competitive nature, large groups of people of different abilities and fitness being able to train together at their individual rates, competing against themselves but also against one another by comparative improvement.

Mobility training

Joint mobility, or the range of movement available at a joint or joint complex is certainly an important determinant of performance (Fig. 4.7). A considerable volume of investigation has been carried out[25,26] which clearly relates above average mobility in relevant joint complexes to top-class performance in many branches of sport, particularly to specific events in athletics and strokes in swimming. The needs of the hurdler are self-evident, as is the need for adequate extension of the ankle in the front crawl swimmer. More complex and subtle but no less important requirements are revealed only by careful analysis of the specific techniques. What is less certain is the degree to which mobility can be effectively modified by training, and indeed the desirability of such training. Mobility, often called flexibility, is not in the same category as the other components of performance so far discussed. Generally speaking there is no limit to the desirable amount of circulo-respiratory endurance to be gained, nor to strength, except perhaps where gains in muscle bulk and weight bring diminishing returns. With mobility, however, in most instances, enough is enough. If the position required by the activity can be reached, for example in hurdling or in a gymnastic movement such as the back flip, then no further mobilization is necessary. Where mobility allows force to be transmitted through a greater range of movement as in throwing events, then again there will be an optimum starting position, and no further mobilizing beyond this point will be required.

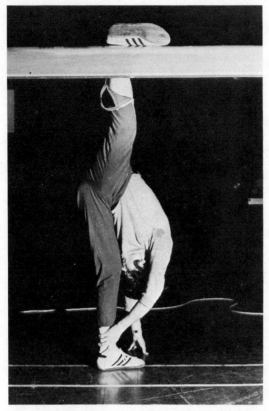

Fig. 4.7 A dramatic demonstration of mobility in more than one plane is given by this near-7-ft. 2·13 m high jumper in training. But to what extent is the mobility endowed or acquired? (Photo: S. K. Joshi.)

Munrow's work[7] is full of sound common sense and shrewd insight concerning the component of mobility; in particular he draws attention to the dangers of vigorous, passive mobilizing exercises. He defines 'passive exercises' as those in which a force external to the muscle group normally responsible for a given movement is used not only to produce that movement but also to attempt to increase it. Such external forces may be applied by a partner or by the individual himself, using for example, body weight and momentum as in the traditional vigorous, bouncing, straight-legged trunk flexion exercises. Munrow underlines the physiological nonsense of adopting a procedure which will at best provoke a limiting contraction of antagonists through the myotatic reflex, and at worst overcome this to produce injury. He claims that 'active' mobilizing exercises, that is those in which the movement is under the control of the active contraction of the protagonist group, are much safer and more effective. More recently, however, Holt, De Vries, and others[27, 28, 29] have described a form of mobilizing or flexibility training which is claimed by them to be effective, both in increasing range of movement, and as a form of therapy for certain conditions of muscle soreness. It is claimed that the system is based on 'proprioceptive neuro-muscular facilitation' techniques developed originally for muscle therapy.[30] Essentially, the method consists of the 'priming' of muscle groups prior to their stretching by a strong isometric contraction against partner resistance at the initial position of ʌull stretch. After this priming, it is claimed that the muscles concerned are amenable to further stretch by a combination of active contraction of muscles on the opposite side of the joint, and partner assistance 'with light pressure'. In practice, experience appears to confirm that the limb concerned can be moved to a new end position in its range of movement after isometric priming. However, the evaluation of this technique is not yet convincingly completed, although some published work gives encouraging evidence for its acceptance.[28] It should be borne in mind that mobility is extremely difficult to measure. If measured by the end position achieved by the extremity of a limb or limb segment, it is essential that the positional relationship of other segments of the body be strictly controlled (e.g. degree of pelvic tilt in hip flexion measures). Also, the achievement of improved mobility scores immediately after such a procedure does not necessarily imply that an increased range of movement will be available during activity.

Whatever method of mobilizing is used, it would seem that caution and the use of physiologically sympathetic procedures should be the keynote, rather than vigorous masochism. Whereas, in the pursuit of endurance, self-inflicted pain and punishment may be end-justifiable means, this is not so for mobility. Indeed, very little is known about the desirability of joint mobilization, except in its therapeutic role where the obviously valid objective is to restore former movement. Even if it is shown that an individual's sports performance is enhanced by increased mobility, it cannot thereby be assumed that the long-term health of the joint mobilized has been improved, or indeed, has not been prejudiced. A great deal of research needs to be done in this important and neglected area, the implications of which are substantial. A number of important questions spring to mind, and there are more. For example, is there an optimum range of movement for a healthy joint or joint complex, such as hip or shoulder; optimum in terms of congruity of articulating surfaces, strength and stability of the joint and endowed anatomy? How amenable to imposed congruity, especially in adulthood, are areas of joint cartilage not previously brought into adjacency? Are muscles in all joint actions the main factors in limitation of movement or are the ligaments of greater importance? Other questions can certainly be added to this list, and the discussion in Munrow[7] is particularly relevant. Finally, whereas there is abundant evidence that strength and endurance improve as a consequence of increased demand (and an increasing conviction that the latter quality is related to health) a certain amount of optimism is needed to assert that human joints thrive on the intense activity indulged in by the modern sportsman.

Conclusion

The foregoing is but a brief review of some of the main objectives of contemporary training methods. Rather than present a detailed description of various individual exercises and elaborate regimes which can be found in coaching and training manuals, an attempt has been made to draw attention to some of the problems and difficulties posed in the prescription of training. A great deal has been left out and the very fault of compartmentalization, referred to in the introduction, has been indulged in. As previously stressed, it is very important that the total situation of the competition or event being trained for should be considered, and all elements which may have an important bearing on performance simulated if possible in the conditioning programme. Acclimatization, whether to heat or altitude, or both, must feature as a large component of a training programme for a sportsman who is to compete in an environment differing in these aspects from his native habitat. Acclimatization to altitude, including the vexed question of altitude training for the improvement of sea level performance, is dealt with in another chapter.

Against this case for the elaboration and complexity of training methods to optimize the preparation of the top-class sportsman must be put the simple questions: 'How much is worthwhile? How much is really in the best interests of sport; or in the best interests of the sportsman?' On the one hand is the point of view that it is a fascinating and valid challenge to tune the human body by all the resources available to explore the ultimate levels of physical performance. On the other hand there is concern that such a large part of a young person's life should be devoted to such narrowly defined objectives, and also concern that such an elaboration of techniques and training separates the élite in each sport even more distantly from the average. For some time too there have been pressing ethical problems concerning what is permissible, or 'fair', in the way of preparation. Such controversial preparation ranges from the exploitation of simple advantages such as type of employment, through the costly procedure of sending athletes to train at altitude for the Olympics, to the use of unnatural dietary regimens to enhance pre-event glycogen reserves, and ultimately to the use of drugs, steroids, autotransfusion and even surgery.

The importance of mental conditioning has been mentioned earlier. This is a subtle, individual business, a matter often for careful understanding by the coach of the personality and state of mind of the athlete or of a whole team. Training can so easily dull rather than sharpen performance. Staleness must be avoided by a variety of challenges and adequate rest. Care must be taken to produce a peak of mental readiness for the vital occasion, a blend of confidence and eagerness to win, rather than apprehension and self-doubts, to give cohesion and purpose to the assembly of trained elements.

W.T.

References

1. (a) Harris, B. (1973) Fitness clinic. *The Squash Player*, **2**, Nos. 10 and 12. (b) Harris, B. (1974) Fitness clinic. *The Squash Player*, **3**, Nos. 3 and 4.
2. Knapp, B. N. (1963) *Skill in Sport*. London: Routledge and Kegan Paul.
3. Tanner, J. M. (1964) *Physique of the Olympic Athlete*. London: George Allan and Unwin.
4. Müller, E. A. (1957) The regulation of muscular strength. *J. Ass. Phys. Med. Rehab.*, **112**, 41.
5. Whitney, R. J. (1958) The strength of the lifting action in man. *Ergonomics*, **1**, 101.
6. Åstrand, P-O. and Rodahl, K. (1970) *Textbook of Work Physiology*. New York: McGraw-Hill.
7. Munrow, A. D. (1962) *Pure and Applied Gymnastics*. London: Edward Arnold.
8. Hettinger, T. (1961) *Physiology of Strength*. Springfield, Ill.: Charles C Thomas.

9. Delorme, T. L. (1945) Restoration of muscle power by heavy resistance exercises. *J. Bone Jt Surg.*, **27B,** 645.

10. Petersen, F. B., Graudal, H., Hansen, J. W. and Hvid, N. (1961) The effect of varying the number of muscle contractions on dynamic muscle training. *Int. Z. Angew. Physiol.*, **18,** 468.

11. Chui, E. (1950) The effect of systematic weight training on athletic power. *Res. Q. Am. Ass. 'lth phys. Educ.*, **21,** 188.

12. McCloy, C. H. (1954) *Tests and Measurements in Health and Physical Education.* New York: Appleton-Century-Crofts.

13. Adamson, G. T. (1959) Milo or Müller II. *Phys. Educ.*, **51,** 59.

14. Berger, R. A. (1963) Comparison between static training and various dynamic training procedures. *Res. Q. Am. Ass. Hlth phys. Educ.*, **34,** 131.

15. Müller, E. A. and Rohmert, W. (1963) Die Geschwindizkeit der Muskelkraft und Zunahme bei Isometrischen Training. *Int. Z. Angew. Physiol.*, **19,** 403.

16. Gardner, G. N. (1963) Specificity of strength changes of the exercised and non-exercised limb following isometric training. *Res. Q. Am. Ass. Hlth phys. Educ.*, **34,** 98.

17. Ikai, M. and Steinhaus, A. H. (1961) Some factors modifying the expression of human strength. *J. Appl. Physiol.*, **16,** 157.

18. Rasch, P. J. and Morehouse, L. E. (1957) Effect of static and dynamic exercises on muscular strength and hypertrophy. *J. Appl. Physiol.*, **11,** 29.

19. Morris, J. M., Lucas, D. R. and Bresler, B. (1961) Role of the trunk in stability of the spine. *J. Bone Jt Surg.*, **43A,** 327.

20. Klein, K. K. and Allman, F. Jr. (1969) *The Knee in Sports.* New York: Pemberton Press.

21. Wilt, F. (1968) in *Exercise Physiology*, ed. Falls, H. B., New York: Academic Press.

22. Doherty, J. K. (1963) *Modern Track and Field.* London: Bailey Bros. and Swinfen.

23. Karvonen, M. J., Kentala, E. and Mustala, O. (1957) The effects of training on heart rate. *Am. Med. Exp. Fenn*, **35,** 307.

24. Morgan, R. E. and Adamson, G. T. (1962) *Circuit Training.* London: Bell.

25. Leighton J. R. (1957) Flexibility characteristics of three specialized skill groups of champion athletes. *Archs Phys. Med.*, **38,** 580.

26. Cureton, T. K. (1951) *Physical Fitness of Champion Athletes.* Urbana, Illinois: University of Illinois Press.

27. Holt, L. E., Train, T. M. and Okita, T. (1970) Comparative study of three stretching techniques. *Percept. Mot. Skills*, **31, 611.**

28. De Vries, H. A. (1962) Evaluation of static stretching procedures for improvement of flexibility. *Res. Q. Am. Ass. Hlth phys. Educ.*, **33,** 222.

29. Holt, L. E. (1974) Scientific Stretching for Sport (3S). Halifax, Nova Scotia: limited publication, Dalhousie University.

30. Knott, M. and Voss, D. E. (1965) *Proprioceptive Neuromuscular Facilitation.* New York: Harper and Row.

31. Åstrand, I., Åstrand, P.-O., Christensen, E. H. and Hedman, R. (1960) Myohemoglobin as an oxygen-store in man. *Acta Physiol. Scand.*, **48,** 454.

5

Environment

Introduction

Extremes of environment create many problems for the athlete and his attending physician, whether the adverse conditions are encountered suddenly on flying to a distant city for an international competition, or are a more incidental feature of normal recreation. In this chapter are considered briefly extremes of heat, cold, and altitude, both as to immediate medical problems, and the potential for acclimatization through such measures as specific training camps. Available literature in the three areas is already extensive,[1] [18] and limitations of space here preclude more than a brief review of the more important topics.

Heat

Practical importance

Even the moderate heat of a north European summer afternoon can impose a dangerous and potentially fatal thermal burden on the endurance competitor—particularly if the weather is humid. The Olympic Games provide several unfortunate illustrations of this hazard. The 1908 marathon contest was run in London; on this occasion Dorando entered the stadium in a dazed condition, turned in the wrong direction, collapsed twice, and remained in semi-coma for two days following the event. In 1912, the Olympic marathon was run in Stockholm; as in London, the day was warm and humid, and one of the contestants (Lazarro) collapsed at the 19th mile, to die on the following day. Again, in Paris (1924), five runners from the 10 000 m track event were admitted to hospital with heat stroke. The British Empire Games in Vancouver (1954) were marred by the near-death of a British marathon contestant, while in the 1960 Rome Olympics, three Danish cyclists developed heat stroke in the 100 km road race, and one subsequently died.

The greater heat of the North American summer provides even more potential for disaster, and although many athletes are at least partially heat acclimatized, the southern 'football' season carries an annual toll of heat illnesses and three or four deaths.[19] [22]

Adverse factors that contribute to needless fatalities include:

(a) failure of the team physician to set appropriate limits of climate for training and competition;
(b) rules that prohibit fluid replacement during a contest;
(c) inadequate monitoring of fluid and salt intake by the team physician;

(d) 'doping' with vasoconstrictor drugs such as the amphetamines;
(e) the wearing of nylon clothing and protective equipment that impede the evaporation of sweat;
(f) lack of heat acclimatization.

Maintaining heat balance

The body is a relatively inefficient machine. It performs best in sports such as distance running and cycling, but even during such activities, 75 per cent or more of the calorie content of the food consumed appears as heat rather than athletic endeavour.

If the activity is brief, this heat can be stored within the body as a rise of temperature. A modest heating of the active muscles is indeed valued by most athletes as a 'warm-up' for competition, but an excessive rise of core temperature is dangerous. If we stipulate that the reactal temperature should not increase more than 3 °C (i.e. from 37 °C to 40 °C), then the potential for heat storage will vary with body weight and initial body heat content, the latter depending on both rectal and skin temperatures; however, possible heat storage will not normally exceed 300–400 kcal (1·26–1·68 MJ) sufficient to accommodate about ten minutes of all-out effort.

If vigorous activity is more prolonged, dangerous hyperthermia can be averted only if heat is dissipated through a combination of evaporation of sweat, convection, conduction, and radiation. Many physiology texts suggest that exercise heat loss occurs largely by sweating. However, the experiments on which such conclusions are based have been conducted either on relatively stationary industrial workers or on a bicycle ergometer, where the effective air movement is close to zero. The data thus obtained have some relevance to sports pursued in a gymnasium or an enclosed arena, but are difficult to extrapolate to the track and the outdoor football stadium. Running in itself creates an effective wind speed of 4–5 m/sec. Given a skin temperature of 35 °C[9] and an air temperature of 20 °C, convective heat loss could amount to 7–8 kcal (0·29–0·32 MJ)/min (more if cycling or running against a stiff breeze). The typical marathon runner operates at some 75 per cent of his aerobic power, and must dissipate about 17 kcal (0·72 MJ)/min to maintain heat balance; thus, if the event is scheduled during the cooler part of the day, almost a half of the body heat production could be dissipated by convection. On the other hand, in a hot desert where air temperature was greater than 35 °C, a runner would gain heat from the environment more quickly than a stationary spectator.

Conduction of heat is usually a minor consideration during competition, although an athlete may gain heat by this route if he collapses on to a hot track.

In bright sunlight, radiant heat adds a further burden not generally encountered in the laboratory; the uptake of this form of energy can be reduced by wearing lightweight white clothing.

Evaporation of a litre of sweat dissipates 580 kcal (2·5 MJ). Thus, depending on the intensity of activity, convective losses, and radiant heat gains, an athlete must evaporate 1–2 litres of sweat per hour to maintain heat balance. Unfortunately, under humid conditions, more than half of the sweat that is secreted may roll to the ground unevaporated.[23] In such circumstances, body cooling is again helped by light and loosely fitting cotton garments that conserve the sweat until it can be evaporated.

Assessment of climate

From the foregoing discussion, an assessment of heat stress should consider not only air temperature, but also humidity, radiant heat load, and effective wind speed. One simple method of synthesizing such information was developed by Minard[24] for the U.S. Marine Corps. His wet bulb globe thermometer index (WBGT) is calculated as follows:

For men outdoors: WBGT $= 0.7$ (WBT) $+ 0.2$ (GT) $+ 0.1$ (DBT)
For men indoors: WBGT $= 0.7$ (WBT) $+ 0.3$ (DBT).

Here, WBT is the 'Wet bulb temperature' recorded from a thermometer where the bulb is surrounded by gauze, moistened with distilled water and ventilated by a fan or a whirling device ('sling psychrometer'); GT is the temperature recorded from a thermometer enclosed in a black or grey metal sphere, and exposed to the intensity of sunlight encountered by the athlete; DBT is the dry bulb temperature indicated by a normal type of thermometer not exposed to direct sunlight.

The index as calculated makes no allowance for air movement. A relative air speed of 4–5 m/sec, can lower the effective temperature by 5–7 °C (less at high air temperatures).

The history of the Olympic Games provides sufficient evidence that no warm summer afternoon can be completely safe for every endurance competitor. Nevertheless, the WBGT provides a simple empirical index of the relative hazard presented by different environments. Minard[24] recommended caution when the WBGT exceeded 82 °F (27.7 °C), with restriction of activity at a WBGT of 85 °F (29.4 °C) (unacclimatized men), or 90 °F (32.3 °C) (fully acclimatized men). Endurance athletes may well exercise more vigorously and for longer periods than the Marines studied by Minard, and for this reason such standards are unduly liberal for many types of competition. Wyndham[9] has proposed that no unacclimatized athlete should compete for more than 30 minutes at a WBGT of 25 °C, and that even acclimatized athletes should not be allowed to compete if the WBGT is above 28 °C. Certainly, such figures indicate that in most countries, distance events should not be scheduled on a summer afternoon.

The apparatus to determine the WBGT is available at most weather stations. However, for those wishing an even simpler climatic indicator, it may be noted that the dominant term of the WBGT is the wet bulb temperature. Murphy and Ashe[21] have suggested that in the context of American 'football', fluids should be given during the game if the WBT exceeds 66 °F (18.9 °C), rest periods should be allowed every 30 minutes if the WBT is over 71 °F (21.7 °C), and practices should be conducted without protective equipment at a WBT of 76 °F (24.4 °C) or above. The U.S. National Road Running Club specifies that no contest should take place if the dry bulb temperature exceeds 95 °F (35 °C); contests should also be cancelled if the dry bulb temperature is 85 °F (29.4 °C) or more and the relative humidity over 60 per cent (WBT 76 °F—24.3 °C), or if the dry bulb temperature is 80 °F (26.7 °C) and the relative humidity is over 75 per cent (WBT 74 °F—23.3 °C).

A third possibility, particularly during training sessions, is to monitor the condition of the players. If the pulse rate is not recovering during rest pauses, this is fairly conclusive evidence that the body is accumulating heat, and rectal temperatures should be checked.

Fluid needs

The weight loss over a marathon run may exceed 5 per cent of body weight, not only in top-level competitors, but also in middle-aged men who cover the 42 km course over five or more hours.[25] Weight losses averaging 3·5 kg are also seen when North American 'football' is practised for 90 minutes under adverse conditions (100 °F (37·7 °C); 80–100 per cent relative humidity). Pugh[23] has estimated that a marathon runner may reach a peak sweat production of up to 1·81/hr.

Fortunately, the immediate fluid requirements are rather less than the simple record of body weights might suggest. On a short-term basis, 1·5–2·0 kg of weight loss is covered by: (a) catabolism (about 0·2 kg); (b) water produced in catabolism (about 0·3 kg); and (c) water liberated by usage of body glycogen stores (up to 1·6 kg). Probably for this reason, the body tolerates a weight loss of up to 3 per cent with no symptoms except thirst. However, larger losses are associated with progressively higher rectal temperatures, the danger zone of 40 °C being reached with a 5 per cent weight loss.

Many marathon runners incur very large water deficits, and for this reason Wyndham[9] has branded as 'criminal folly' the international rule prohibiting the drinking of fluid over the first 10 miles (15 km) of a competition.* A variety of replacement fluids have been proposed, ranging from water to commercial solutions of flavoured salts with or without added glucose. The main practical considerations are (a) palatability, and (b) absorption. Gastric emptying is delayed by hypertonic solutions of glucose, and Costill[26] has found that in marathon events other preparations have no advantage relative to water. However, if the athlete is competing in an under-developed country it is vital to check the potability of the water supply; an attack of gastroenteritis has disastrous effects upon performance.

The athlete who is left to follow his personal inclination rarely drinks sufficient fluid to maintain a water balance, either during an endurance contest, or immediately afterwards.[26] The maximum possible intake of an active man is still debated, but is probably about 200 ml (one glass) of fluid every 15 minutes. Costill's subjects were required to drink 100 ml every 5 minutes during a simulated marathon. After about an hour, they began to find difficulty in sustaining this schedule, and at 110 min reportedly could drink no more. At this stage, the stomach contained 200–600 ml of unabsorbed fluid. Despite this ceiling of absorptive capacity, much can be done to avoid dehydration. Given a modest pre-loading with fluid (several days of a high salt diet, with two or three glasses of fluid shortly before competition), and regular 200 ml drinks every 15 minutes, Kavanagh and Shephard have succeeded in avoiding haemo-concentration, and have even sustained a modest urine formation over several hours of marathon running.[27] The

* In fact, the usually accepted International rule has been no fluids for 11 km. Because of representations from the Canadian Association of Sports Sciences and the American College of Sports Medicine, the rule is changed for Montreal (1976).

early demand for sweating can be curbed by applying ice or cold water to the clothing. It is more effective to wet the thighs than the trunk, since the former have a greater surface area, are the main source of heat production, and are exposed to a greater relative air movement during running.

Mineral needs

Sweat contains less sodium chloride (0·1–0·4 per cent) than blood (0·9 per cent). Thus, unless fluid intake is large, the sodium content of the plasma tends to rise during competition. Potassium ions 'leak' from the active muscles, partly as a consequence of glycogen depletion, and there is thus some tendency to hyperkalaemia.[25] Commercial replacement fluids with a high content of sodium and potassium ions are plainly contraindicated at this stage.

Mineral deficiencies are incurred in the hours following competition, when muscle potassium is restored and the body is rehydrated. A single contest in a hot environment is rarely sufficient to cause any problem, but a cumulative mineral deficit can arise from an extended exposure in training or a succession of heats. The normal salt loss in a temperate climate is 12 g/day, but a man who sweats hard can lose up to 8 g/hour from a total body pool of 175 g. A loss of 0·5 g/kg causes lassitude, weakness, giddiness, fainting, and muscle cramps, while a deficit of 0·75 g/kg leads to apathy, stupor, and a marked fall of blood pressure.[9] In the absence of supervision, more acute salt deficiency may occasionally develop, with marked weight loss, constipation, scanty urine, and other signs of dehydration such as nausea, vomiting, sunken eyes, inelastic skin, and circulatory failure. Once vomiting has begun, this leads to a vicious circle of further salt loss and dehydration.

Difficulties are most likely on first arriving in a warm climate. Hormonal adjustments in sweat and urinary salt losses are incomplete, and the athlete has not yet become accustomed to adding more salt to his food. Given proper supervision of the training table, an adequate mineral intake can be attained by additional salting of soups, vegetables and salads. Proprietary flavoured salt solutions can also be provided, but plain salt tablets should be avoided. These can cause gastric irritation or pass through the bowels without absorption. Alternatively, they may produce a transient peak of plasma sodium, forcing the kidneys to excrete additional water in an attempt to restore plasma electrolyte balance.

Heat and performance

The performance of most events suffers in hot weather. It is easy to envisage how progressive dehydration, mineral loss, and a rising body temperature can impede a gruelling all-day bicycle race. On the other hand, it is less easy to demonstrate physiological changes in brief effort. There is no change of efficiency or cardiac output when sub-maximal exercise is carried out in a hot room;[28–30] the maximum oxygen intake also remains unchanged,[30 32] and some gains of physical performance might be anticipated from 'warm-up'.

Why, then, does performance deteriorate? The answer is probably that in real life, heat exposure is not the brief affair examined by the experimental physiologist. The hot weather has persisted through several days of arduous training, and has continued into a series of sleepless nights. Loss of sleep has impaired reaction time, co-ordination, and vigilance. The unaccustomed climate has overaroused an already excited competitor. The circulating blood volume has been depleted by a progressive peripheral displacement of fluid, possibly compounded by inadequate replacement of water and salts.

There may be mild heat exhaustion, marked by symptoms of circulatory inadequacy such as dizziness, black-outs, and fainting spells, and psychological reactions such as loss of initiative, fatigue, and irritability. If uncorrected, there can be progression to a chronic neurosis (heat neurasthenia), with apathy, hysteria, or aggression.[9] The team physician should be alert for such manifestations with a view to preserving the team spirit, avoiding unnecessary combat and irrational assaults upon other players or officials, and preventing unwarranted penalization of a sick contestant (see also Chapter 9).

Dehydration and mineral loss sufficient to produce such severe symptoms generally reflect poor team management. In a hot climate, body weight should be checked on rising each morning (after emptying the bladder!). A Fantus test of urinary chlorides should also be carried out at least weekly, more often under extreme conditions. Where possible, air-conditioned quarters should be secured. Finally, all team members must be exhorted frequently to take extra salt and enough fluids to sustain a normal urine flow.

Acclimatization

Repeated exposures to a hot climate lead to a progressive acclimatization to the adverse environment. Physiological adjustments include an increase of blood volume, an augmentation of venous tone, earlier and more vigorous sweating, a decrease in the mineral content of the sweat and the urine, and dramatic gains of subjective comfort. The athlete feels better, sleeps better, and performs better. Benefits are naturally greatest for endurance competitors, but even a sprint runner profits from acclimatization, particularly if he has to compete in many preliminary heats.

There are superficial similarities between heat acclimatization and endurance training, and perhaps for this reason adjustment is realized most rapidly in individuals who are relatively fit. Nevertheless, the full potential of heat acclimatization can only be acquired through a combination of physical activity and heat exposure.[33] The ideal pattern of activity has yet to be resolved, but in the absence of more precise information, a normal training programme may be adopted under increasingly rigorous climatic conditions. Much of the total course of acclimatization is seen in the first week, and after two weeks further gains are relatively slow.[9] The course of acclimatization is speeded if fluid and salt balances are carefully monitored over this period. Some tricks of tropical life can only be learnt by a period of residence at the site of competition.[6] Nevertheless, there is a wide overlap between acclimatization to dry (desert) heat and humid (jungle) heat, and if the athlete cannot leave home for a long stay in a tropical training camp, he can develop many of the necessary adjustments through wearing impermeable clothing[34] or exercising in an over-heated gymnasium.

Most of the benefits of acclimatization are lost within two months of return to a temperate region. However, the adjustments of body physiology can be largely sustained if the athlete is prepared to undertake several hours of activity in an over-heated gymnasium at least once per fortnight. Reacclimatization also proceeds more rapidly in those who have previous tropical experience.[35]

International-class athletes are increasingly required to voyage between very hot and very cold parts of the world. Fortunately, it seems possible to develop a simultaneous acclimatization to heat and cold.[35]

It might finally be enquired whether natives of tropical regions have an unfair advantage over competitors from temperate regions. Ladell[36] examined this point some years ago, and concluded that the natives of a hot region fared no better than well-acclimatized visitors when hard work was performed in the heat.

Heat collapse (syncope)

Heat collapse is probably the commonest medical problem of competition on a hot day, shown equally by the athlete who omits an adequate 'warm down', and by members of the watching crowd who have stood for a long period. The loss of consciousness reflects an inadequate cerebral blood flow. There is evidence of a progressive loss of fluid from the central circulation, associated with: (a) relaxation of the peripheral veins; (b) sweating; (c) extravascular oedema (particularly in the legs of the watching crowd); and (d) intramuscular accumulation of fluid (particularly in the active limbs of the athlete). The effects of a falling cardiac stroke volume are compounded by a drop in systemic blood pressure due to cutaneous vasodilation, and there may be a superimposed vasovagal attack with slowing of the heart and general muscular vasodilatation.

It is important to check that the loss of consciousness is not a manifestation of progressive heat exhaustion (see above), or a dangerous heat stroke. One important warning criterion is rectal temperature. Unfortunately, readings of 104 °F (40 °C) are common in distance runners.[9, 23] Nevertheless, a combination of impaired consciousness and a temperature of over 41 °C must be treated as heat stroke until the diagnosis is disproved.

An uncomplicated case of heat collapse responds rapidly to adoption of a supine position with elevation of the legs, tepid sponging, and oral administration of fluids.

Heat stroke

Suspected heat stroke is not uncommon. However, a true and potentially fatal failure of the heat regulating mechanisms of the body occurs much more rarely. The presenting symptom may be a clouding rather than a complete loss of consciousness. The contestant may be stuporose and roused with difficulty, but equally can be wildly excited; there may also be hallucinations, muscle twitching, and even convulsions with loss of control of body sphincters. On examination, there may be profuse sweating, but the skin is more often hot and dry, with diminished sweat production (anhidrotic heat exhaustion). If the patient is stuporose, reflexes are depressed, but if he is excited the reflexes also are exaggerated.

If untreated, the rising core temperature and diminishing cardiac output can lead to irreversible damage in the brain, the kidneys, the liver, and the adrenal cortex ('heat shock'). Emergency treatment is directed to reducing body temperature as rapidly as possible by a combination of tepid sponging and fanning. Iced fluids or ice baths should not be used. These may initially cause cutaneous vasoconstriction and thus further difficulty in heat elimination; later, there is a danger of transition from hyper- to hypothermia.

During the recovery period, metabolic acidosis should be countered by intravenous bicarbonates.[9] Hydrocortisone and intravenous fluids may also be needed to sustain the systemic blood pressure, and up to 25 per cent of cases may require dialysis to counter renal failure. With such complications, early admission to hospital is mandatory. Sponging and fanning should continue in the ambulance until the core temperature has dropped to 38 °C or less.

If treated energetically, the prognosis for a complete restoration of function in all affected organs is good. However, if officials allow the case to linger until the rectal temperature has reached 42 °C, the probability of death is high. Wyndham[9] has recommended assaying blood enzyme levels (SGOT—Serum Glutamic Oxaloacetic Transaminase, SGPT—Serum Glutamic Pyruvic Transaminase and LDH—Lactic Dehydrogenase). A twofold increase of enzyme levels is normal during sustained activity such as marathon running,[9,25] but if heat stroke is accompanied by organ damage, ten- to twentyfold increments may be observed together with a massive haematuria, proteinuria, and rapidly rising blood urea. If good biochemical facilities are available, it is helpful to fractionate the LDH.[37] Normal runners show increments of the LDH-3, LDH-4, and LDH-5 fractions, whereas patients with cardiac and renal damage show increases of LDH-1 and LDH-2.

Swimming

A hot climate may direct the attention of the athlete towards unsuitable bathing places. An alert physician will thus check the bacterial content and other hazards of potential swimming areas.

Medical conditions

Many medical conditions are aggravated by hot weather, and a level of physical activity well tolerated under cool conditions may become dangerous and/or impractical if it is hot and humid. The increase in cardiac deaths during heat waves is well-documented.[38] Presumably, the added demands on the heart from cutaneous vasodilation push many patients with congenital, rheumatic, or atherosclerotic heart disease into decompensation. Kavanagh and Shephard have also noted an increased frequency of cardiac arrhythmias in a post-coronary exercise programme when the weather is hot; the lowering of systemic blood pressure should help this group of patients, and the difficulties presumably arise from disturbances of electrolyte balance with heavy sweating. The ease with which body heat is dissipated depends not only on skin blood flow but also on the thickness of the insulating layer of subcutaneous fat. Grossly obese patients have great difficulty in losing heat,[39] and for this reason should not undertake extended exercise when the weather is particularly hot and humid.

Saunas

Saunas are becoming increasingly popular, not only in Scandinavia, but also in North America. Many are home-made affairs with poorly controlled climatic conditions. Commonly, the user is first exposed to dry air at anything from 160 °F (71 °C) to 200 °F (93 °C); he then directs water on to heated rocks, increasing the humidity. Many saunas remain quite warm with a humidity of only 10–20 per cent, but if humid heat is produced, the limit is about 127 °F (53 °C). The user then goes outside into the snow or a cold lake to cool off.

Since it is possible to leave the sauna room at any time, and the user is sitting at rest, excessive heating of the body is unlikely. Practical hazards include: (a) fungal infection of the sauna benches; (b) heat collapse on standing to leave; (c) a remote possibility of ventricular fibrillation from the shock of the sudden change in temperature; and (d) scalding, electrocution, and fire from improper operation of the sauna.

Cold

Practical importance

As with the problems of heat, there is some danger of thinking that cold emergencies arise only in extreme climates such as those found in the circumpolar regions of Canada, Russia, and Alaska. In fact, permanent residents of the Arctic are well-equipped to deal with the cold, having not only appropriate clothing but also a substantial measure of acclimatization, and a wealth of practical experience. Medical problems are much more likely to arise in the visitor to the Arctic and in the hill-walker, the cave explorer, or the dinghy sailor who encounters adverse conditions in an ostensibly temperate zone.

Pugh[40] has described 23 incidents in the United Kingdom involving hill-walkers from the armed services, schools, youth organizations, and private groups, with 25 deaths, a further 5 cases of unconsciousness followed by recovery, and 58 milder cases of hypothermia. Perhaps the most dramatic episode was the annual Four Inns walk in March of 1964.[41] The walk covers 45 miles of the English Derbyshire hillside, and in that year attracted 240 entrants. The weather commenced with a light wind and drizzle, the reported valley temperatures being in the range 4–7 °C. Later, the rain became heavy, and valley winds reached 25 knots (46·25 km/hr). The fittest competitors completed the course in approximately normal times. However, many normally healthy young men were unable to develop a high enough metabolic rate to avoid chilling over the course. The rescue team brought down five exhausted walkers (two in a state of collapse), one further participant died of hypothermia shortly after being carried to a hill farm on a stretcher, and two others were dead when discovered.

Despite the publicity attending these unfortunate accidents, there were several further deaths among a party of inadequately clothed schoolchildren walking in the Scottish Cairngorm mountains in the spring of 1972. Equally, each Canadian winter sees fatalities from hypothermia in and around the major metropolitan centres, while in the spring a number of people are lethally chilled when boats capsize into ice-cold lakes.

Factors contributing to a fatal outcome include (a) a limitation of body heat production (through injury, lack of food, poor initial physical fitness, and exhaustion by high winds or more vigorous colleagues), (b) high winds and a lack of wind-proof clothing (winds are usually higher, and temperatures 2–3 °C cooler on the hillside), (c) virtual loss of insulation (due to saturation of clothing by rain, mist, spray, or sweat), (d) mental confusion (due to hypothermia, hypogly-caemia, ketosis, and/or alcohol), and (e) cutaneous vasodilation (due to alcohol).

Maintaining heat balance

The principles governing heat balance in a cold environment are much the same as those described for the heat. A brief exposure to cold can be tolerated by depleting body stores of heat. However, there is a loss of physical efficiency if the core temperature drops by as little as 2 °F (1 °C), and in general the heat lost in the cold must be made good by either a high rate of voluntary physical activity, or by involuntary movements (shivering).

Convective heat loss is normally limited mainly by a thin film of still air surrounding the body. The thickness of this barrier, and thus the rate of heat transfer, is influenced markedly by relative windspeed. If clothing were not increased, and skin temperature remained at 35 °C, then the rate of heat loss by convection could reach 17–18 kcal (0·072–0·075 MJ)/min at an air temperature of 0 °C and a wind speed of 4–5 m/sec. Much higher wind speeds than this are often encountered in hill-walking, and much higher relative velocities are developed by sports such as snow-mobiling, downhill skiing, speed skating, cycling, and dinghy sailing. Thus, it is easy to envisage how heat losses can engender fatigue and eventually exceed the body's potential for heat production.

The first line of defence is to reduce skin temperatures by vasoconstriction. This adjustment commences at an air temperature of about 88 °F (31 °C), and is normally relatively complete at 75 °F (24 °C). However, constriction of the subcutaneous blood vessels may fail to occur in the skier who has spent the lunch hour at the bar, or in the snow-mobiler who is weaving an erratic course from one ski chalet to another on the local cocktail circuit. Under the type of conditions that have caused hill deaths in England, skin temperature drops to about 20 °C.[42] With more extreme conditions, a lower limit of skin temperature is set by the metabolic needs of the skin and the danger of frostbite (which can occur if skin temperature drops below 30 °F, (−1 °C). Often, even if a person is exercising hard, it is necessary to supplement natural insulation by increased thicknesses of clothing.

Conduction of heat is usually a local problem. Hands may be numbed by contact with an ice-pick or rudder bar, and if the boots provide inadequate insulation, the feet may be chilled by contact with cold ground. However, if a climber sinks to the ground exhausted, more rapid and general body cooling can occur. If rest is necessary, a knapsack or other available gear should be used to keep the body out of direct contact with the ground.

Radiant heat exchange depends on the temperature gradient between the sportsman and surrounding objects. On a bright winter afternoon, radiant heating from the sun can be as effective as in the summer. However, in a shaded and windowless hillside shelter, heat may pass rapidly from a man and his clothing to the walls. On a clear evening, radiant heat loss develops rapidly as the sun sets, a phenomenon well known at autumn barbecue parties in Canada.

Evaporation of sweat may occur even in a cold climate if vigorous activity is undertaken while wearing excessive clothing; indeed, some recent studies of circumpolar parties have suggested that the active man may be exposed to a microclimate that leads to heat stress! Such sweating should be avoided by using clothing with adjustable insulation. Once garments become sodden with sweat, their insulation is destroyed, and local frostbite or general hypothermia may develop during rest pauses. Even in the absence of frank sweating, there can be considerable water loss in dry cold, both through the skin (insensible perspiration) and the respiratory tract (where a litre or more of fluid can be exhaled every day). Pugh has suggested that much of the deterioration in physical condition of mountain climbers may reflect a high rate of fluid loss and difficulty in melting snow to maintain fluid balance. The heavy rate of water loss compounds the problem of sustaining thermal balance. Each litre of water evaporated (whether derived from the body or from external sources such as rain) costs the body 580 kcal (2·5 MJ) of heat.

Assessment of climate
It is clear from the long winter journeys undertaken by the Eskimo that given adequate experience, a suitable level of acclimatization, moderate physical fitness, and appropriate clothing, man can withstand even extreme Arctic conditions. However, if temperatures are below 10 °C it is necessary to insist on adequate protection against rain, and if temperatures are below 0 °C, precautions must be taken to avoid frostbite of the extremities. At temperatures of −30 to −40 °C, the equivalent of many layers of normal clothing may be required, particularly if it is necessary to shelter out of doors overnight. The effect of wind speed is indicated in Table 5.1.

Table 5.1 The influence of wind velocity on thermal comfort in dry air.

Air speed (m/sec)	Pleasant	Cool	Very cold	Bitterly cold
0	10 °C	0 °C	−14 °C	−50 °C
5	26 °C	19 °C	11 °C	−11 °C
10	27 °C	21 °C	14 °C	−4 °C
20	28 °C	21·5°C	16 °C	0 °C

Clothing
Clothing increases natural insulation by trapping still air within its fibres. Natural fibres are more effective than nylon, and the warmest clothing of all is provided by animal skins such as the caribou garments of the Eskimo. The insulation is largely lost if the still air is displaced by a strong wind or by relative air movement (as in downhill skiing). In dry cold, the most effective clothing assembly thus includes an outer tightly woven, wind-proof garment such as sail-cloth, and a layer of loosely woven, air-trapping fibres such as a woollen blanket underneath; this arrangement is well-illustrated by the double-layered Eskimo parka. However, if a high rate of metabolism is anticipated (as in cross-country skiing), it may be appropriate to limit the wind-excluding fabric to the front, and leave the rear more permeable to allow evaporation of sweat. In wet, or potentially wet cold (0–10 °C), the outer layer should be fully waterproof, since insulation is rapidly degraded by rain or wet snow. Pugh[42] examined the properties of one lethal outfit from the Four Inns walk; this included anorak with hood, woollen jersey, shirt, string vest, short cotton drawers, cotton jeans, socks, boots, and gloves. Sitting

in still air, with the clothing dry, the air around the body contributed an insulation of 1 CLO unit,* and the garments a further 1·5 CLO. However, when exercising in wet clothing and with a 9 mile/h (14·4 km/h) wind, the total insulation was only 0·40 CLO units, with the clothing contributing no more than 0·15 CLO. Modern silicone-proofed garments, although convenient in city showers, are largely ineffective when exposed to several hours of heavy rain on the hillside. Mountain rescue teams currently place their faith in heavy oilskin garments, although in view of the potential for accumulation of sweat, such clothing remains far from ideal.

In extremes of dry cold, fleece-lined outer boots and additional socks are advisable, although care must be taken that the latter are not so tight as to impede the circulation. However, if the rate of metabolism is high (as in cross-country skiing), a single pair of shoes with snow-excluding cuffs will suffice. Excessive local cooling can occur if the shoes become filled with sweat or melted snow, and if water penetrates from the exterior. Under slushy conditions, many skiers choose to reinforce water-repellant creams by a plastic sleeve fitted over their shoes.

For local protection of the hands, mittens are much more effective than gloves, particularly if fitted with long gauntlets and loosely fitting air seals at the wrists.

A fur-trimmed hood traps enough air to protect the face during light activities, but for skiing under Arctic conditions it is necessary to provide added protection for the nose, cheeks, and ears by a woollen face mask. Male cross-country enthusiasts also find a need for added local protection of the genitalia.

Cold and performance

Performance of short-term events is much influenced by what is in essence the opposite of a 'warm-up'. Muscle functions best at a temperature of 40–41 °C,[43] but in Pugh's laboratory simulation of the Four Inns walk, many of the leg muscles had cooled to 32 °C or lower.[42] Such cooling increases muscle tone and viscosity, the speed of contraction is slowed, and there is delayed relaxation of antagonist muscles. Speed and power events are performed poorly, and there is an increased risk of muscle tears and other injuries due to: (a) failure of relaxation, (b) impaired function of cutaneous sense organs and muscle proprioceptors, and (c) hypoglycaemic or hypothermic degradation of cerebral co-ordination.

The normal pre-contest 'warm-up' should be extended as necessary, and if it is very cold it may be helpful to wear additional clothing during this period. Both muscle stiffness and shivering affect the execution of most tasks. Coarse movements may be performed with increased speed and diminished accuracy (although slow relaxation hampers such ballistic movements as the swing of a cricket bat). Delicate movements, whether the repair of a defunct snow-mobile or sinking a putt on the golf green, become almost impossible with numbing of the hands and the onset of frank shivering.

In more long term events, a small increase of maximum oxygen intake might be anticipated to result from exposure to moderate cold. Venous return is

*The protection afforded by clothing is commonly expressed in CLO units. British indoor clothing has a CLO value of one, and Arctic clothing may provide an insulation of 4–10 CLO units.

improved by constriction of superficial veins, while constriction of the subcutaneous arteries directs the available cardiac output towards the active muscles.[44] On the other hand, the increase of systemic blood pressure increases the work of the heart, while bronchoconstriction and an increase of muscle viscosity could also augment the work of breathing. Beneficial effects of cold are most likely when venous return is severely compromised (sustained exercise performed mainly with the arms). In practice, gains of maximum oxygen intake are negligible, and their potential to improve endurance performance is outweighed by (a) increased muscle viscosity, (b) the metabolic cost of shivering (which can increase the metabolic cost of moderate work up to 50 per cent,[42, 45] (c) the added weight of clothing carried, and (d) the added cost of moving over wet or snow-covered terrain against high winds.[42, 46]

Acclimatization

It is less easy to demonstrate acclimatization to cold than to heat. Over 1–2 weeks of experimental exposures, subjects shiver less, perform fine motor tasks more accurately, and have fewer complaints. However, their deep body temperatures may be lower than in unacclimatized men exposed to the same stress, suggesting that part at least of the apparent adaptation to cold is merely habituation to an unpleasant situation.[47]

The general level of skin blood flow is commonly reduced with acclimatization in order to conserve body heat, but there may be a secondary increase of flow to the extremities, restoring manual dexterity, and reducing liability to chilblains and frostbite.

Leblanc[48] has discussed local acclimatization that can occur with repeated exposure of the hands or face to intense cold, whether from wind or icy water. The normal body response is a brisk rise of pulse rate and systemic blood pressure, cutaneous vasoconstriction, and loss of dexterity in the hands. However, with acclimatization, the hypertensive reaction is much reduced, and dexterity is better sustained.

Prolonged residence in an Arctic region teaches many tricks that help in conserving body temperature. Clothing is better chosen (see above), a more forceful pattern of activity is adopted, windy spots are avoided, and the skin is kept well-covered. Although not physiological acclimatization, these modifications of behaviour do much to extend the tolerable range of environmental conditions. A high level of physical fitness,[49] good intramuscular stores of glycogen and fat, and adequate food supplies[42] are all important pre-requisites of maintaining sufficient activity to sustain thermal equilibrium when the climate is adverse.

Canada has had some success in selecting winter sports teams from populations indigenous to the Arctic, such as the Eskimos. With respect to cold, such groups combine extensive experience with a high level of physical fitness, and above average acclimatization to cold, both local[48] and general.[11, 13, 50] At one time, it was held that the Eskimos—and possibly other groups exposed to cold for long periods—gained some protection from an increase of basal metabolism; however, this may have reflected not acclimatization but a high fat diet. Certainly, recent studies of Eskimos[51] and of 'white' volunteers[52] do not confirm this phenomenon.

Cold exhaustion, collapse

Cold exhaustion and/or collapse usually occurs as a combined response to falling blood sugar and decreasing body temperatures; cerebral function begins to fail if the rectal temperature drops below 95 °F (35 °C). At this stage, intramuscular reserves of glycogen have been exhausted by (a) battling high winds, (b) attempting to match the climbing pace of fitter colleagues, and (c) the added metabolic demands of shivering and other attempts to sustain body temperature ('non-shivering thermogenesis').

The earliest signs of difficulty are a slowing of pace, unsteadiness, clumsiness, muscle weakness or cramps, and stumbling. If shelter and food are sought at this stage, recovery is rapid. However, if such symptoms are ignored, the body has increasing difficulty in sustaining heat balance. Mental symptoms[42] appear—anxiety, irritability, apathy, or loss of purpose—and collapse occurs within 1–2 hours. Evacuation by stretcher is dangerously slow, and if a person is capable of walking, the best emergency treatment probably includes removal of water from drenched clothing by rolling in dry snow (if available), a brief rest in a temporary wind shelter, administration of hot sweet fluids and provision of additional clothing, with subsequent escort to a place of safety. Although cerebral manifestations are a late feature, it is dangerous to leave such patients unaccompanied. They may (a) lose their way, (b) sustain injury, or (c) remove their clothing from a combination of confusion and a paradoxical feeling of warmth.

Hypothermia

Cooling to a rectal temperature of less than 95 °F (35 °C) is associated with a progressive failure of both cerebral and muscular function.[42] As in surgical hypothermia, acid/base regulation is disturbed, and there is a risk of cardiac arrest or ventricular fibrillation. Heat regulating mechanisms of the brain begin to fail around 90 °F (32 °C), and at still lower temperatures death becomes increasingly likely.[5]

The choice of emergency treatment depends on the isolation of the victim. If far from safety, perhaps the most effective approach is to share a well-insulated sleeping-bag with the rescuer. The five unconscious patients retrieved from the Four Inns episode all recovered in hospital beds, with or without added heat. If the patient is conscious, a hot bath rapidly restores body temperature, but if unconscious a risk of convulsions makes this a dangerous therapy; if hypothermia is severe, it is in any event desirable to rewarm the body slowly.

There is an appreciable risk of later circulatory, respiratory, and renal failure, and the patient should be evacuated to a hospital as soon as he can withstand the journey.[53] Hydrocortisone injections may be needed to counter hypotension, with oxygen or assisted ventilation to meet respiratory complications. The electrocardiogram should be monitored continuously for arrhythmia until rewarming is completed, and metabolic acidosis and electrolyte imbalance should be corrected as necessary.

Frostbite

Frostbite is a form of local and superficial tissue destruction caused by freezing of exposed parts. Since the tissue fluids have a substantial osmotic pressure, freezing is unlikely until the part has cooled to about 30 °F (−1 °C).

Contributory factors are contact with cold metal, intense local vasoconstriction (more likely in an unacclimatized person), a very low air temperature (-20 to -30 °C) and/or an excessive air movement over the exposed part (a high wind or downhill skiing). Protuberances such as the tip of the nose and the tips of the ears are particularly vulnerable. If the footwear is of poor quality or its insulation is destroyed by wetting, the feet may also reach the critical temperature for frostbite.

Prevention is simple if vulnerable areas are adequately protected. However, patients with peripheral vascular disorders may benefit from prophylactic vasodilator drugs. Treatment consists of a brief rewarming of the affected part by warm (42 °C) water, body heat or expired air. After the temperature is increased sufficiently to avert further tissue destruction, it should be kept cool to lessen the metabolic demand on damaged tissues, and reduce the risk of secondary vascular occlusion by oedema. If areas of skin are destroyed, measures will be needed to prevent secondary infection; this is particularly important if there is extensive tissue destruction progressing to dry gangrene. Occasionally, the recovery process may be complicated by vascular thrombosis.

Cold water

A fall into near-freezing water can be fatal in as little as 15 minutes, and even if the water temperature is around 40 °F (4–5 °C), survival may be no more than one hour. The reason is that heat loss by conduction and convection proceeds much more rapidly in water than in air. There has been some discussion as to whether swimming is desirable in such circumstances.[54, 55, 56] In an obese person, the added metabolism may help sustain body temperature, but in the average athlete the resultant stirring of the water hastens heat loss and ultimate disaster; the best advice is to minimize the cooling surface by keeping the limbs pressed close together. The use of a life-jacket in dinghy sailing is a vital precaution even for a strong swimmer, since normal swimming patterns are impeded by reflex hyperventilation,[57] viscous muscles, malfunction of sensory receptors, and disturbed judgement. When developed, life-jackets that incorporate insulation will be the safety equipment of choice. The skater or snow-mobiler who ventures on to thin ice has the added encumbrance of heavy clothing.

Injuries

Recreational skiing carries a high toll of injuries.[58] These are commonly blamed on poorly-tended slopes, inexperience, and excessive enthusiasm on the part of the skier. However, the role of cold exposure and associated viscous muscles, vigorous exercise without any limbering-up, and impaired sensory perception should not be ignored. If a skier is feeling cold, he should avoid making a descent that would be close to his capacity when warmed up.

Medical conditions

Exercise rehabilitation following myocardial infarction must continue through the cold winter months. Those patients with a tendency to angina of effort find their condition worsened in cold weather. This is partly because the oxygen cost of carrying out a given exercise prescription is increased by the need to wear heavier clothing, cross snow-covered terrain, and initiate shivering or non-shivering thermogenesis. Other contributory factors are the hypertensive reaction to local or generalized cold,[48] which increases cardiac work load, and possibly also a reflex coronary spasm induced by the impingement of Arctic air upon bronchial nerve endings. Myocardial oxygen lack can progress to the point of initiating infarction, particularly if the exercise is of isometric type. In one series of 204 non-fatal infarctions, 8 cases were found where infarction developed during or immediately following the shovelling of wet snow.[59] The best practical suggestion for the patient with angina is to avoid exercise in the cold by moving indoors. At the same time, the pattern of activity should not be modified if intensity is to be sustained without risk of musculo-tendinous injuries. Thus, if the summer prescription calls for jogging and an indoor track is not available, jogging can continue in the corridors of schools, offices, or warehouses. Alternative possibilities are to minimize cold exposure of skin (wearing a woollen face mask under extreme conditions), to adopt nose breathing where possible and, if the vigour of activity makes mouth-breathing mandatory, to use an air-warming device such as a hose-pipe coming from under the sweat suit or a face mask with copper mesh heat-exchanger.[60]

Cold air may also induce intense bronchitis and bronchospasm, particularly in patients with chronic chest disease and/or hyperreactive airways. There has been speculation that with repeated exposure, this may contribute to the development of pulmonary hypertension and heart block.[61] The obvious remedy is to insist on nose-breathing. However, in a normal person this is impractical if effort exceeds 7 kcal (0·029 MJ)/min and in patients with nasal obstruction mouth-breathing may develop even during brisk walking. The remedy is then to recommend some form of air-warming device, as for the anginal patients.

Patients with peripheral vascular disorders are naturally particularly vulnerable to such problems as frostbite and chilblains. Greater than average care should be taken in protecting the extremities, and peripheral vasodilator drugs may be used with advantage. If there is a history of the Raynaud phenomenon, patients are well advised to avoid the vibration and passive cold of snow-mobiling.

Altitude

Practical importance

Since the Mexico City Olympics were completed without serious medical problems, some physicians may consider a discussion of altitude and the athlete a dated concern. In fact, this is not the case. Cities at even greater altitudes than Mexico City now vie for International Contests, and there is a danger that such requests may be granted by regulating agencies on the basis of the Mexican experience. It is thus vital to establish how far the risk of such hazards as pulmonary oedema and myocardial infarction would be increased on moving from Mexico City (7350 ft; 2240 m) to 9000 or even 10 000 ft (2743 or 3048 m).

Again, the brilliant endurance performance of high altitude natives such as Keino has drawn attentioon to the possibility that all competitors might profit from a period spent in high altitude training camps.

Lastly, mass air travel has extended the many problems of high altitudes from the specialist to the general practitioner, as vast numbers of middle-aged, poorly-conditioned adults fly without any acclimatization to the mountain peaks of the Alps, the Rockies, and even the Himalayas.

Maintaining oxygen transport

The oxygen partial pressure of the atmosphere diminishes progressively with altitude. Near sea-level, it is about 149 mm Hg. The body must sustain a normal delivery of oxygen to the tissues in the face of these diminishing partial pressures. Much is gained from the normal S-shape of the oxygen dissociation curve; the drop in arterial oxygen saturation is substantially less than if there were a linear relationship between blood oxygen content and alveolar gas pressures.[62, 63] Nevertheless, in Mexico City, arterial saturation drops by 7–8 per cent unless there is a compensatory increase of alveolar ventilation.[64] In sub-maximal exercise, the deficit of arterial oxygenation is made good by an equivalent increase of heart rate, but in maximum effort, there is inevitably a 7–8 per cent impairment of oxygen transport.

Several other points of physiology deserve emphasis. Firstly, the chest muscles encounter little difficulty in producing an increase of ventilation (BTPS) since the air is thin.[65] However, it is not practical to sustain a compensatory increase of ventilation over the first few days at altitude, because adjustments of body buffers are incomplete. Attempts at hyperventilation lead to a drop of arterial P_{CO_2}, intermittent breathing, a reduction of cerebral blood flow, and other disturbances that contribute to the picture of mountain sickness.

Secondly, the relative resistance to oxygen transport across the pulmonary membrane (diffusing capacity, ml O_2/min per mm Hg concentration gradient) decreases in direct proportion to the drop in atmospheric pressure.[66] At sea-level, the athlete finds little difficulty in sustaining full oxygenation of arterial blood, even during maximum effort. However, unsaturation develops progressively more easily as the altitude is raised.

Finally, Mexico City is at rather a critical height for those who wish to undertake vigorous exercise.[66] The maximum advantage has been gained from the normal shape of the oxygen dissociation curve. At greater altitudes, substantial arterial unsaturation is inevitable, particularly when large volumes of oxygen are demanded by the active tissues.

Assessment of altitude

As with cold exposure, most authors are reluctant to make a categorical definition of 'safe' altitudes. Much depends on environmental temperatures, on the type and intensity of activity that is contemplated, and on the fitness, acclimatization and general health of the individual concerned. At moderate altitudes, problems of oxygen transport can be accommodated by the very simple expedient of moving a little more slowly, and an added risk to health can arise only if the individual attempts to sustain the pace he would adopt at sea-level. Difficulty is more likely in oxygen-demanding endurance events than in sprint competitions, but even in brief contests recovery is slowed, and a series of heats may lead to cumulative fatigue.

It is difficult to demonstrate impairment of oxygen transport below 5000 ft (1524 m). At still greater heights, the newcomer shows a progressive loss of aerobic power, 3·2 per cent for each additional 1000 ft (305 m) of altitude.[67] The recent World Congress of Sports Medicine (FIMS, Melbourne, 1974) passed a resolution urging caution above 7500 ft (2286 m) with an absolute prohibition of competition at altitudes over 10 000 ft (3048 m). In the present state of knowledge, these figures seem realistic. The threshold for pulmonary oedema ranges from 8500 to 12 000 ft (2591 to 3658 m),[68, 69] vulnerability being greatest when vigorous activity is sustained for long periods under cold conditions. Even slight reductions of arterial saturation increase the likelihood of cardiac arrhythmias,[70] and manifestations of cerebral hypoxia (for example, central scotoma, impairment of colour vision and disturbances of co-ordination[71]). Somewhat broader limits of altitude can be set for recreational purposes; vast numbers of holidaymakers walk in the Rocky Mountain National Park (12 000 ft; 3658 m) with little ill effect. However, even recreational exercise must be pursued with discretion. Some of the population have medical conditions aggravated by oxygen lack and some of the reported episodes of pulmonary oedema have arisen in young and ostensibly healthy recreational skiers at altitudes of only 3500 m (11 500 ft).[68]

Altitude and performance

Performances in Mexico City were better than predicted by physiologists.[17, 72] Previous winning Olympic performances had averaged 2·9 per cent poorer than world records,[72] yet in Mexico, 29 per cent of the successful competitors exceeded the best world marks, and the average of all winning scores was only 0·9 per cent below world records. Records were generally broken in brief events, with a progressive deterioration of performance in events lasting longer than one minute (3 per cent for a four-minute contest, 8 per cent for a one-hour event).

Most competitors, except the swimmers, benefited from diminished wind resistance.[70, 73, 74] At sea-level, wind resistance accounts for 11 per cent of the energy expended in running three miles; much of this resistance is turbulent, and thus varies directly with atmospheric density. The burden of the distance runners was diminished by 24 per cent in Mexico City, boosting their potential performance by 2·5 per cent; competitors in short distance and throwing events such as discus and javelin[74] were helped even more. This effect, coupled in some instances with preliminary periods of altitude acclimatization, accounts for much of the discrepancy between the physiological decrements found in pre-Olympic trials and actual track performances at the games.

In very short events, the main physiological concern is the rate at which an oxygen debt can be developed, the so-called anaerobic power (see Chapter 2). Such races are concluded before the athlete has had opportunity to develop his maximum tolerated oxygen debt; nevertheless, recovery at altitude may be somewhat slower than that at sea-level. Performance can thus deteriorate if there are a succession of closely spaced heats. Some sprint athletes who visited Mexico City complained of unusual stiffness on the day following competition.[75] It is difficult to envisage anaerobic metabolites such as lactate persisting for more than an hour, even at altitude, and an increased exudation of fluid into the active tissues may be suspected. Where possible, it seems prudent to allow longer than usual between heats, and to reduce the daily volume of training at least until a measure of acclimatization has been attained.

Some 50 per cent of the energy needed for medium distance events such as the 400 and 800 m track contests may be based on the build-up of an oxygen debt. The size of this debt should remain unchanged with acute exposure to altitude. However, it may diminish as the athlete becomes acclimatized and the bicarbonate reserves of the tissues are depleted.[76,77]

If a just sub-maximal exercise is performed over a distance of 1–3 miles (1·6–4·8 km), lactate will accumulate faster at altitude than at sea-level. The result is a premature and distressing shortness of breath, and the remedy is a compensatory slowing of pace. The training should emphasize not only the change of pace, but also any needed alteration of breathing pattern. In some sports such as swimming and rowing the respiratory rate is necessarily linked to the rhythm of arm movement, and in other activities such as cycling and running the athlete may relate breathing frequency and limb movements.

The main physiological determinant of endurance events is the maximum oxygen intake. Many authors compared maximum oxygen intake at altitude and at sea-level when advising national teams on preparations for the 1968 Olympics. Two summary reports,[17, 67] predicted respectively a 7 per cent and a 16 per cent reduction of aerobic power in Mexico City. The present author accepts the 7 per cent estimate as the true physiological decrement; however, larger losses can result from extraneous factors such as a disruption of the normal training routine, fear of altitude, and intercurrent gastrointestinal infections. Certainly, distance performances in the 1968 Olympics (3 per cent loss over 1 mile (1·6 km), 8 per cent over one hour) support a relatively small deterioration.

Acclimatization

Unlike adjustments to heat and cold, acclimatization to high altitude includes certain slow components that continue over several months. The optimum period to be spent at the site of competition thus presents a problem for team managers. While there are physiological gains from prolonged residence at altitude, these must be nicely weighed against the costs of such a camp—not only the financial burden placed on the athlete and his supporting organization, but also cumulative adverse effects from the unaccustomed environment, the boredom and emotional strain of absence from family and friends, a possible reduction in the volume and intensity of training, discouragement from poor track times, and infection by unfamiliar microorganisms.

Physiological adaptations include a reduction in tissue bicarbonate levels, an increase of haemoglobin, restoration of blood volume, and increases in tissue enzyme activities.[78]

The bicarbonate content of cerebrospinal fluid is reduced within a few hours of reaching altitude; this allows some hyperventilation without the onset of intermittent ventilation, and in consequence the arterial oxygen saturation is improved. Adjustments in the buffering capacity of the blood and other tissues occur over the following week.[79]

An increase in the haemoglobin level of the blood provides a second valuable adaptation to high altitudes. In Mexico City, for example, the 7 per cent decrease in arterial oxygen saturation could be made good by an equivalent increase of haemoglobin concentration, provided that the maximum cardiac output was not diminished by the associated rise of blood viscosity. Red cell count and haemo-globin concentration increase within a few days of reaching altitude, but this seems due to haemo-concentration;[17] red cell mass develops more slowly over several months.[80] The oxygen affinity of the haemoglobin may also change with alterations in the acid/base status of the blood, and an increase in the diphospho-glycerate concentration of the red cell membranes. Irrespective of whether red cell formation is stimulated by a brief period at altitude, it is important for the team physician to check the sea-level haemoglobin concentration of competitors. Fads of diet, iron loss in the sweat, depressed formation of red cells, and increased breakdown may contribute to the development of anaemia in the athlete. Iron therapy is helpful only if serum iron figures are low.

There is a progressive diminution of plasma volumes over the first few weeks at altitude, more obvious at 10 000 to 12 000 ft (3048–3658 m) than at 7000 to 8000 ft (2134–2438 m). Contributory factors include hyperventilation in dry mountain air, disturbances of fluid regulation secondary to mountain sickness, and possibly a deliberate attempt by the body to increase haemoglobin levels by haemo-concentration. The stroke volume of the heart is reduced by both the diminution of plasma volume and also a deterioration in myocardial con-tractility; the maximum cardiac output is depressed even more by the high blood viscosity, and some diminution of maximum heart rate. Ultimately, the plasma volume is restored, but nevertheless over the first few weeks at altitude the fluid loss and the associated deterioration in performance are cumulative.[67, 81, 82]

Tissue adaptations such as an increase in myoglobin and in the activity of cer-tain enzyme systems, develop over 1–2 weeks.[83–86] One important gain is a speed-ing of lactate utilization, and thus the rate of recovery from exhausting exercise.

Is it possible to base an overall recommendation on the time courses of these several adaptive changes? Most of the physiologists consulted in connection with the Mexico City Olympics recommended at least 3–4 weeks of acclimatization.[87] This seems appropriate at 7350 ft (2240 m), where there is little deterioration of stroke volume. However, at 10 000 ft (3048 m) loss of plasma fluid cannot be ignored; an athlete may be in a worse physiological condition in the third than in the first week after arrival. Thus, unless time, money, and contest rules permit a lengthy residence, the wise plan for contestants who are visiting altitudes over 8000 ft (2438 m) might be to compete *before* they incur a substantial loss of plasma, that is within 72 hours of arrival. Such a schedule would permit recuperation from the journey, adjustments of cerebrospinal fluid bicarbonate, and recovery from the worst effects of mountain sickness, while anticipating un-welcome decreases of blood buffers and cardiac stroke volume. Little time would be allowed to learn correct pacing, and it would thus be an advantage to gain ex-perience of this aspect of the event from a pre-conquest visit to the competition site.

Adaptations peculiar to the person born at altitude are a little hard to pin-point. Two obvious features are a high haemoglobin level,[88] and a diminution in sensitivity of the carotid body chemoreceptors.[89] Barcroft[90] also noted dif-ferences of body build, including larger chest dimensions.

Mountain sickness
Railway passengers in the Andes regularly develop mountain sickness around 14 000 ft (4267 m). Symptoms are non-specific but nevertheless very unpleasant,

including headache, insomnia, irritability, and a variety of gastrointestinal disturbances.[90]

A healthy person undertaking moderate recreational activity is unlikely to develop mountain sickness at altitudes of less than 10 000 ft (3048 m). A group of physiologists carried out daily maximum effort tests during their first week in Mexico City without noticing any unusual symptoms. However, some investigators have argued that the heavy training schedule of the athlete places him at greater risk, leading to the development of typical symptoms at altitudes of only 6000 to 7000 ft (1829 to 2134 m).[91] The headache reflects an increase of extracellular fluid, while the gastrointestinal symptoms seem associated with an alteration in the volume and composition of the pancreatic juice,[92] on the other hand gastric secretion and motility remain unchanged.[92]

At the altitudes under discussion, mountain sickness is usually a transient disorder, and most patients recover within two days. Conservative treatment is thus quite effective—a temporary lightening of training schedules, general encouragement, and symptomatic therapy for headache and sleeplessness. Immediate symptoms can be reduced by carbonic anhydrase inhibitors such as acetazolamide (250 mg four times daily); the excessive CO_2 wash-out from the lungs is stopped, thereby permitting the patient to sustain a larger ventilation and a better cerebral blood flow. However, the advantage is temporary and won at the expense of slowing acclimatization, since the wash-out of CO_2 provides the stimulus to the adaptive diminution of tissue bicarbonate levels. Acetazolamide also has a diuretic action. Although not large enough to account for its value in the treatment of mountain sickness, the diuresis can have a negative effect on the performance of an endurance athlete who is finding difficulty in maintaining plasma volumes during his first few weeks at altitude.

Chronic forms of mountain sickness have been described, but are difficult to diagnose with certainty. Residual effects of acute exposure are compounded with symptoms from intercurrent gastrointestinal infections, irrational fears of altitude, discouragement from poor trial times, and a real loss of condition secondary to a reduction in the volume and intensity of training.

Pulmonary oedema

An intense pulmonary oedema can develop 9–36 hours after reaching high altitude. The Indian army experienced many casualties from this condition when recruits were rushed to the Tibetan border to counter the Chinese threat; well-documented cases have also developed among recreational skiers at altitudes of less than 9000 ft (2743 m).

The physiopathology is still unclear. Often, there is a history of recent respiratory infection. Pulmonary congestion is favoured by peripheral vasoconstriction (secondary to CO_2 wash-out), pulmonary venous constriction (secondary to the low alveolar oxygen pressure), an increase of total blood volume and pulmonary hypertension (secondary to previous altitude exposure), and an increase of left ventricular diastolic pressure (secondary to myocardial oxygen lack). The permeability of the pulmonary capillaries may be increased by the combined effects of recent respiratory disease and oxygen lack, and the net result is a rapid and potentially fatal flooding of the lungs, usually initiated by vigorous effort.

Presenting symptoms include acute dyspnoea, a blood-stained watery phlegm, chest discomfort and cough, nausea, and vomiting. On examination, there are the usual signs of alveolar exudate, electrocardiographic evidence of right ventricular strain, and intense pulmonary vascular congestion on chest radiographs.

Most cases respond well to bed rest, oxygen, and antibiotics for the prevention of secondary infection.

Medical conditions

The small reduction of oxygen pressure at altitudes of 8000 to 10 000 ft (2438 to 3048 m) can be critical for patients with diseases affecting the oxygen transport system—angina, anaemia, heart failure, and chronic respiratory disease. Exercise prescriptions for cases of this type should be reduced while spending a holiday at a mountain resort.

Negro athletes should be checked for sickle-cell disease before departing for altitude; several deaths from splenic rupture have occurred at or around 8000 ft (2438 m).

Patients with a history of epilepsy may require additional sedation while at altitude.

Altitude training camps

Since the athlete ultimately adapts well to moderate altitudes, and the permanent resident apparently has an advantage in endurance competitions at sea-level, it is tempting to recommend that all athletes should spend a period at an altitude training camp in preparation for major international competitions. The objective would be to return to sea-level at such a time that the polycythaemia was largely preserved for the day of contest, but body buffers had returned to their standard sea-level values.

In practice, this is difficult to organize. It is by no means certain that polycythaemia develops with a few weeks at a mountain camp; often, the rise of red cell count is no more than haemo-concentration. But even the true polycythaemia of the long-term altitude resident is dissipated within 2–3 weeks of return to sea-level through the combined effects of increased erytholysis, decreased red cell production, and expansion of plasma volume. There are other disadvantages. The training schedule may be curtailed while at altitude, and in the crucial final weeks of preparation, the athlete learns an incorrect pace of running and a breathing technique that will be inappropriate for sea-level conditions.

For these reasons, the value of altitude training camps is disputed.[18] Some exercise physiologists such as Faulkner and Mellerowicz have succeeded in augmenting the maximum oxygen intake of average young men relative to values observed before attendance at the altitude camp. However, where subjects were initially in peak condition, the net result of the mountain sojourn has been either no change or a small deterioration of both maximum oxygen intake and track times.[18] A number of national teams used mountain camps in preparation for the 1972 Munich games. While there has been no detailed analysis of results, the general consensus seems a disillusionment with altitude training, and it is likely that this measure will be used much less freely in preparations for the Montreal games of 1976.

R.J.S.

Underwater*

Introduction

It must always be borne in mind that when the sportsman is placed in an unusual physical environment (such as altitude or under water) the whole body is affected and not just the particular functional system that is his immediate concern.[93] For example, it is not enough for the cross-channel swimmer to worry about his stroke and his technique, he must know his thermal capability and his fluid requirements. Training at altitude may benefit the blood constituents but may have adverse effects on gas diffusion in the lungs.

Drowning

Diving in the sense of underwater activities is a sport, recreation, and occupation in which the environmental hazard is most obvious. The greatest hazard and the most urgent is drowning. For all practical purposes water, salt or fresh, is an irrespirable medium for man, and death from asphyxia results from the physical and chemical effects of inhalation of appreciable quantities. The minimum quantity that has to be inspired to produce a fatal result has not been determined, as cases have been recorded of clinical drowning fatalities with no obvious foreign fluid in the respiratory system. However, there is no doubt that small amounts inhaled deeply can be fatal. Theoretically, fresh water drowning will lead to dilution of the blood and sea water drowning to excess fluid in the lung. These are, however, delayed effects in individuals rapidly recovered from immersion. The problem is primarily one of resuscitation by adequate forced ventilation and of maintenance or restoration of cardiac function. As a general guide, a rescuer should not waste time trying to drain the victim of water. This is only of value where copious quantities of water are in the air passages—and even then water will still be in the narrower tubes. The emphasis must be on ventilation of the unaffected lung segments.

Once initial resuscitation has been successful, subsequent management is a skilled matter involving biochemical control. Research in various centres is presently testing methods of treatment of those immersion casualties who reach hospital, in order to determine the most successful and exclude the less desirable methods. Reports cover all degrees of severity of drowning and their management, from a need for no action to exchange blood transfusions.

Table 5.2 Categories of diving activity

Type of dive	Gas in lungs	Apparatus
(1) Skin	Air	None, breath holding
(2) Snorkel	Air	Simple tube to surface
(3) (a) SCUBA	Air	Supply and valves carried by divers
(b) Surface supply	Air/others	Supply on support vessel valving on diver
(c) Mixture	Oxygen with others	Highly specialized

* Thanks to the Medical Director General (Navy) for permission to publish this material.

Diving

Diving activities can be divided into various categories according to the need for specialized breathing equipment (Table 5.2).

Skin diving

Skin diving is carried out by taking a deep breath and then going under water. Underwater swims for distance and spear fishing are competitive forms of this type of diving. With training, individuals can cover distances of 60–70 yards (54·6–63·7 m) and can descend to depths greater than 100 ft (30·5 m). These activities are highly dangerous and record breaking should be actively and vehemently discouraged. Preliminary hyperventilation leads to hypocapnia ('washing-out' of carbon dioxide) and hyperoxia (excessive oxygenation) of the blood. Exercise then alters this state gradually to hypercapnia and hypoxia—but not exactly in step. In distance swims, tragedies have arisen where the hypercapnia has not reached a level to stimulate respiration before hypoxia has resulted in loss of consciousness. Add a psychological drive to suppress respiration, and the respiratory stimulus may fail to produce a response until the individual is unconscious and the inhalation of water is inevitable.

In spear fishing, the hyperoxia is increased by the rise in ambient pressure and this may suppress the response to slight hypercapnia—in fact the best divers can all tolerate raised blood CO_2 levels. However, as the ambient pressure decreases during ascent to the surface, the hyperoxia rapidly falls and may become hypoxia (depending on time and oxygen consumption)—and once again unconsciousness may supervene.[94] In general, time and depth should not be elements in any skin diving competitions. Pre-dive hyperventilation must be discouraged and stringent safety precautions should be in force. Furthermore, it should be obvious that such activities should not be carried out unaccompanied.

Snorkel diving

Snorkel diving is not usually a competitive activity, although this may happen in organized clubs as part of progressive diving training. The snorkel is used primarily to allow a skin diver to survey the area below him on a continuous basis by providing a short airway from his mouth to the air above the back of his head. A secondary use enables the scuba diver to conserve or supplement his cylinder supply when he is on the surface.

Tubes may be of any firm material, usually a plastic, and vary from a simple U-tube with legs of different length to tubes of sophisticated shapes and/or with various valves. There is only one serious problem with snorkel tubes and that concerns the 'dead space'. Accidents have occurred to youngsters using adult tubes who have got into respiratory difficulties, and instead of abandoning the tube have gripped it even harder, till fainting occurred—a dangerous event when in the water. This is due to the fact that the length and bore of the adult tube may contain such a volume of air that the child's respiratory turnover is insufficient to ensure that used air is blown out of the system and replaced by enough fresh air. Thus in effect, all the child is doing is to breathe the same air in and out over and over again (see Fig. 5.1). In the early stages, beginners may take some time to develop the habit of keeping enough air in the chest during a skin

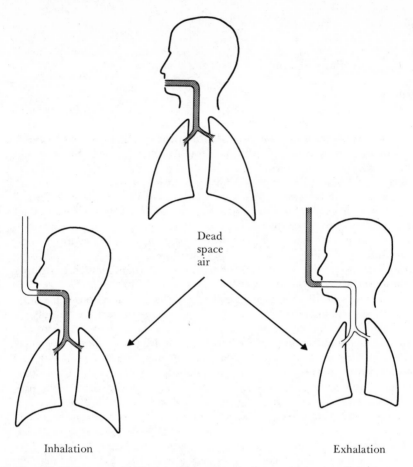

Dead
space
air

Inhalation   Exhalation

Fig. 5.1 If the snorkel tube is too large in relation to tidal volume, no air exchange is possible.

dive with snorkel so as to make the first action on surfacing a further exhalation to expel the water that has entered the tube. Failure is, however, rarely more than a salutary reminder of good practice!

SCUBA*
In using self-contained underwater breathing apparatus (SCUBA), in which breathing gases are supplied to the diver from some apparatus, a new set of problems arise. These will depend on the physiological effects of each gas at the various partial pressures at which it may be inhaled; on the effects of changes of ambient pressures on physical factors such as volume and solubility; on the sophistication of the equipment used and especially on the basic design and on the maintenance problems; and on the physical capabilities of the diver himself. It cannot be too strongly urged that individuals should be properly taught by certified instruc-

*Thanks to the Medical Director General (Navy) for permission to reproduce this material.

tors, and thereafter should dive in groups whose capabilities are known to be adequate for the particular expedition. All diving manuals have been, metaphorically, written in blood, and most problems have arisen from human error either by slip in drill or poor maintenance.

It is not intended to review every problem, for example the acute and chronic toxicity[95] of oxygen or oxy-helium saturation diving, since many have no place in the activities of the sportsman or individual diving for recreation. However, some points need to be made for the individual using air in simple equipment. The diver must be fit, because diving is physically demanding. He should not be suffering from any acute condition or infection. Chronic conditions may be acceptable if therapy has produced a stable controlled state, but chronic bronchitis or chronic sinusitis would almost never be in such a controlled state. In doubt, each case should be referred for advice to a doctor experienced in diving conditions.

The equipment must be well maintained and cared for; a pin hole in a demand valve diaphragm may permit a jet of water to enter the pharynx and cause laryngospasm; a hidden cut may weaken the cylinder; the compressor may contaminate the air with oil and carbon monoxide; and unusual sources of compressed air may have a very low oxygen content.

During the dive, gas will dissolve in the tissue fluids and will enter body cavities to maintain their volume. At depths deeper than 100 ft (30·5 m), nitrogen absorption leads to a euphoric condition, the severity varying with experience and increasing with depth. The diver may become irresponsible concerning his own safety. During the return to the surface the dissolved nitrogen may form bubbles and cause local symptoms by pressure distortion or by embolisation—the condition known as 'bends' or decompression sickness. If access and egress of gas to body cavities is restricted, signs and symptoms will occur and vary with the site, from earache during the descent to cerebral air embolism on the ascent.

It should be obvious that proper training for, and organization of, are the only sure ways of safely enjoying all diving activities.

Other metabolic problems

The problems of respiration under water have been mentioned: other problems are also under investigation. Diving produces blood changes, some of which are psychosomatic indicators of stress; others resemble those seen in massive trauma. Research has shown that the physiological effects of gases are altered (e.g. nitrous oxide loses its anaesthetic properties at great depths for equivalent concentrations, thus showing nervous system effects). The blood distribution is altered and kidney function is affected. Bacteria seem to be affected and antibiotic sensitivity may be altered.

However, the most important control system after external and internal respiration is thermoregulation. It is a fruitless exercise for divers to try to warm up the sea on their own. So far it has been found adequate to insulate the individual by suitable clothing. At one time, rubberized canvas suits were worn over normal woollen clothing. Now, foam neoprene suits that permit a layer of water between skin and suit are popular and effective at shallow depths—at greater depths the foam collapses and the suit is as good as wet tissue paper! The ideal insulated suit has not been found but many solutions have been advocated.

Functional suits have been produced which are electrically or chemically heated and even nuclear heat exchangers have been tried. The definitive answer is still awaited.

External risks

It would be wrong to omit the risks of dangerous marine life. Around Britain this is of minor concern where the jelly-fish and occasional weaver fish are less of a problem than abrasions on barnacles and mishandled boats. This makes it easy to forget that in other waters the risks run from corals through molluscs (such as the blue ringed octopus) and jelly-fish (such as the seawasp) to predators such as sharks. The wise diver will discover the local fauna problems at the same time as he investigates local tides, currents and byelaws—and of course will prepare the appropriate antidote or preventive measure. Some marine mammals are dangerous purely by reason of their size, and human beings have to remember this. One particular danger is another human being driving a power boat—who rarely seems to keep watch for any obstruction in his path, be it floating wood or a diver.

The world beneath the surface is utterly inimical to human life. It can only safely be entered by the individual who is in all respects properly equipped—and then only with care.

D.E.M.

References

1. Adolph, E. F. (1947) *Physiology of Man in the Desert.* New York: Interscience.
2. Burch, G. E. and de Pasquale, N. P. (1962) *Hot Climates, Man and his Heart.* Springfield, Ill.: Charles C Thomas.
3. Leithead, C. S. and Lind, A. R. (1964) *Heat Stress and Heat Disorders.* London: Cassell.
4. Dill, D. B. (1964) Adaptation to the environment. In *Handbook of Physiology*, ed. Dill, D. B., Adolph, E. F. and Wilber, C. G., Section 4. Washington, D.C.: American Physiological Society.
5. Kerslake, D. McK. (1965) The effects of thermal stress on the human body. In *A Textbook of Aviation Physiology*, ed. Gillies, J. A., Oxford: Pergamon Press.
6. Edholm, O. G. and Bacharach, A. L. (1965) *The Physiology of Human Survival.* London: Academic Press.
7. Folk, G. E. (1966) *Introduction to Environmental Physiology.* Philadelphia: Lea and Febiger.
8. Lee, D. H. K. and Minard, D. (1970) *Physiology, Environment and Man.* New York: Academic Press.
9. Wyndham, C. H. and Strydom, N. B. (1972) Korperliche Arbeit bei hoher Temperatur. In *Zentrale Themen des Sportmedizin.* Berlin: Springer.
10. Kerslake, D. McK. (1972) *The Stress of Hot Environments.* Cambridge: Cambridge University Press.
11. Itoh, S., Ogata, K. and Yoshimura, H. (1972) *Advances in Climatic Physiology.* Tokyo: Shoin.
12. Edholm, O. G. and Gunderson, E. K. E. (1973) *Human Polar Biology.* London: Heinemann.
13. Itoh, S. (1974) Physiology of cold-adapted man. *Hokkaido University Medical Library Series*, **7**, 1.
14. Goddard, R. F. (1967) *International Symposium on the Effects of Altitude on Physical Performance.* Chicago: Athletic Institute.

15. Margaria, R. (1967) *Exercise at Altitude*. Dordrecht: Excerpta Medica Foundation.
16. Jokl, E. and Jokl, P. (1968) *Exercise and Altitude*. Basel: Karger.
17. Faulkner, J. A. (1971) Maximum exercise at medium altitude. In *Frontiers of Fitness*, ed. Shephard, R. J., Springfield, Ill.: Charles C Thomas.
18. Richardson, R. G. (1974) ed. Symposium on altitude training. Special Issue, *Br. J. sports Med.*, **8**, 1.
19. Buskirk, E. R. (1968) Problems related to conduct of athletes in hot environments. In *Physiological Aspects of Sports and Physical Fitness*. Chicago: Athletic Institute.
20. Goodman, R. F. (1968) The effects of football equipment on heat transfer. In *Physiological Aspects of Sports and Physical Fitness*. Chicago: Athletic Institute.
21. Murphy, R. J. and Ashe, W. F. (1965) Prevention of heat illness in football players. *J. Am. med. Ass.*, **194**, 650.
22. Spickard, A. (1968) Heat stroke in college football and suggestions for its prevention. *Sth. med. J.*, **61**, 791.
23. Pugh, L. G. C. E., Corbett, J. L. and Johnson, R. H. (1967) Rectal temperatures, weight losses and sweat rates in marathon runners. *J. appl. Physiol.*, **23**, 347.
24. Minard, D. (1961) Prevention of heat casualties in Marine Corps recruits. *Milit. Med.*, **126**, 261.
25. Kavanagh, T. and Shephard, R. J. (1975) Biochemical changes with marathon running—observations on post-coronary patients. In *Proceedings of 2nd International Symposium of Exercise Biochemistry*, Magglingen. Basel: Birkhauser Verlag.
26. Costill, D. L. (1972) Fluid replacement during and following exercise. In *Fitness and Exercise*, ed. Alexander, J. F., Serfass, R. C. and Tipton, C. M., Chicago: Athletic Institute.
27. Kavanagh, T. and Shephard, R. J. (1975.) On the maintenance of fluid balance during marathon running—observations on post-coronary patients. *Brit. J. Sports med.* **9**, 130.
28. Wyndham, C. H., Bredell, G. A. G., Williams, C. G., Strydom, N. B., Morrison, J. F., Peter, J., Fleming, P. W. and Ward, J. S. (1962) Circulatory and metabolic reactions to work in heat. *J. appl. Physiol.*, **17**, 625.
29. Rowell, L. B., Kraning, K. K., Kennedy, J. W. and Evans, T. O. (1967) Central circulatory responses to work in dry heat before and after acclimatization. *J. appl. Physiol.*, **22**, 509.
30. Rowell, L. B. (1974) Human cardiovascular adjustments to exercise and thermal stress. *Physiol. Rev.*, **54**, 1.
31. Pirnay, F., Deroanne, P. and Petit, J. M. (1970) Maximum oxygen consumption in hot atmospheres. *J. appl. Physiol.*, **28**, 642.
32. Saltin, B. (1964) Aerobic and anaerobic work capacity after dehydration. *J. appl. Physiol.*, **19**, 1114.
33. Strydom, N. B. and Williams, C. G. (1969) Effect of physical conditioning on state of heat acclimatization. *J. appl. Physiol.*, **27**, 262.
34. Fox, R. H., Goldsmith, R., Kidd, D. J. and Lewis, H. E. (1963) Acclimatization to heat in man by controlled elevation of body temperature. *J. Physiol.*, **166**, 530.
35. Glaser, E. M. (1966) *The Physiological Basis of Habituation*. London: Oxford University Press.
36. Ladell, W. S. S. (1964) Terrestrial animals in humid heat: man. In *Handbook of Physiology*, ed. Dill, D. B., Adolph, E. F. and Wilber, C. G., Section 4. Washington, D.C.: American Physiological Society.
37. Rose, L. I., Bousser, J. E. and Cooper, K. E. (1970) Serum enzymes after marathon running. *J. appl. Physiol.*, **29**, 355.
38. Berenson, G. S. and Burch, G. E. (1952) The response of patients with congestive heart failure to a rapid elevation in atmospheric temperature and humidity. *Am. J. med. Sci.*, **223**, 45.

39. Bar-Or, O., Skinner, J. S., Buskirk, E. R. and Borg, G. (1972) Physiological and perceptual indicators of physical stress in 41- to 60-year-old men who vary in conditioning level and in body fatness. *Med. Sci. Sports*, **4**, 96.
40. Pugh, L. G. C. E. (1966) Accidental hypothermia in walkers, climbers, and campers. Report to the Medical Commission on Accident Prevention. *Br. med. J.*, **i**, 123.
41. Pugh, L. G. C. E. (1971) Deaths from exposure on Four Inns walking competition, March 14–15th, 1964. In *Exercise and Cardiac Death*, ed. Jokl, E and McClellan, J. T., Baltimore: University Park Press.
42. Pugh, L. G. C. E. (1972) Accidental hypothermia among hill-walkers. In *Environmental effects on Work Performance*, ed. Cumming, G. R., Snidal, D. and Taylor, A. W., Toronto: Canadian Association of Sports Sciences.
43. Asmussen E. and Bøje, O. (1945) Body temperature and capacity for work. *Acta physiol. scand.*, **10**, 1.
44. Bryan, A. C. (1967) Commentary. *Can. med. Ass. J.*, **96**, 804.
45. Hart, J. S. (1967) Commentary. *Can. med. Ass. J.*, **96**, 803.
46. Christensen, E. H. and Högberg, P. (1950) Physiology of skiing. *Int. Z. angew. Physiol.*, **14**, 292.
47. Glaser, E. M. and Shephard, R. J. (1963) Simultaneous experimental acclimatization to heat and cold in man. *J. Physiol.*, **169**, 592.
48. Leblanc, J. (1973) Evaluation of adaptation to the polar environment by autonomic system responses. In *Polar Human Biology*, ed. Edholm, O. G. and Gunderson, E. K. E., London: Heinemann.
49. Andersen, K. L. (1967) The effect of physical training with and without cold exposure upon physiological indices of fitness for work. *Can. med. Ass. J.*, **96**, 801.
50. Irving, L. (1968) Adaptations of native populations to cold. *A.M.A. Arch Envir. Hlth*, **17**, 592.
51. Shephard, R. J. and Godin, G. (1973) Activity patterns in the Canadian Eskimo. In *Polar Human Biology*, ed. Edholm, O. G. and Gunderson, E. K. E., London: Heinemann.
52. Keatinge, W. R. (1961) The effect of repeated daily exposure to cold and of improved physical fitness on the metabolic and vascular response to cold air. *J. Physiol.*, **157**, 209.
53. de Villota, E. D., Barat, G., Peral, P., Juffe, A., de Miguel, J. M. F. and Avello, F. (1973) Recovery from profound hypothermia and cardiac arrest after immersion. *Br. med. J.*, **iv**, 394.
54. Cannon, P. and Keatinge, W. R. (1960) The metabolic rate and heat loss of fat and thin men in heat balance in cold and warm water. *J. Physiol.*, **154**, 329.
55. Editor. (1968) Survival in arctic waters. *Br. med. J.*, **i**, 399.
56. Keatinge, W. R., Prys-Roberts, C., Cooper, K. E., Honour, A. J. and Haight, J. (1969) Sudden failure of swimming in cold water. *Br. med. J.*, **i**, 480.
57. Canabac, M., Lacaisse, A., Pasquis, P. and Dejours, P. (1964) Charactères et mecanisme des réactions ventilatoires au frisson thermique chez l'homme. *C. R. Soc. Biol., Paris*, **157**, 80.
58. Toney, J. M., Garrick, J. G. and Requa, R. K. (1974) Reportability of ski injuries to ski patrols and physicians. *Med. Sci. Sports*, **6**, 78.
59. Shephard, R. J. (1973/4) *Can Exercise Cause Cardiac Death?* Illinois: Hermes, **8**, 343.
60. Kavanagh, T. (1970) A cold-weather 'jogging mask' for angina patients'. *Can. med. Ass. J.*, **103**, 1290.
61. Shephard, R. J. (In press) Work physiology and activity patterns. In *A Synthesis of I.B.P. Data on the Human Adaptability of Circumpolar Populations*, ed. Milan, F.
62. Houston, C. S. and Riley, R. L. (1947) Respiratory and circulatory changes during acclimitization to high altitude. *Am. J. Physiol.*, **149**, 565.

63. Ernsting, J. and Shephard, R. J. (1951) Respiratory adaptations in congenital heart disease. *J. Physiol.*, **112**, 332.
64. Shephard, R. J. (1967) Physical performance in Mexico City. In *The Effects of Altitude on Athletic Performance*, ed. Goddard, R., Chicago: Athletic Institute.
65. Cotes, J. E. (1954) Ventilatory capacity at altitude and its relation to mask design. *Proc. R. Soc.* B, **143**, 32.
66. Shephard, R. J. (1971) The oxygen conductance equation. In *Frontiers of Fitness*, ed. Shephard, R. J., Springfield, Ill.: Charles C Thomas.
67. Buskirk, E. R., Kollias, J., Picon-Reategui, E., Akers, R. F., Prokop, E. K. and Baker, P. (1967) Physiology and performance of track athletes at various altitudes in the United States and in Peru. In *The Effects of Altitude on Athletic Performance*, ed. Goddard, R., Chicago: Athletic Institute.
68. Houston, C. S. (1960) Acute pulmonary oedema of high altitude. *New Engl. J. Med.*, **263**, 964.
69. Singh, I., Kapila, C. C., Khanna, P. K., Nanda, R. B. and Rao, B. D. P. (1965) High altitude pulmonary oedema. *Lancet*, **i**, 229.
70. Pugh, L. G. C. E. (1967) Athletes at altitude, *J. Physiol.*, **192**, 619.
71. Jokl, E., Frucht, A. H., Brauer, H. and Simon, E. (1968) Interpretation of performance predictions for Tokyo Olympic Games, 1964, with extrapolations for Mexico City Olympic Games, 1968. In *Exercise at Altitude*, ed. Jokl, E. and Jokl, P., Basel: Karger.
72. Craig, A. B. (1969) Olympics, 1968—a post-mortem. *Med. Sci. Sports*, **1**, 177.
73. Hill, A. V. (1927) The air resistance to a runner. *Proc. R. Soc.* B, **102**, 380.
74. Dickinson, E. R., Piddington, M. J. and Bain, T. (1966) Project Olympics. *Schweiz Z. Sportmed.*, **14**, 305.
75. Shephard, R. J. (1967) A possible deterioration in performance of short-term Olympic events at altitude. *Can. med. Ass. J.*, **97**, 1414.
76. Durand, J., Paunier, Cl., de Lattre, J., Martineaud, J. P. and Verpillat, J. M. (1967) The cost of the oxygen debt at altitude. In *Exercise at Altitude*, ed. Margaria, R., Dordrecht: Excerpta Medica Foundation.
77. Edwards, H. T. (1968) Lactic acid in rest and work at high altitudes. *Am. J. Physiol.*, **116**, 367.
78. Shephard, R. J. (1973) Athletic performance at moderate altitudes. *Med. dell. Sport*, **26**, 36.
79. Severinghaus, J. W. and Mitchell, R. A. (1964) The role of cerebrospinal fluid in the respiratory acclimatization to high altitude in man. In *The Physiological Effects of High Altitude*, ed. Weihe, W. H., Oxford: Pergamon Press.
80. Reynafarje, B. (1964) *Haematologic Changes During Rest and Physical Activity in Man at High Altitude*. New York: MacMillan.
81. Buhlmann, A. A., Spiegel, M. and Straub, P. W. (1969) Hyperventilation und Hypovolaemia bei Leistungsport in mittleren Hohen. *Schweiz. med. Wschr.*, **99**, 1886.
82. Vogel, J. A. and Hansen, J. E. (1967) Cardiovascular function during exercise at altitude. In *International Symposium on the Effects of Altitude on Physical Performance*, ed. Goddard, R. F., Chicago: Athletic Institute.
83. Bischoff, M. B., Dean, W. D., Bucci, T. J. and Frics, L. A. (1969) Ultra-structural changes in myocardium of animals after five months' residence at 14 110 feet. *Fedn Proc. Fedn Am. Socs exp. Biol.* **28**, 1268.
84. Mager, M., Blatt, W. F., Natale, P. J. and Blatteis, C. M. (1968) Effect of high altitude on lactic dehydrogenase isozymes of neonatal and adult rats. *Am. J. Physiol.*, **215**, 8.
85. Reynafarje, B. (1962) Myoglobin content and enzymic activity of muscle and altitude adaptation. *J. appl. Physiol.*, **17**, 301.

86. Reynafarje, B. and Velasquez, T. (1966) Metabolic and physiological aspects of exercise at high altitude: Kinetics of blood lactate, pyruvate and inorganic phosphate during exercise and recovery and their relation with oxygen debt. *Fedn Proc. Fedn Am. Socs exp. Biol.* **25,** 1397.

87. Mach, R. S. (1967) Acceleration of acclimatization to work at high altitudes. *Progress Rep., U.S. Army Contract* DA–79–193–MD–2446.

88. Hurtado, A. (1964) Acclimatization to high altitudes. In *The Physiological Effects of High Altitude*, ed. Weihe, W. H., New York: MacMillan.

89. Byrne-Quinn, E., Sodal, I. E. and Weil, J. V. (1972) Hypoxic and hypercapnic ventilatory drives in children native to high altitude. *J. appl. Physiol.*, **32,** 44.

90. Barcroft, J. (1914) *The Respiratory Function of the Blood.* Cambridge: Cambridge University Press.

91. Jokl, E. (1968) Indisposition after running. In *Exercise and Altitude*, ed. Jokl, E. and Jokl, P., Basel: Karger.

92. Hartiala, K. (1967) Digestive functions in altitude conditions. In *International Symposium on the Effects of Altitude on Physical Performance*, ed. Goddard, R. F., Chicago: Athletic Institute.

93. Miles, S. (1966) *Underwater Medicine.* London: Staples Press.

94. Cabarron, P. (1960) The work of the committee for the prevention of free diving accidents, *Sous Marine*, Feb./March 25.

95. Donald, K. W. (1947) Oxygen poisoning in man, *Br. med. J.*, **i,** 172.

6

Biomechanics and physique

Introduction

Biomechanics is the study of mechanical movement in the human and animal organism. Man's movements are extremely complex, reflecting both locomotor activity and cerebral function. Human motion acquires its sophisticated character from the association of the mechanical with the biological forms of movement. Biological mechanics (biomechanics) deals with that association and the laws which govern it.[1]

Since man acts consciously, he is interested in the outcome of his movements and is continually seeking ways to improve his performance in executing them. In physical education and sport, biomechanics deals with the peculiarities of the specific movements involved and hence the means of improving efficiency, precision and energy saving, as well as with the optimal manner of training.

Basic concepts in biomechanics

Before mechanical motion in the human or animal body can be studied, it is necessary to define certain terms that are used in biomechanics.

Biomechanical events take place in Euclidean three-dimensional (E_3) *space* with a reference system consisting of a rectangular trihedral of axes X, Y, and Z, and O as the origin.

Time
Time in biomechanics is extended to the universe as a whole and is an independent variable (t); other physical magnitudes are expressed in terms of it. The origin in time can be any arbitrarily selected instant; negative values refer to events occurring before, and positive values to those subsequent to that instant.

Mass
Matter is distributed into bodies each having a physical magnitude called Mass (M). The practical unit of measure of mass is the kilogram (kg).

Centre of mass (CM)
The human body or its segments can be considered to be devoid of linear dimensions, with the centre of mass acting as a single point in space representing the mass of the body or the segment under consideration.

Movement
Movement is the change in position of the body, body segment, or centre of mass in relation to the reference system.

Force
Mechanical stress on the mass is characterized by force (F). In biomechanics, force may be either external (gravity) or internal (muscular effort) in origin, and is measured in Newtons.

Gravity
Bodies on earth are influenced by a force which is proportional to their mass, called gravitational acceleration (g) and it is effectively constant though showing slight geographical variations. Just as the centre of the mass concentrates the mass of the body or body segment, so does gravity concentrate the weight of the body or any body segment to become the centre of gravity.

Force in biomechanics
Force applied to a body is a vector and as such possesses magnitude, direction, and a point of application and so can be represented graphically. In graphic representation it is customary to use a standard scale for the magnitude of the force and the length of the arrow representing it (Fig. 6.1).

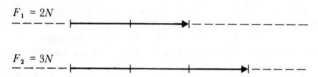

$F_1 = 2N$

$F_2 = 3N$

Fig. 6.1 The common graphic vector representation of forces, with magnitude and direction.

The fundamental laws in biomechanics

Biomechanics applies the basic laws formulated by Isaac Newton to the study of mechanical motion in the human and animal body.

The fundamental problems in biomechanics consist of: (a) explaining the way in which the human body or any of its segments vary their movements, and (b) establishing the quantitative relationship of such actions. For the human body and its larger parts, biomechanical movement is identical with the mechanical movement of systems functioning according to Newton's three fundamental laws.

Newton's first law—the law of inertia
'A body will remain in a state of rest or uniform motion in a straight line unless it is compelled to change from these states by external force(s) acting upon it.'

According to this law material objects are inert whether at rest or in uniform motion in a straight line until acted upon by a force (F). When such a force operates it applies the acceleration $a = F/M$ (Fig. 6.2).

If the external force is zero the fundamental equation $F = M \times a$ becomes $0 = M \times a$, and so no acceleration takes place; therefore the body will remain at rest or in uniform motion in a straight line.

For example the shot putter (Fig. 6.3) acts with a muscular force (F) upon the shot which changes its speed from rest to $14\,\text{m/sec}$. At the same time the shot is subject to the gravitational force G which is tending to change the motion of the

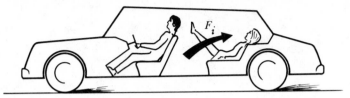

Fig. 6.2 Inertial force resists acceleration.

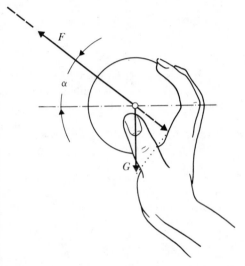

Fig. 6.3 Inertial force, shot putt. *F*, throwing force; *G*, weight of shot; α, throwing angle.

shot. Clearly neither of these forces is acting directly on the centre of the mass (gravity) but each can be resolved for purposes of study so to do, thus obeying Newton's fundamental equation.

Newton's second law—Law of proportionality

As was stated in the first law, a body will remain in a state of rest or uniform motion in a straight line, unless acted upon by an external force. The second law now expands this and states that when such a force does operate 'the resulting change in velocity will be directly proportional to the amount of force causing the change', and inversely proportional to the mass of the body.

For example (see Fig. 6.4) if a force (F_2) is applied to a mass (M) at rest (i.e. $V_1 = 0$) the mass acquires speed V_2. If the force applied is twice as great (F_3) then the resulting speed will also be twice as great (V_3).

Newton's third law—law of interaction

'To every action there is an equal and opposite reaction'. In nature the various bodies act on one another reciprocally (Fig. 6.5).

Inertia is manifest as a reaction equal and opposite to the action which produced the acceleration (that is $M \times a$).

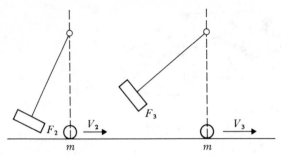

Fig. 6.4 The law of proportionality represented by a stroke in croquet (for explanation see text).

The reaction $M \times a$ is called inertial force. It does not act on the CM itself but resists the agent exercising its action on the CM. Inertial force manifests itself whenever an external force causes the body to move in the direction of that external force (Fig. 6.2).

In Fig. 6.6, if G is the weight of a body resting on a horizontal plane, the body apart from the influence of its weight also undergoes a reaction from the plane, so the total force on the body, $= R + G$.

In equilibrium the reaction of the plane is equal to the weight of the body, the latter acting in the opposite way, thus $R = G$. Similarly in shooting the kick of the gun represents the reaction (R) of the gas distention force (F) which ejects the bullet, so $F = R$.

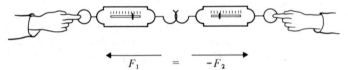

Fig. 6.5 Action and reaction are equal and opposite.

The locomotive concept of the body

All mechanical devices, no matter how perfectly made, are subject to wear and tear in the course of use. In other words they reflect their past and present by the destructive component of evolution.

In living matter, evolution involves not only a destructive component but also a constructive component. Thus during exercise a muscle will show hypertrophy or improvement in its contractile qualities as well as wear and tear. This continuous and contradictory 'dialogue' between the destructive and constructive components is resolved either downwards (with a degrading of the appropriate qualities as in overtraining) or upwards (as when increased physical fitness improves performance).

Like mechanical devices or engines, human muscle produces mechanical energy. Machines transform thermal or electrical power into mechanical energy whereas the human muscle converts chemicals into mechanical energy directly without a thermal intermediary. This process is not encountered in technology and has yet to be fully elucidated.

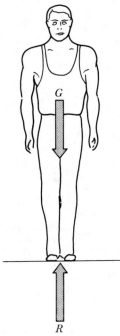

Fig. 6.6 The reaction of the horizontal plane (R) on the weight of the body at rest (G).

Mechanical energy

The energy of a body is defined as that property of a body which enables it to overcome resistance to motion, to do work, or to produce a physical effect. Kinetic energy is the energy possessed by a body by virtue of its velocity, whereas potential energy is the energy possessed by virtue of its position. Work is done when a force acts through a distance, and power relates work done to unit time.

Through a series of equations, Lloyd and Moran[2] and also Fidelus[3] calculated the work done in different sports activities. Fidelus showed the close comparability of the work done by a sprinter and a weight lifter in unit time.

Muscle as an energy convertor
The useful mechanical work performed by a muscle during contraction represents consumption of mechanical energy. Thus to move an object at a speed V the muscle must act with force F over a time interval t. The mechanical energy (W_n) expended in this case originates in the muscle and is: $W_n = F \times V \times t$.

Not all the mechanical energy developed in the muscle is utilized to produce useful mechanical work (Fig. 6.7). Some of it is wasted in counteracting forces which do not relate to useful mechanical work, e.g. internal frictional forces. Another part of the mechanical energy is stored in the viscous and elastic elements of the contractile system. The part which is accumulated in the elastic elements re-enters the circuit and is not considered as wasted mechanical energy.

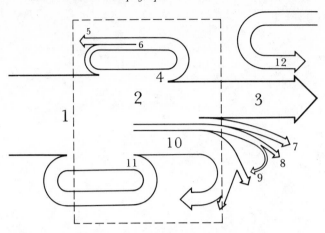

Fig. 6.7 Energy flow in muscle as an energy converter. 1, chemical energy input; 2, mechanical energy; 3, useful mechanical energy; 4, mechanical energy consumption in muscle; 5, mechanical energy of viscous elements; 6, mechanical energy of elastic elements; 7, friction; 8, radiant electrical power; 9, electrical power; 10, caloric energy; 11, chemical energy returned to converter; 12, external mechanical energy.

However, not all the useful mechanical work done derives from mechanical energy supplied by muscle; some may also come from elements which are external to the biomechanical system, e.g. the weight of the object moved.

The mechanical energy produced in muscle originates from chemical energy. Part of the energy yield of adenosine triphosphate (ATP) is available for direct use in the contraction–relaxation process, while another part is indirectly used for the energy supply, i.e. in the transformation of phosphorylase b into the a form, in the phosphorylation of glucose and of fructose-6-phosphate, and in the 'activation of the free fatty acids'. Finally ATP is needed in the cell for 'maintaining the labile protein structures'. This explains why only part of the ATP is used in the muscle for the performance of mechanical work.[4] Chemical energy also supplies the thermal energy dissipated in the muscle as well as a relatively small amount of electrical and radiant energy.

According to the principle of conservation of energy, the sum of all the forms of energy supplied by the muscle is equal to the energy received by the muscle.

The mathematical pattern of muscular conversion of energy

It is clear that no waste of energy occurs in the muscle, but from the mechanical point of view, interest is confined to the mechanical energy which produces useful mechanical work. Thus, it is possible to discuss a conversion efficiency[5] W_u/W_t where W_u is the useful mechanical energy and W_t the total mechanical energy produced by chemical changes. This efficiency reflects the mode of utilization of mechanical energy rather than the functional potentialities of the muscle.[6]

Movement

Movement of the human body or of its segments can be analysed in terms of theories relating to machines and engines. Those segments of the human body with mobile links are studied as kinematic couples or kinematic chains. Kinematic couples are binary systems involving the contact of two rigid segments which secure the transmission of forces. The kinematic chain includes the mobile connection between the rigid element or links which allow a range of movement.

Kinematic chains consist of couples which are connected successively or by branching. When the final link is free, the link is *open* permitting isolated move-

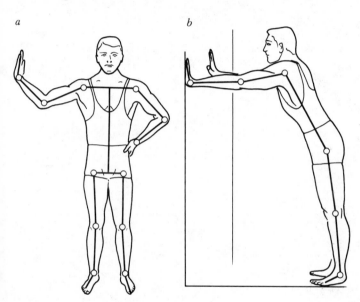

Fig. 6.8 Kinematic chains of the body, (a) open, (b) closed.

ments, which, geometrically, are independent of the movements of other links (Fig. 6.8a).

Within a *closed* link no isolated or irregular movement (i.e. motion through a single joint) is possible. An example of a closed link within the human body is the spinal column–rib–sternum link. In Fig. 6.8b, flexion of the elbows produces movement in the other joints also, such as the ankle and wrist. The transmission of muscle action to adjacent or distant articulations is characteristic of closed links. Within closed links the possibilities of motion are less than with open links, but those of control are greater.

The degrees of freedom of movement

A body which can move in any direction is a free body. In relation to the X, Y, and Z axes a free body may execute three linear movements along the axes and three rotational movements around the same axes (Fig. 6.9). Therefore a free body is said to possess six degrees of freedom. The degree of freedom corresponds to the number of possible independent movements of the body, whether linear or rotational.

The segments of the body possess fewer degrees of freedom because of their articulations. Thus in the case of the leg, three degrees of linear freedom disappear as it is unable to move independently along the three co-ordinate axes. However, it is able to rotate around these axes (as for example at the hip joint).

If two points of the segment are attached, rotation is only possible around the axis passing through the two points. The uniaxial bones are articulated in this way and possess only one degree of freedom. The articulations, therefore, are

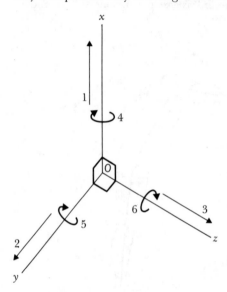

Fig. 6.9 Possible movements in relation to O, X, Y, Z axes.

divided into six orders, with the order (S) and the degree of freedom (H) related thus: $S = 6 - H$. It should, however, be noted that the joints do not have perfect geometrical shapes and that the reference axes of these joints are therefore not fixed.

Joint mobility is measured by range of movement, which coincides with the maximum value of the angle between the two segments adjacent to the articulation. The range of movement may also refer to the movement of several links of the kinematic chain. For example, the range of movement of the vertebral column is measured by the angle between the first link and the other end of the chain.

Lever systems in the limbs

In biomechanics the skeleton (consisting of rigid bones and mobile joints) and the forces acting upon it represent a system of levers.

A lever is a simple machine which transmits force and motion at a distance. All levers possess an axis or fulcrum (O), a point F where the force is applied, and a point R where the resistance is applied. Conventionally the force F is considered to produce useful motion and the force R to be the force of resistance or weight.

The portion of the lever between the fulcrum and the force point is known as the force arm (a) and similarly the portion between the fulcrum and the resistance point is known as the resistance arm (b). If the force and resistance do not act perpendicularly upon the lever their arms are measured on the perpendiculars passing through the points of support (Fig. 6.10).

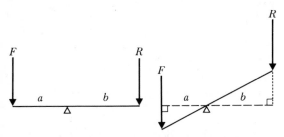

Fig. 6.10 Application of force and resistance to a lever.

The principle of levers

A lever will balance or turn uniformly about the point of support when the product of the force and force arm equals the product of the resistance and resistance arm.

From the relation $F \times a = R \times b$ it emerges that the usual function of a lever is to gain a mechanical advantage whereby a small force applied over a large distance at one end of the lever produces a greater force operating over a smaller distance at the other end of the lever, or whereby a given speed of movement at one end of the lever is greatly increased at the other.

In the human body, the action of the contracting muscles normally constitutes the force, and the resistance is furnished by the centre of gravity of the segment being moved plus any additional weight which may be in contact with the segment. The axis is the joint around which the movement takes place. In the human body the force arm is generally shorter than the resistance arm, resulting in a mechanical disadvantage. However, in accordance with the law of conservation of energy, what is lost in force is gained in speed and range of movement.

The classification of levers

Levers are divided into three classes or orders according to the point of support (fulcrum) and points of application of the force F and the resistance R.

First-class levers

In the first-class lever, the fulcrum lies between the force and resistance points. For example, the action of the triceps (F) upon the olecranon process of the ulna (G) produces extension of the forearm (Fig. 6.11).

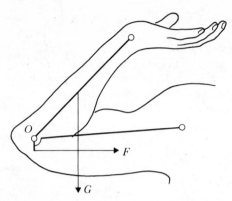

Fig. 6.11 Example of class one lever. *F*, force; *G*, resistance; *O*, fulcrum.

Second-class levers

In levers of the second order the resistance lies between the fulcrum and the force. Here speed is sacrificed to gain power. For example, in push-up exercises, the body held in a prone position with hands pointed forward and approximately under the shoulders may be compared with a second-class lever in which the force

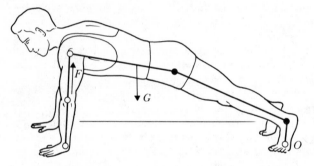

Fig. 6.12 Example of class two lever. *F*, force; *G*, resistance; *O*, fulcrum.

of the muscles producing extension of the elbow joint (*F*) lifts the weight *G* of the body in relation to the fulcrum represented by the ankle joint (Fig. 6.12).

Although the presence of second-class levers in the human body is still doubted, numerous situations involving external forces or even the weight of body segments can be described as examples of second-class levers.

Third-class levers

In the third-class lever the force is applied between the fulcrum and the resistance. This class of lever is the one most common in the limbs; it permits the muscle to be inserted near the joint and to produce range and speed of movement, although at a sacrifice of force. A typical example is found in the biceps flexing the forearm against the resistance of the forearm weight (Fig. 6.13). The same class of lever is demonstrated in flexion of the wrist, of the leg at the knee and in dorsiflexion of the foot.

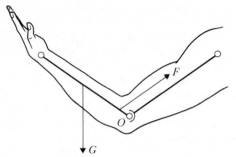

Fig. 6.13 Example of class three lever. *F*, force; *G*, resistance; *O*, fulcrum.

This classification of levers into three classes is conventional and does not consider the mode of action of forces. The lever is in a state of equilibrium when the torques are equal. By simply turning the resistance torque in first-class levers through 180° they become second- and third-class ones.

Lever systems

In the example of kicking a football (Fig. 6.14), the movement is for simplicity considered to be executed only by the agonists, namely the anterior tibial, quadriceps and psoas muscles.

The inertia of the ball represents the resistance of the third-class lever which

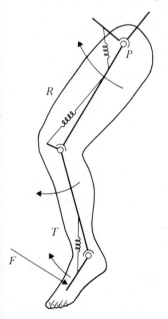

Fig. 6.14 Lever systems kicking a football. *T*, contraction force—anterior tibials; *R*, contraction force—quadriceps; *P*, contraction force—psoas; *F*, inertial force of ball.

is the ankle joint, where the force is by convention the action of the anterior tibial muscles.

This kinematic chain with two links is itself a third-class lever in relation to the knee joint. Here the momentum created by the inertial force is overcome by the momentum of the active force of contraction of the quadriceps.

In its turn, the kinematic chain consisting of three links is itself a third-class lever in relation to the hip joint. This time the acting force (which produces rotation) is the resultant of the contraction of the hip flexors. Thus, the force of the kick is the product of the successive summation of the torques for each of the three joints, it being considered that one end and subsequently two of them become rigid.

Limb movements may be extremely complex. In studying situations such as these, excessive simplification can invalidate the biomechanical analysis.

Use of synergist muscles to diminish inertia

The movement of kinematic chains occurs through the actions of groups of muscles and not through the contractions of single muscles.

Muscles which act separately but produce a single movement (determined by the type of joint) are synergists. For example adduction of the shoulder is executed by simultaneous contraction of the pectoralis major and the latissimus dorsi. The muscles which oppose movement in the joints are antagonists. They play a part not only in retarding movement, but also in improving co-ordination.

Synergism may exist at the level both of the single joint and in complex movements that involve several links of a kinematic chain.

In the limbs, certain long muscles act simultaneously on two joints. Lombard's paradox is well known, that while the rectus femoris tends to flex the hip and extend the knee, the hamstring tends to extend the hip and flex the knee. It might be expected that the rectus femoris and the hamstrings would mutually neutralize each other's action at both the hip and knee joints when their torques were balanced, and this they do in the process of synergistic stabilization.

Programming the work of the synergist and antagonist muscles is done by the central nervous system in four modes of contraction grading:

(1) qualitatively by innervation of the phasic or tonic muscles;
(2) intensively by raising the intrinsic muscular tension;
(3) spatially through the action in various zones of movement (optimal zones of contraction);
(4) temporally by desynchronizing the action of the various muscular bundles or of the muscles within the group.

All these ways of grading the contraction determine the 'quality' of movement, that is, the dynamics of counteracting the resistive force. If the resistive force itself decreases during movement, antagonist muscles start to act to brake the movement so that disruption of the ligaments or of the articular capsule of neighbouring joints does not occur.

Since the attachments of synergist muscles vary, the relative force characteristics of their torques change during motion. These torque variations together with the non-linearity of the contractile characteristics of the muscle (the relation of force to the contraction of a muscle is not constant), produce fluctuations in the resultant torque. (Resultant torque is produced by vectorial summation against time of the torques created by each separate synergist muscle for its optimal zone of action, the latter being defined both by the lengthening/force characteristic and the angle between the direction of the muscular force and the direction of movement). As a consequence of the variation in the resultant torque, acceleration occurs in the joint, i.e. a change in speed within the link of the kinematic chain.

Whether the link was initially at rest or at constant speed, its change of pace signifies a diminution in inertia resulting from the action of the synergist and the antagonist muscles.

Mass and centre of gravity of the body

Commonly, the term biomechanical system means the human body. Sometimes in studying biomechanical events it is more helpful to consider the human body as being made up of several biomechanical systems, while at other times it is preferable to consider certain objects together with the human body as forming a single system. For example, in studying spring-board diving the diver's body is considered to be made up of two connected systems, i.e. the upper trunk and arms, and the lower trunk and legs, while in the case of ski jumpers the biomechanical system comprises the jumper and his skis together.

Because of its heterogeneous structure the mass of the human body is unevenly distributed. From the biomechanical standpoint the masses of the mobile body segments are theoretically regarded as being concentrated in centres of mass of the respective segments.

These fictitious centres of mass may stand in different positions relative to one another, depending on the position of the mobile body segments, but do not essentially vary (in position) with time. Therefore, the biomechanical system is a non-deformable system.

Denoting by m_1, m_2 ... m_n the masses concentrated in the centres of mass 1, 2 ... n of the segments of system, then

$$m = \frac{\sum m_1, m_2 \ldots m_n}{n}$$

in the mass of the biomechanical system (the human body) which is concentrated in the centre of mass m of the biomechanical system as a whole.

The forces acting on the system can be divided into those that are external and those that are internal to it. The forces external to the human body (considered as a biomechanical system) are the body's own weight, the reaction of its supports, the resistance of the environment, the inertial forces of distant bodies, and the elastic-deformation forces. The forces internal to the human body are the muscle contraction forces, but in the case of the spring-board diver (as mentioned above), the muscle power that connects the upper and lower parts of the diver's body, which are considered as two connected biomechanical systems, is considered an external force.

Gravitational force and weight

Because of gravitational acceleration g, the mass m of the biochemical system is attracted to the earth by a force G (where $G = m \times g$), which stands for the weight force of the biomechanical system (the human body).

The weight force is equal to the vectorial sum of the gravitational (attraction) and centrifugal (inertial) forces which act upon the human body at the earth's surface because of its daily revolutions.

The centre of gravity

The point of application of the gravitational (vectorial) force acting upon the human body is known as its centre of gravity. The centre of gravity coincides spatially with the centre of mass.

Since the difference between the gravitational force and the weight force applied to the human body is insignificant the term centre of gravity is used throughout.

Given centres of mass for segments and parts of the human body, it is then reasonable to refer also to centres of gravity of those segments or parts. The position of these centres of gravity is determined experimentally on the human body or on models of it under equilibrium conditions. The centres of gravity of segments or parts of the body are related to their length. The axes of rotation and, in general, mechanical articulations do not coincide with the hinge points of the bones.

The link in the biomechanical system, in the anthropologist's acceptance of the term, is defined as 'a straight line through the body segment between adjacent hinge points'.

Table 6.1 The relative weights of the human body segments

Body Segment	Braune and Fischer[9]	According to Borelli[8]		Dempster[10]	Acceptable Approximation
		Males	Females		
	%	%	%	%	%
Head	7·06	6·72	8·12	6·9	7
Trunk	42·70	46·30	43·90	46·1	43
Hip	11·58	12·21	12·89	10·7	12
Leg	5·27	4·65	4·34	4·7	5
Foot	1·79	1·56	1·29	1·7	2
Shoulder	3·36	2·65	2·60	3·3	3
Forearm	2·28	1·82	1·82	2·1	2
Hand	0·84	0·70	0·55	0·8	1
Total Body weight	100	100	100	100	100

Williams and Lissner[7] consider the length of the link to be easily recognizable when adjacent segments change their angle, by the line of the skin flexure. Although such a determination of the length introduces error, this is acceptable as far as biomechanical accuracy is concerned.

The gravitational (weight) forces of the links are determined by direct or indirect measurement. Direct weighing, which introduces the least measuring error, can be done only once, i.e. after the subject's death! The weights of the links are also expressed in units or per cent relative to the weight of the human body as a whole (Table 6.1).

The weights as well as the centres of gravity differ from subject to subject, depending on age, sex, body build and size. The positions of the centres of gravity of the links also change under the influence of sports training or of the blood supply, and sometimes also because of excessive feeding. These latter modifications are relatively unimportant and are therefore negligible.

Determination of the centre of gravity of the human body

The centre of gravity of the human body can be measured in effect by weighing the human body in three perpendicular planes.

Many authors of studies of the centre of gravity have reported original methods. The results illustrated are those of Borelli,[8] Braune and Fischer,[9] and Dempster.[10]

For determination of the centre of gravity of the human body in various (dynamic) positions using calculus, the relative (per cent) data of Table 6.1 are used, as well as the arrangement of the centres of gravity of the links.

The graphic method of determination of the centre of gravity

The centre of gravity of the body (the biomechanical system) may be determined graphically by resolving the moments of the centres of gravity of the constituent links.

In the example shown (Fig. 6.15), the position of the combined centre of gravity of two adjacent segments G_1 and G_2 (respectively representing 3 per cent and 2 per cent of body weight) is found to be a point two-fifths of the way along a straight line drawn between them (i.e. the point at which their respective moments balance out). The combined centre of gravity for the segments G_1, G_2 and G_3 together (1 per cent of body weight) is similarly calculated as being one-sixth of the way along the line joining the combined centre of gravity for G_1 and G_2 (total 5 per cent of body weight) with G_3.

The progressive application of this method of resolving the moments of the centres of gravity of the constituent segments of the body up to 100 per cent body weight ultimately defines the centre of gravity of the body as a whole.

The analytic method of determination of the centre of gravity of the human body

This method is based on Varignon's theorum: 'The sum of the moments of a force in relation to any pole is equal to the moment of those forces in relation to the same pole' (Fig. 6.16).

The determination of the centre of gravity of the human body by calculation

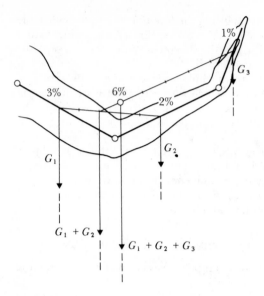

Fig. 6.15 Graphic calculation of centre of gravity of adjacent segments (see text).

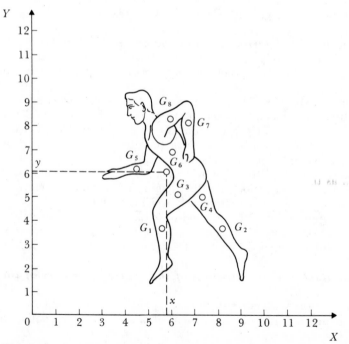

Fig. 6.16 Analytic method of determining the centre of gravity of the human body.

introduces great errors. According to Donskoi[1]: both the relative weights of the human body links, and the siting of the centres of gravity of the links, are variable. This is because firstly, the centres of gravity of the links are not situated exactly on their longitudinal axes, secondly there are in any case wide individual differences, and thirdly the links of the biomechanical system change their shape (and by implication the positions of their centres of gravity) during movement.

For example, in the vertical position of the vertebral column, the centre of gravity of the trunk is not situated on its axis, but is situated on the line which joins the centres of gravity of the two halves of the body which are of equal weight. It should be noted that in the case of movements of the shoulder girdle, the axis of the shoulder joints from which the distance is measured to the centre of gravity of the trunk suddenly changes position. As a consequence of this, the position of the centre of gravity of the trunk is no longer acceptable for calculation, since great errors are introduced.

Further centres of the human body

For events taking place in water or in an airflow the position of two other centres should be known: the centre of volume, and the centre of surface of the human body.

The centre of volume (or centre of buoyancy) is the point of application of the resultant of the downward pushing forces in the case of complete submersion of the body in water. The centre of volume is situated in the centre of gravity of the volume of water removed by the contour of the diving body. Donskoi[1] maintains that with the human body in a vertical position the centre of volume is situated 2–6 cm higher than the centre of gravity.

The centre of surface (or centre of pressure) is the point of application of the resultant of the reacting forces generated by the environment. For example, in the free fall of parachutists, the centre of surface is not coincident with the centre of gravity, and the forces applied to these form a couple which rotates the body. By movement of the arms and legs the position of the centre of gravity can be changed, so permitting acrobatic performances.

The centre of gravity outside the human body

In certain positions of the links of the biomechanical system, the centre of gravity may be situated outside the body.

This situation permits good performance by high jumpers and pole vaulters. The latter, for instance, by a bar wrapping movement succeed in jumping over the bar though the centre of gravity passes *under* it (Fig. 6.17).

The trajectory of the centre of gravity

In the flying phase of the high jumper the centre of gravity is acted upon by the force G of the body weight, and force R of the resistance of the milieu or environment. In this case the resistance of the milieu (air) is negligible as the centre of gravity is moving at a low speed.

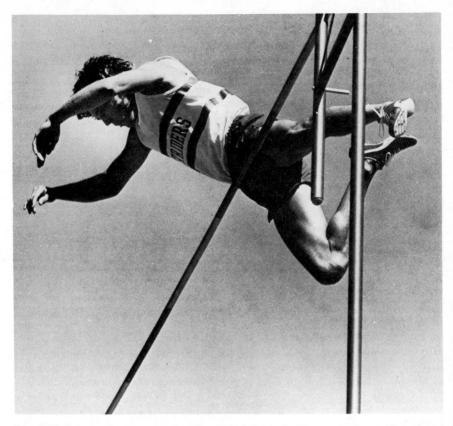

Fig. 6.17 Pole vaulter at top of vault. Although the body passes above the bar, the centre of gravity passes beneath it. (Photo: E. D. Lacey.)

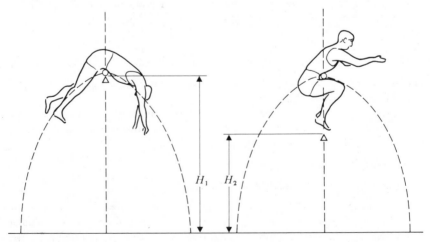

Fig. 6.18 Ballistic trajectory of centre of gravity.

The maximum height of the jump depends on the initial speed, the take-off angle, and the gravitational acceleration (paradoxically the height of the jump does *not* depend on the mass (weight) of the jumper). The trajectory of the centre of gravity is thus a ballistic trajectory.

The ballistic trajectory of the centre of gravity cannot be modified by the jumper during flight (Fig. 6.18), and the movements of the jumper are due to the internal forces of the system. These have no external resultant and do not

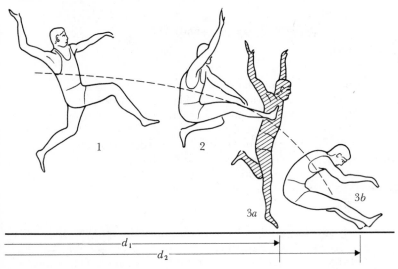

Fig. 6.19 Compensatory movements of arms and feet in long jumping produce distance gain $(d_2 - d_1)$.

modify the trajectory. The descent of one segment automatically entails the compensatory ascent of another. By appropriate movements of the body segments, it is possible to obtain rotation of the body round its centre of gravity. For example, the long jumper can get a considerable gain of distance (Fig. 6.19) during the landing phase by raising his feet through compensatory movements of the arms and trunk.

Rotational movement

Rotation takes place when the line of action of a force applied to an object passes at a distance from the point of support of the object. The torque or turning moment is the product of this force applied (f) and the perpendicular distance (r) of the line of action from the support point (or fulcrum) (Fig. 6.20). Rotation takes place about an axis (which may be fixed or free) which lies perpendicular to the plane of the movement.

In diving from a spring-board the diver's whole body rotates about an axis which passes through his centre of gravity. The axis of rotation moves along the trajectory of the centre of gravity of the body. In this case, the axis of rotation of the body is free. The linear speed and linear acceleration of the segments

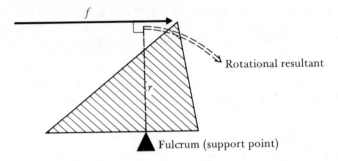

Fig. 6.20 Rotation—basic mechanics.

of the rotating body depend on the distance between their centres of gravity and the axis of rotation. This distance is called the radius of rotation (r).

In rotational movement, the velocity vector changes continuously because of centripetal acceleration. This acceleration is brought about by the restraining centripetal force which prevents the rotating body from flying off at a tangent and keeps it moving at a fixed distance (r) from the axis of rotation. Centripetal acceleration A_n is proportional to the square of the velocity of the rotating body and inversely proportional to its radius of rotation.

thus
$$A_n \propto V^2/r$$

The restraining centripetal force is counteracted by the centrifugal (inertial) force which seeks to keep the rotating body moving in a straight line. This force is the product of the mass of the body (m) and the centripetal acceleration (A_n). (It is to counteract this force that race track bends are banked (Figure 6.21).)

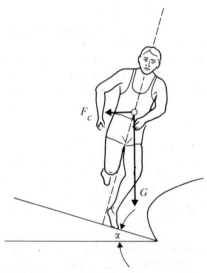

Fig. 6.21 Centrifugal force running round bend on indoor track. G, athlete's weight; F_c, centrifugal force; α, inclination of track.

Applied biomechanics

The ankle as a torque convertor

The ankle is the most distinctively 'human' part of man's anatomy.[11] It is a trochlear joint, the articular surfaces being the tibiofibular clamp, and the upper and lateral surfaces of the talus.

The articular surfaces of the talus are like a reel with a central groove, which is anteriorly and outwardly oblique at 30° to the sagittal plane, so that movements are executed not anteroposteriorly but slightly obliquely, the toes being adducted in dorsiflexion. The articular surfaces are connected by a fibrous capsule reinforced by medial and lateral ligaments.

The lateral ligament is made up of three independent bundles (the anterior talofibular ligaments, the calcaneofibular ligament, and the posterior talofibular ligament), which during various movements undergo different degrees of stress. In the intermediate position, it is only the middle bundle that is stretched. In dorsiflexion of the foot the posterior bundle stretches while during plantar flexion the anterior bundles are stretched.

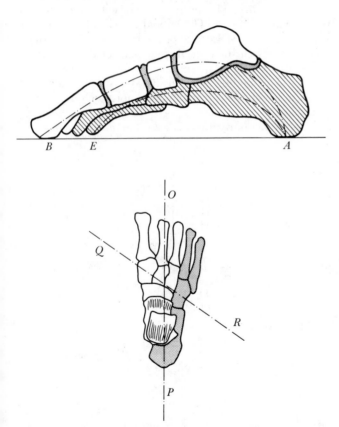

Fig. 6.22 Arches of the foot, AB, medial longitudinal; AE, lateral longitudinal; BE, anterior transverse; OP, longitudinal axis; QR, transverse axis.

The biomechanics of the ankle joint cannot be discussed without reference to the foot. The structural arrangement of the foot as a whole depends on two complex fibrous formations, the superficial and the deep plantar aponeuroses of which the superficial is the more important. It is extremely solid and helps to support the arch of the foot in the standing position.

There are three arches of the foot: two longitudinal (medial and lateral) arches, and a short anterior transverse one (Fig. 6.22). The external arch serves as a support while the internal one serves motion.[12]

The action of these elements of the arches facilitates the foot's complicated biomechanical actions in walking, running, jumping, dancing, and weight carrying. Note that the talus must be included in the plantar arch and may be considered as its key. The talonavicular joint is essentially 'ball and socket' allowing three degrees of rotational freedom while the linked sub-talar joint allows only one type of rotation. In consequence, rotation of the leg about the tibial long axis is converted into rotation of the plantigrade foot (pronation/supination) as the talonavicular joint moves in relation to the calcaneocuboid (Fig. 6.23).

The standing position implies alternate pronation and supination of the foot, with each of the arches stressed in turn. The arches are, however, not functionally isolated as their structure unites them. (The cuboid is partially involved in the structures of the instep, while the lateral side of the vault is linked through the talus with the medial one.) With such an arrangement of the arches, the middle metatarsals support the weight at the moment when the weight shifts from one arch to the other. The middle metatarsals also support the vault anteriorly in those instances in which the calcaneum does not touch the ground, as in tiptoeing or wearing high heels.

Thus in weight-bearing by the plantar vault it is seen that *all* the heads of the

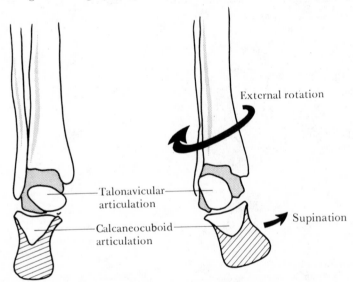

External rotation

Talonavicular articulation

Calcaneocuboid articulation

Supination

Fig. 6.23 The ankle as a torque converter. As the leg externally rotates, the relationship between the talonavicular and calcaneocuboid articulation alters and the foot supinates.

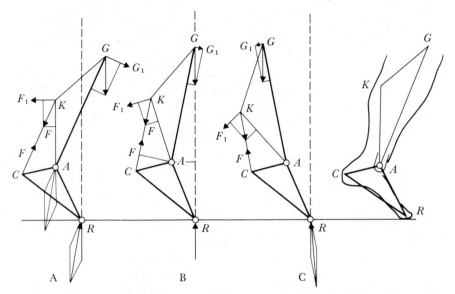

Fig. 6.24 Ankle joint torques (see text). A, In forward propulsion; B, in stable support position; C, in backward falling.

metatarsals become, in turn, points of support.[12] In walking, running, jumping, going downstairs and other 'toe-down' activities, the weight is successively transmitted from the talus to the navicular and then to the metatarsal heads. The posterior pillar of the plantar vault (the calcaneum) provides insertion on the one hand for the triceps surae to counteract gravity, and on the other for the plantar muscles to maintain the foot in the plantigrade position.

Under conditions of passive stabilization of the lower limb, the iliofemoral ligament of the hip joint and the capsule and posterior ligaments of the knee are tense. The projection of the centre of gravity of the body passes a short distance behind the transverse axis of the ankle joint. From this position plantar flexion (involving the lifting of the heels from the ground and the transfer of the point of body support to the metatarsal heads) is possible in three situations:

(1) with the body falling forwards;
(2) the body held upright;
(3) with the body falling backwards.

For the sake of simplicity, plantar flexion is considered to take place by contraction of the triceps surae, and the movement to occur in the saggital plane (Fig. 6.24). Contraction of the triceps surae means application of a force F to the posterior surface of the calcaneum C and of the same force F applied reciprocally to the posterior aspect of the condyles of the femur and to the posterior surface of the tibia and fibula K. The weight force G is applied to the centre of gravity G of the body. For description purposes the other body joints are regarded as stiffened when the ankle joint represents the connection with a single degree of free rotation, of two rigid triangular structures, ARC (the foot) and AKG (the body).

Plantar flexion with forward propulsion of the body is only possible when the projection of the centre of gravity passes in front of the point of support R. At this point two inversely applied torques are acting on the ankle joint, F_1 and G_1. As $G_1 > F_1$, forward rotation of the body takes place.

When the turning moments F_1 and G_1 balance out, the body remains upright, as long as the projection of the centre of gravity G passes through the point of support R. In leaping backwards the situation is more complicated since the foot is still rotating *forward* in relation to the point of support R while the body is rotating *backwards* over the ankle joint. Such a movement can only

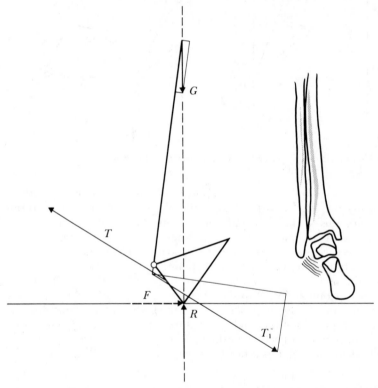

Fig. 6.25 Torques in ankle joint sprain mechanism (see text). G=weight force R=point of support F=force tending to displace heel horizontally T_1 and T=torque and reaction of medial malleolus.

take place therefore when the projection of the centre of gravity falls behind the ankle joint.

This process of torque conversion occurs in the sagittal plane as well. In this case weight bearing in eversion or inversion develops significant torque effects which are compensated by pronation and supination of the foot in the inner range and resisted by the malleoli in the outer (Fig. 6.25).

Stresses in the ankle mortice will therefore depend upon the extent of inversion/eversion of the foot in combination with the degree of tibial rotation, and the mechanisms of injury at the ankle joint are thus apparent.

Twisting

Twisting of the biomechanical system is a complex movement of rotation round two or three axes. In the case of diving for example, the body may rotate round its own transverse axis (the body's own rotation); the body's own axis of rotation may describe a curve round another axis (precession); and finally the angle between these axes (of the body's own rotation and of precession) may vary (nutation—or oscillation).

The biomechanical system may twist in two ways:

(1) with modification of the kinetic moment;
(2) with preservation of the kinetic moment.

Modification of the kinetic moment of the system requires the action of an external force. Such a force may be the weight force, the resistance force of the environment, or another man's muscular force. Modification of the kinetic moment is most frequently encountered in twisting when supported, as for example in gymnastics on the horizontal bar.

Twisting (or modification of the angular speed of rotation of the system) with preservation of the kinetic moment is based on the law of preservation of the kinetic moment: '*If the sum of the moments of the external forces which act upon an isolated body is zero, the kinetic moment of the body remains unchanged.*'

In the case of biomechanical systems, two modes of application of this law exist:

(1) If the moment of an external force is applied to the body, then for a constant moment of inertia (I) the body's angular speed is modified.
(2) If the body reduces the moment of inertia (I), the angular speed increases proportionally.

In the case of preliminary rotation, that is when the kinetic moment is not equal to zero, modification of inertia takes place through variation in the radius of inertia. For example, by folding the arms and legs during dives, the moment of inertia of the body is reduced and the speed of initial rotation increases— unfolding produces an opposite effect.

In the absence of support, folding and unfolding are always preparatory movements. Examples of preparatory movements are rotation of the body and flexion of the trunk. These are due to the inertial forces of the system, i.e. the muscular forces. Rotation of the limbs and flexion of the trunk are likely to produce essential modifications of the orientation of the body as a whole which may exceed 360°.

Angular acceleration of the link or of the system as a whole depends on the relation between the moment of the external forces which are acting upon it and the system's own moment of inertia in relation to the axis of rotation. Accordingly, in creating angular acceleration it is possible to use variations in the moment of external forces or in the moment of inertia or both simultaneously.

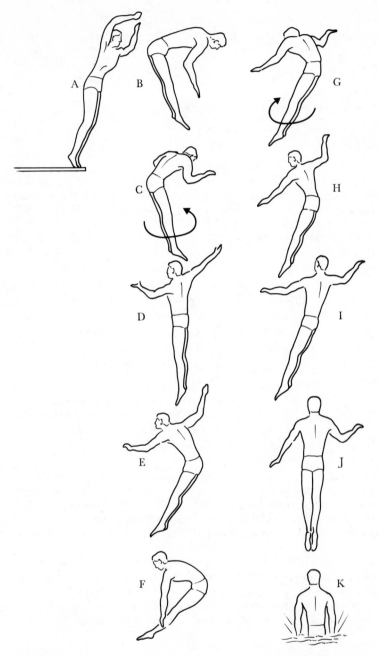

Fig. 6.26 Example of spring-board jumping with complex twisting (after Donskoi[1]) (see text).

Examples of twisting without support

This type of twisting is used by the cat or rabbit when dropped with its back to the floor. The body pikes and, using the extended lower segment of the body to get some action/reaction, the upper segment twists. This body segment is then fixed, and the lower segment again by action/reaction completes the half-twist as the body extends. As long as these actions are repeated the body will continue to twist.[13]

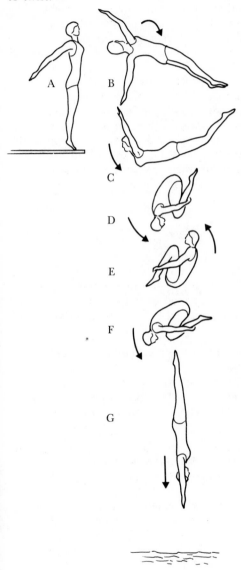

Fig. 6.27 Example of reverse one-and-a-half somersault with half-twist dive (after Donskoi[1]) (see text).

In jumping from a spring-board, complex twisting (Fig. 6.26) starts by preparatory nutation of the body segments. The body bends forwards (B) and simultaneously turns about its longitudinal axis (C). Subsequently, rotation of the upper and lower segments of the body takes place concomitantly to precession. There follows an inverse nutation, i.e. straightening of the body (D). The kinetic moments of the body segments, which are rotating in the course of such twisting, balance one another reciprocally. There is again nutation, this time concomitantly with the upper and lower segments' own rotation the other way round (E–G). Twisting is completed by straightening of the trunk with unfolding of arms, so that the speed of rotation is reduced by an increase in the moment of inertia (H–J). At the moment of entry the body is in the vertical position with the arms at the sides (K).

In the reverse one-and-a-half somersault with half-twist dive from the spring-board (Fig. 6.27), the body is given initial rotation around the transverse axis and also rotation around the longitudinal axis (B). After completing 180° of rotation around the longitudinal axis, the body is now in a face-downwards position and is still rotating about its transverse axis (C). At this point the body tucks up (D), thus increasing its angular velocity around the transverse axis (E–F). Prior to entry into the water the angular velocity is then decreased by straightening out the body once more (G). In this dive both rotations are taken by action/reaction with the board.

Pendular effects

Running is a cyclic movement, each cycle involving a series of actions and intermediate positions between two identical positions in which the body is resting on the same foot. Each cycle thus consists of two consecutive running steps.

Pendular effects may be more easily understood by considering each period to include three phases. These are delineated by the following four instants (Figs. 6.28 and 6.29):

(1) The instant when the pendular movement begins, the supporting foot being no longer in contact with the ground;
(2) The instant when the leg changes from one direction of rotation to another;
(3) The instant when the thigh changes its direction of rotation;
(4) The instant when the pendular movement ceases, the other foot being brought in contact with the ground.

The pendular movement of the leg is extremely complex, not only because the three links are in simultaneous rotation and translation, but also because it depends on the speeds at the other links of the kinematic chain (and on the external forces and their torques).

In an attempt to outline the principal pendular effects, it must be accepted *a priori* that pendular motion is an indispensable and useful component of running:

(1) By its contribution to increasing the speed of the centre of gravity of the body;
(2) by a redistribution of speeds at the other links of the kinematic chain.

The relative position of the links with the foot at the instant of impulsion depends on the running speed, the anatomical properties of the runner, the power of certain muscle groups, the mobility of the joints, and many other factors. This makes it difficult to delineate the phases of pendular motion using the foot as a reference point.

However, in the case of a fixed landmark such as the hip joint, the swinging phases are well marked and are characterized as follows:

1–2. The *first phase* begins with flexing of the hip thus bringing the thigh forwards from its maximally posterior (extended) position, as, simultaneously, the lower leg is rotated (flexed) backwards. This produces a 'whipping' effect that causes the knee to flex more rapidly and thus, rotation of the leg backwards results in raising the centre of gravity of the swinging foot. The acceleration of the links summate algebraically.

2–3. The *second phase* begins when the leg alters its direction of rotation while the thigh is still in rotation forwards. At the onset of this phase the centre of gravity of the foot is situated at the shortest distance from the reference point at the hip joint. Initially, acceleration of the ankle joint is zero but it then increases due to change in the moment of inertia and to the action of the thigh flexors.

The second phase ends when the thigh is in its highest anterior position, at which point the acceleration at the knee becomes zero. The leg is meanwhile continuing its rotation forwards. The centre of gravity of the foot which is in pendular motion moves away from the axis of rotation of the hip joint.

3–4. The *third phase* of pendular motion begins with a change in the direction of rotation of the thigh. Angular acceleration increases such that it appears that the leg itself has changed its direction of rotation.

This phase ends when the foot is again in contact with the ground but the foot may, before it is grounded, be in plantar flexion. The centre of gravity of the foot in pendular motion quickly moves away from the axis of rotation of the hip joint modifying the moment of inertia of the kinematic chain. Whether the foot or heel is first grounded depends upon the algebraic sum of the foot acceleration.

4. Across the phases of the pendular period rapid changes of speed of the foot segments occur. These changes are transmitted to the whole biomechanical system and especially to the support foot. Slowing down of speed produces acceleration in the support foot and vice versa.

Long leg carriage in middle-distance runners

The pendular period in middle-distance running differs from that seen in sprinting in respect of duration, general amplitude, and relative position of the links at the moments of change from one to the next phase of the pendular motion. Thus, the duration of the period of pendular motion as compared to that of grounding is about 2·15 : 1. Rotation in the hip joint is at an angle of about 95–100°.

Pendular movement of the foot may show very different positions of the links in the trailing leg across the four instants of pendular oscillation. These positions depend on many factors, such as relative lengths of the body segments, the

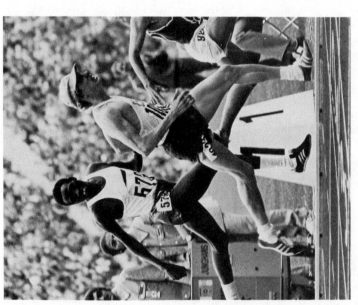

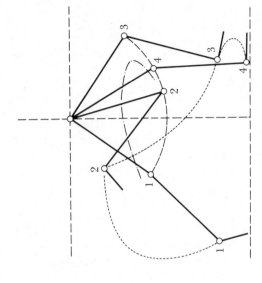

Fig. 6.28(a) Example of pendular motion in middle-distance running.—Wortle. (Photo: E. D. Lacey.)

(a)

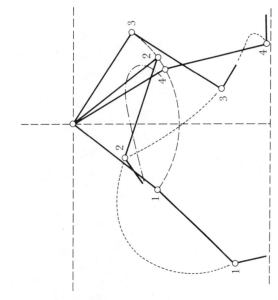

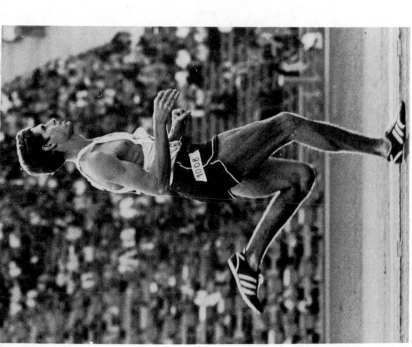

(b)

Fig. 6.28(b) Example of pendular motion in middle-distance running.—Ryun. (Photo: E. D. Lacey.)

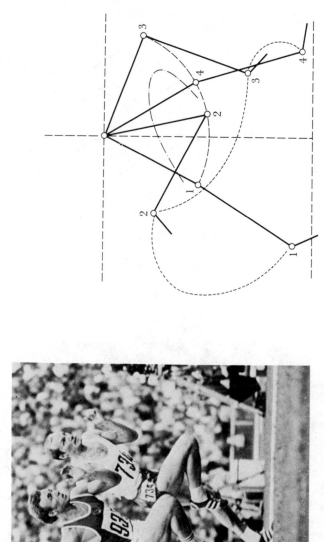

Fig. 6.29(a) Example of pendular motion in sprinters.—Borzov. (Photo: E. D. Lacey.)

(a)

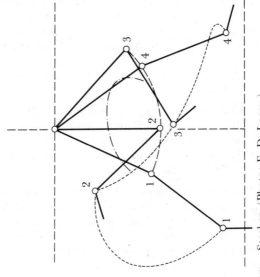

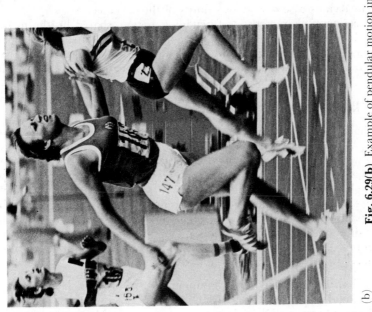

(b)

Fig. 6.29(b) Example of pendular motion in sprinters.—Stecher. (Photo: E. D. Lacey.)

runner's body weight, the forces of the muscles, and mobility of the joints, and often vary even during a single run by the same runner.

No significant correlation has been found between the total or partial amplitude of the pendular motion and the athletic performance. It seems that the amplitude and relative position of the segments of the foot in pendular motion are indirectly related to the running speed through impulsion of the supporting foot.

Figure 6.28 shows the phases of pendular motion in two famous middle-distance runners:

(a) David Wottle—Olympic champion in the 1972 Olympic Games in Munich at 800 m, when he ran 1 min 45·9 sec; and former world record holder of the 800 m with the time 1 min 44·3 sec.
(b) Jim Ryun—former world holder for the 800 m (1 min 44·9 sec) 1500 m (3 min 33·1 sec) and 1 mile (3 min 51·1 sec).

The four instants of pendular motion are obtained by graphical analysis of kinograms. The films are taken from the side, and the O, X, Y reference plane is the hip joint. The pendular motion is considered to take place in a plane parallel to the running plane and not in several planes. (The oscillations of the trunk in the sagittal plane are negligible and the movements of the hip joint are therefore regarded as pure rotation.)

It is at the second instant of pendular motion of the foot that the two runners appear to differ most in the way they change the direction of the leg's rotation. For Wottle this instant is located midway through the thigh oscillation, while in Ryun's case it is at two-thirds of this distance.

The common characteristic of pendular motion, shared by the majority of famous international runners, is the long duration of the first phase of pendular movement (mostly through maintenance of the leg at a short distance from the centre of rotation), and small extension of the knee joints in the last phase.

High knee pick-up in sprinters

The characteristic of sprinters is a period of pendular motion, about 1·85 times as long as the set-down. The thigh is raised at an angle of about 90–95°. Compared with long-distance running, pendular motion in sprinting is of shorter duration and the upwards movement of the thigh is of lesser amplitude. Although the angle at which the thigh is raised is less than that in middle-distance runners, the knee pick-up movement is greater in sprinters because when pendular motion starts, the angle between the thigh and the vertical is less than in middle-distance runners.

Figure 6.29 shows the phases of pendular motion in two world-famous sprinters:

(a) Valerii Borzov—Olympic champion in 1972 in Munich at 100 m in 10·1 sec, and at 200 m in 20·0 (19·99) sec.
(b) Renate Stecher—Olympic champion in 1972 in Munich at 100 m in 11·07 sec, and at 200 m in 22·4 sec; world record holder at 100 m run in 10·8 sec, and at 200 m in 22·1 sec.

The *first phase* is characterized by angular acceleration which is higher at the leg than at the thigh. At the instant of zero acceleration of the leg, the position of the thigh is scarcely beyond the vertical and the thigh is not even halfway through the angle of rotation. The *second phase* characteristic of sprinters ends with a knee pick-up movement of relatively great amplitude, accentuated by a more marked inclination of the trunk than in middle-distance runners. The *third phase* of pendular motion is characterized by a relatively great angle of rotation of the thigh (preparatory movement).

Significance of biomechanics to understanding the mechanism of injury

Athletic performances today draw nearer and nearer to physiological limits and to the maximal human capacity for adaptation to effort. Besides contributing greatly to an understanding of the best way in which mechanical energy can be applied to an objective, biomechanics provides insight into the mechanisms of sports accidents. These have first to be clarified before it is possible (a) to prevent injury, and (b) restore functional integrity.

The body's levers are known to transmit forces and motion at a distance but they also favour injuries (for example, sprains and fractures) by amplifying the external forces (and occasionally also the internal forces) acting in the biomechanical system.

Statistics of the frequency of injuries to the various segments of the body vary from one sport to another. It is difficult to discern any common biomechanical factors in the large number of groups classified on criteria such as age, sport, site, and aetiology. Statistical information is still lacking which could relate site of injury to the transmission and interaction of external forces upon the joints and segments of the body through the various lever mechanisms. It does appear, however, that injuries due to excessive stress appear especially on the short arm of first-class levers.

For example, the mechanism of disruption of the medial collateral ligament of the knee consists most frequently in the overstressing of the valgus knee. In extension the point of application of the external force (in this instance the body weight acts as an external force) is situated at a distance from the fulcrum several times that between the fulcrum and the ligament.

Dobosin and co-workers[14] describe how in the mechanism of disruption of the anterior cruciate ligament, internal rotation of the femur with the knee slightly bent produces a relaxation of the cruciate ligaments as they untwist. With forced external rotation of the femur the cruciate ligaments become tense again and the anterior cruciate ligament, being weaker than the posterior, gives way. As twisting of the knee also disrupts the meniscus this explains the coincidence of the two lesions.

Like the knee sprain, the ankle sprain produces various degrees of damage, according to which ligament is stretched, or partially or totally torn. The commonest of all forms of tarsotibial sprain is produced by twisting the leg when in varus, which leads to injury of the talofibular bundle of the lateral ligament. This is also an instance of a class one lever amplifying by five or six times the external force to a level above the limit of resistance of the ligaments or bones.

Diagnosis can be more easily and accurately made if the mechanism of production of the injury is understood. Biomechanics plays an important part in elucidating the mechanism of the injuries and thus in their prevention and management.

A. D.
A. G.
A. McC.

Physique

The Oxford English Dictionary defines 'Physique' as

'The physical or bodily structure, organization and development; the characteristic appearance or physical power of an individual or a race.'

During the early 'twenties Ernst Kretschmer published *Korperbau und Charakter*[15] which was destined to exert a profound and lasting influence on clinical medicine and anthropology. The theme was derived from the then new classification of mental disease into 'endogenous' and 'exogenous' proposed by Emil Kraepelin (1856–1926). The two main forms of 'endogenous' psychoses, schizophrenia and manic-depressive madness are, as Kraepelin pointed out, genetically determined. This places them apart from 'exogenous' psychoses, chief among which are those caused by infections (such as syphilis), toxins (such as alcohol and drugs), brain disease (such as tumours and degenerative processes), and injuries.

Kretschmer's key observation was that 'schizophrenic' patients were usually lean, while 'manic-depressive' patients were stout. The question was whether the linkage between 'physique and character' revealed by the different bodily design of the two groups of patients was but a special instance, or a general law that applied to the human species as a whole.

The first edition of Kretschmer's book begins with the well known passage from Shakespeare's *Julius Caesar*:

Caes: Let me have men about me that are fat;
      Sleek-headed men and such as sleep o' nights;
      Yon Cassius has a lean and hungry look;
      He thinks too much: such men are dangerous.

A central feature of Kretschmer's book was that it looked upon human physique as individualized composites from three prototypes: 'asthenic', 'athletic', and 'pyknic' (lean, muscular, and round). Over the years Kretschmer identified a variety of psychological, physiological, and pathological variants that corresponded to his bodily prototypes.

Sheldon introduced the term 'somatotyping' for the classification of physiques in 1940 in *The Varieties of Human Physique*.[16] In 1954 he published an atlas of men's physiques.[17] To Kretschmer's prototypes asthenic, athletic, and pyknic, Sheldon gave new names: ectomorph, mesomorph, and endomorph (Fig. 6.30). These names have been accepted in the English and American literature, notwithstanding the serious criticism to which Kretschmer subjected them, namely that Sheldon's nomenclature implied that leanness reflected a dominant influence upon body development of the ectoderm, and that corresponding influences of mesoderm and ectoderm were responsible for the development of muscularity and roundness.

The most original feature of Sheldon's system of somatotyping is the use of his triangular pattern of recording individual physiques (Fig. 6.31). Sheldon also tried to identify 'temperamental scales' which he thought corresponded with somatotypes, but his findings have not been generally accepted. No correlation between the two parameters, somatic and psychosomatic, has as yet been demonstrated with athletes' physiques or with athletic performances.

As a result of Tanner's studies the Sheldon system of somatotyping has been

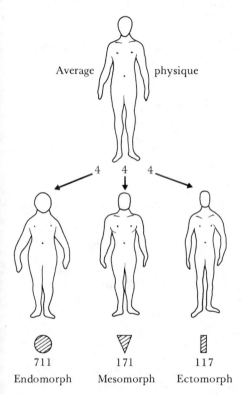

Fig. 6.30 The Sheldon body types.

developed to facilitate the precise assessment of body form, and thus its modifiability through hereditary endowment and extraneous influences, including training. These findings proved of considerable value in the study of problems of sports physiology and sports psychology. Tanner took body measurements from participants at the 1960 Olympic Games in Rome[18] and reported on numbers of athletes he had examined, described the anthropometric methods applied in the study, and presented representative illustrations of the different somatotypes observed. Tanner's studies of the physique of athletes were supplemented by those obtained in earlier investigations by Parnell,[19] and by recent researches

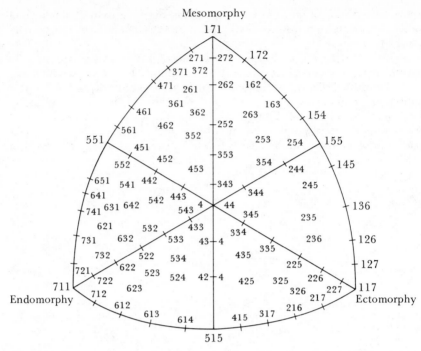

Fig. 6.31 Somatogram showing body types plotted by three-point classification system.

by De Garay and Lindsay Carter[20] who examined participants in the Olympic Games at Mexico City in 1968.

Special insight into the problem of physique and performance was afforded by work on 'body composition', a term introduced by Behnke.[21] Originally, Behnke's studies (1942) were undertaken without reference to 'somatotyping'. During the ensuing years, however, body composition became a subject of major importance for the understanding of physique, and especially its modifiability through sport; also body composition is seen to determine many kinds of athletic performance.

Recently, attention has been directed to the correlation between physical performance in various fields of sporting activity and body type—this is remarkably close. Study of international athletes and games players has shown that the best performers in each event appear to be drawn from a closely circumscribed area on the somatogram (Figure 6.31). Thus, for example, shot putters and discus throwers will be found in the area 361 to 262, and swimmers in the area 543 to 334. The majority of champion sportsmen and women will be found along the meso-ectomorph axis. Except among long-distance swimmers, a high degree of endomorphy is inimical to the achievement of high levels of physical performance. Although there are exceptions (and these are seldom very extreme) there would seem to be a high degree of specificity in suitability of body type for particular forms of physical activity. This specificity is doubly significant. In the first place it means that there must be many athletes and sportsmen taking part in events for which they are physically unsuited and in which therefore they probably cannot aspire to a high level of performance; further a large proportion of the population (some authorities put it as high as 80 per cent) can *never* aspire to any great height in terms of purely physical level of performance. In the second place it means that the technique of champions, upon which are based the standard performance techniques for any event, may be more or less unsuitable for others of different physique in the same events.

It now seems certain that somatotyping could play an important part in the selection of individuals for training in various sports events. Just because an individual has a suitable physique he will not necessarily become a champion or a high-class performer, but persons of unsuitable physique may be directed into some other event for which they are better equipped in terms of body type.

Somatotype is largely determined by genetic factors, that is it would seem to be hereditary and to a great extent immutable. Heredity may well play a part in potential capacity for physical performance in other ways.

Heredity

As yet there have been only a few deliberate attempts to breed humans to bring forward specific physical characteristics, but it is possible that more such attempts may be made, particularly under the aegis of a totalitarian regime. Certainly, breeding is considered to be of extreme importance in racing horses and dogs, and indeed in animal farming generally. Instances of families whose members have all made an impact in various sports are legion, but it is difficult to be sure that this has been due to physical (genetic) rather than environmental factors, and perhaps also a degree of nepotism. Certainly the achievement of high levels of performance in some events and sports, particularly team games, may often be determined by the opportunities available both for coaching and experience rather than by innate ability, and certainly there have been many members of sporting families who have shown no aptitude despite their 'breeding'. Sporting prowess in families may therefore be a psychological sequel of conditioning rather than a physical sequel of the interaction of genetic factors, although of course top-class performance cannot be achieved by the physically unsuitable.

Acceleration of growth, selection of athletes, and adaptation of organ systems

Referring again to the definition of 'physique' as 'The physical or bodily structure, organization and development', three factors of special relevance require consideration:

(1) There has been a continuous growth of maximal performances in sport during the past 100 years. This necessitates consideration of results obtained alongside comparative analysis of patterns of physique, because a conspicuous 'acceleration of growth and development' has occurred during the period under review (Fig. 6.32).
(2) There is a tendency to select athletes endowed with physique which facilitates special athletic performances, e.g. tallness for basket-ball playing,

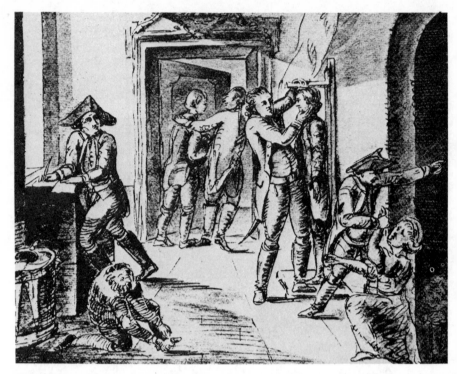

Fig. 6.32 Drawing by Goethe made prior to the turn of the eighteenth-century. The scene depicts examination of military recruits. Body measurements taken at the time are available and can be compared with present data. Youths of 18 measured in Goethe's time were about 3 inches shorter and weighed 30–40 pounds less than they do today.

muscularity for shot putting and discus throwing, or daintiness for gymnastics and long-distance running (Fig. 6.33).

(3) There is evidence that physique is a determinant of performance excellence in sport in terms of adaptation of different organ systems[22] chiefly of: (a) skeletal muscle, (b) heart, (c) bone, (d) liver, (e) body water, and (f) fat.

That Kretschmer's and Sheldon's investigations have been of major relevance in sports medicine is beyond doubt—Kretschmer's in that he was the first to recognize the nature of the threefold prototypical design of physiques as well as of their linkage to 'character'; Sheldon's in that he rendered Kretschmer's concept suitable for statistical evaluation and enumerated a variety of personality parameters amenable to correlation with morphological entities. However, the voluminous literature on 'somatotyping' contains as yet little concerning the assumed interdependence between physique and character on the one hand, and sport and physical education on the other. A conspicuous lack of knowledge about relations between physique, character, and sport stands in sharp contrast to the ample information available on anthropometry of athletes.

As early as 1949 Tanner in an article in the *British Medical Student's Journal*

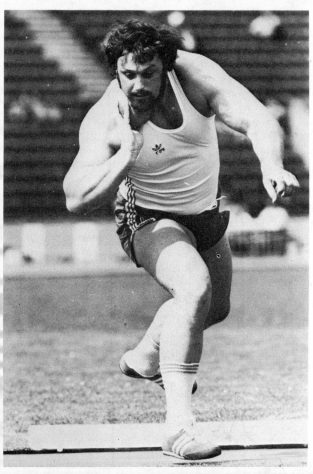

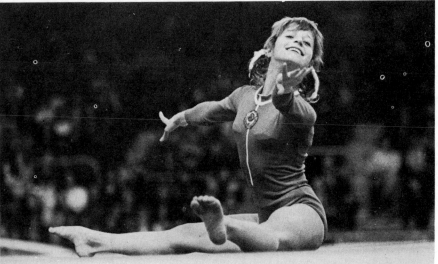

Fig. 6.33 Extremes of body build in champion athletes. (a) The massive bulk of the shot putter Geoff Capes, (b) the elfin grace of the gymnast Olga Korbut. (Photos: E. D. Lacey.)

pointed out that general views on the relation of physique and behaviour are not necessarily reliable. He quoted Francis Galton to the effect that 'general impressions are never to be trusted', and cited Charles Darwin's saying 'I have no faith in anything short of actual measurement' quoted on the cover of a journal founded by Karl Pearson, co-worker of, and successor to, Galton. In respect of the relationship between physique and personality in sport, Tanner pointed out that the juxtaposition of these terms can be studied on the anatomical, physiological, psychological, and sociological levels. What measurements, he asked, at the morphological level of personality link up with, and are translatable to, personality? What measurements at other levels of personality are thus translatable? Can measures of physique be devised which will be related to measures of intelligence, or of instinct, or of blood constituents, or what else?

Tanner's questions raised 25 years ago have remained unanswered. Many descriptive accounts of somatotypes of athletes have been presented since then, but their supposed psychological and sociological correlates have not been demonstrated. The validity of the latter statement is detailed[23] in Kane's *Psychological Aspects of Physical Education and Sport*, which contains a chapter of

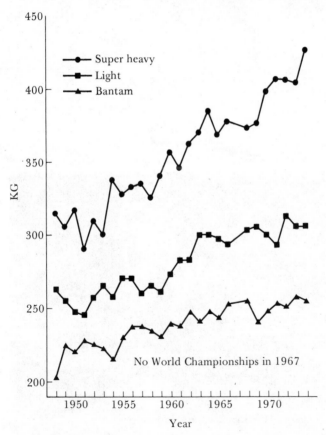

Fig. 6.34 Weight lifting, World Championships' results 1948–74.

'Personality, Body Concept, and Performance'. Kane refers to psychological counterparts of the three 'somatotype-dimensions', endomorphy (fat), meso-morphy (muscle), and ectomorphy (linearity) which, he writes, are 'significantly related to the three Sheldonian temperamental scales, namely viscerotonia (relaxed), somatotonia (energetic) and cerebrotonia (detached). This statement, however, is justified only as a general statistical pronouncement: it is of no relevance to sports psychology as such. The issue of somatotype and personality in relation to sport remains unexplored. Sheldon's 'temperamental scales' were not evaluated in terms of variants of physique and performance of athletes.

Major personality changes must have accompanied the sustained performance improvements that have occurred in all sports since the beginning of this century. The latter process is well documented through growth curves of world records. Figure 6.34 shows weight lifting world records since 1948 for three body weight classes, bantam-, light-, and super heavy-weight. The data are of relevance since the curves for the bantam- and light-weight classes apply to athletes of like body weights throughout, reflecting the participation during recent years of athletes of exceptional physique.

Assuming a definable interrelation between physique and personality along lines such as those discussed in Kane's book, it would be interesting to know what changes have taken place in the bantam- and light-weight champions between the years 1948 and 1974. The weight lifter who became world champion in the bantam-class in 1948 with an aggregate of 202·5 kg may have been been a different personality from the competitor who won the same event in 1974 with an aggregate of 255 kg. Even more puzzling would be the same question in as far as it pertains to the world champion in the super heavy-weight class, who in 1948 won with a total lift of 215 kg, as compared with the champion in the 1974, who won with a total lift of 425 kg.

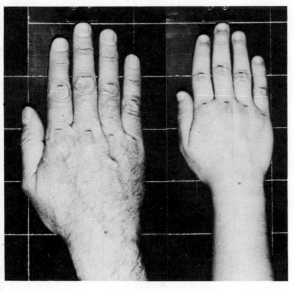

Fig. 6.35 The hands shown above belong to two equally outstanding pianists.

There is no information whatever about this issue. Evidence is available concerning cause-and-effect correlation between physical fitness on the one hand, and modification of personality features in the intellectual, social, and psychological sectors on the other. However, none of the studies under reference contain information on somatotypes of the subjects included in the tests. No conclusion can therefore be drawn from them as to the role of physique as a possible determinant of the personality shifts that took place under the influence of training during these investigations.

A reference must be made to the role played by physique in respect of performances of power, in comparison with that of the integrative action of the central nervous system as a determinant of performance of skill. Buytendijk has pointed out that in the design of language and manual tasks (both represent exclusively human capabilities), size, weight, and other morphological attributes are of little importance. Figure 6.35 serves as an example. The hand on the left is that of the German pianist Wilhelm Backhaus, that on the right of the Polish artist Wanda Landowska. Many concert programmes played by these two distinguished artists were the same. Thus in terms of the quoted definition, physique in its diverse manifestations reflects bodily power but does not (or not necessarily) correlate with variants of skill and character.

E.J.

References

1. Donskoi, D. (1973) *Biomechanica bazele Technicii Sportive*. Bucharest: Stadion.
2. Lloyd, B. B. and Morgan, P. T. (1966) Analogue computer simulation of the equation of motion of a runner. *J. Physiol.*, **186**, 18.
3. Fidelus, K. (1974) *Propozycje Jednolitego Pomiaru Obciazenia Treningowego*. Warsaw: Sport Wyczynowy.
4. Hultman, E., Bergström, I. and McLennan-Anderson, N. (1967) Breakdown and resynthesis of phosphoryl-creatine and adenosine triphosphate in connection with muscular work in man. *Scand. J. clin. Lab. Invest.*, **19**, 55.
5. Demeter, A., Gagea, A. and Iliescu, A. (1974) Relatia forta-viteza in atletism. *Rev. Ed. Fiz. si Sport*, **1.**
6. Hochmuth, G. (1967) *Biomechanik Sportlicher Bewegungen*. Frankfurth am Main: Wilhelm Limpert-Verlag Gmbh.
7. Williams, M. and Lissner, H. (1972) *Biomechanics of Human Motion*. Philadelphia: W. B. Saunders.
8. Borelli (1608–79) *De motu animalium*.
9. Braune, W. and Fischer, O. (1889) Über den Schwerpunkt des Menschlichen Körpers mit Sicht auf die Ausrüstung des Deutschen Infantelisten. *Abh. sächs Akad. Wiss.*, **15**, 11.
10. Dempster, W. (1955) Space requirements of a seated operator. *W.A.D.C. Technical Report*, **55**, 159.
11. Jones, R. L. (1941) The human foot; an experimental study of its mechanics and the role of its muscles and its ligaments in the support of the arch. *Am. J. Anat.*, **68**, 1.
12. Baciu, C. (1967) *Anatomia Fonctionala a Aparatului Locomotor*. Bucharest: National Centre for Physical Education and Sport.
13. Dyson, G. H. G. (1973) *Mechanics of Athletics*, 6th Edn. London: University of London Press.

14. Dobosin, C., Baciu, C. and Tomescu, D. (1958) *Traumatologia Sportiva*. Bucharest: Tineretului.
15. Kretschmer, E. (1921) *Körperbau und Charakter*. Berlin: Springer Verlag.
16. Sheldon, W. H. (1940) *The Varieties of Human Physique*. New York: Harper Bros.
17. Sheldon, W. H. (1954) *Atlas of Man*. New York: Gramery.
18. Tanner, J. M. (1964) *The Physique of the Olympic Athlete*. London: George Allen and Unwin.
19. Parnell, R. W. (1958) *Behaviour and Physique*. London: Edward Arnold.
20. De Garay, A. and Lindsay Carter, J. E. (1974) *Genetic and Anthropological Studies of Olympic Athletes*. New York: Academic Press.
21. Behnke, A. R. and Wilmore, J. H. (1974) *Evaluation and Regulation of Body Build and Composition*. Englewood Cliffs, N.J.: Prentice Hall.
22. Jokl, E. (1973) Physique and performance. *Am. corrective Ther. J.*, **27**, 4.
23. Kane, J. E. (1972) *Psychological Aspects of Physical Education and Sport*. London: Routledge and Kegan Paul.

7

General medical aspects of sport

However 'Sports Medicine' is defined there is a substantial interface between general internal medicine and sport. Any doctor can, by applying his basic discipline to a sporting context, find immediately a whole new range of interesting clinical challenges and experiences open to him. The demand from sportsmen for advice and help with all aspects of general medical care and preparation is insatiable, and the response of the medical profession has in the past failed almost totally to meet this challenge.

While for most doctors interested in sport, involvement may be confined to individual patients or small groups of sportsmen, a number of doctors find themselves involved with clubs or area organizations in sport and a privileged few with the governing bodies of sport themselves. It is important to emphasize the co-operation which should exist between the general physician looking after sportsmen and the team physician involved in the more limited context of the occasional championship situation away from home. Major championships should be the focal point of a carefully planned programme of medical and technical surveillance of a team or squad, and the problems of the team in the championship situation cannot be dissociated from the basic problems between major championships. The prime function of the team physician will be in caring for his sportsmen from year to year on a 'constant surveillance' basis, with episodes of specialized preparation for specific major events. The team physician should be able to co-operate closely with his team's manager and coaches.

General screening

The physician will aim to screen his sports population—be it club, event or national squad—on a regular basis in order to establish a good clinical relationship of trust at a time when there is least stress; to look for the early prevention and diagnosis of disabilities, and to arrange any necessary treatments; as well as to check on routine procedures such as inoculations (which should never be left to the last minute before major championships because of possible side-effects).

A close relationship should exist with the sportsman's own family doctor so that any clinical activities are clearly specified and co-ordinated between the interested parties involved. While some doctors object to what they regard as external clinical interference with their patients, it is unusual to find such objections when a reasonable degree of courtesy and communication has been shown. In fact, the average doctor should warmly welcome the special interest being taken in his patients by properly qualified doctors looking after specific groups of sportsmen, because of their greater experience in these problems.

While a number of sports medical examination proformas exist, and no doubt each clinician will prefer his own, Fig. 7.1 (see pp. 164–7) represents a typical form used with male track and field athletes. A sports medical examination must include full personal details including both competition and training performances. Similarly, the clinical examination must include both general medical (similar to the routine life assurance) and locomotor examinations with event-specific emphasis. To omit either part would clearly invalidate the whole. During the interview necessary to take a full medical and training history, a useful rapport can be established and the physician can gain valuable insight into the athlete's attitudes, as well as merely into his training loads. Each sport will wish to devise its own specific questions of interest, and the form illustrated is one derived by trial and error for one particular situation only. Such factors as sleep or travel problems, undue difficulties in acclimatization to heat or altitude on past occasions, and the question of regular medication will clearly be of major importance should the physician find the athlete in his team on a future occasion. Adverse effects on team efficiency and morale can be prevented by judicious handling at this stage. It is especially important that the physician should know of such problems as epilepsy, asthma or major allergy not only because of the possibility of acute disabling episodes which may occur under stress, but also because of the question of drug therapy in relation to the statutory doping control requirements. Any necessary changes in essential maintenance or emergency therapy can be made under optimum conditions allowing the possibility of a spell of trial and error in advance of a crisis situation so that the athlete is not caught unawares at a major competition.

Inoculations

Today's top sportsmen are liable to travel considerably to compete, often at short notice. It is therefore absurd to leave any foreseeable inoculation requirements until the last minute. While most sportsmen will have had diphtheria, pertussis, and tetanus inoculation together with polio oral vaccine in childhood, and a number will have had primary smallpox vaccination, this may not be certain. If there is any doubt, arrangements should be made for further inoculation. The ideal time to do this is in the off-season when there is no impending competition. Many sports arrange that on admission to a major training or national squad, the sportsman is brought fully up-to-date with protective inoculations. Where smallpox is not a mandatory vaccination the requirement for it is liable to fluctuate rapidly, and the variation in different countries' requirements is so great that it is obviously simpler to vaccinate routinely any sportsmen liable to travel internationally. Though medical opinion may be divided on the effectiveness of the TAB and cholera inoculation, the globe-trotting sportsman certainly has nothing to lose from this procedure and disability is usually minimized if the two injections are given intradermally rather than subcutaneously. Yellow Fever inoculation is a statutory requirement only in a limited range of tropical countries, but with the strong emergence of the tropical African and American nations in sport, an increasing number of European sportsmen will be likely to require this protection as well. However, the most important of all the inoculations are the oral polio and the tetanus toxoid. As avoidable sports deaths are still occurring in all countries in the world because of tetanus in unprotected players, it must be the responsibility of every sports doctor to insist upon this elementary and harmless protection for his sportsmen.

Clinical examination
The routine clinical examination of the sportsman will not vary from any other thoroughly conducted clinical examination. Recent examples in Great Britain of the discovery of gross cardiac valvular disorders may suffice to illustrate both the athlete's capacity to overcome extreme physical disability on occasion, and the personal health services' inability to detect gross pathology through sheer neglect to organize the necessary routine examinations. Clearly the finding of unexpected pathology will require the utmost tact on the part of the sports doctor. His is not the simple role of the insurance medical officer who gives no reason for rejecting a candidate. His is the special relationship of a privileged clinician who stands close to his patient in an area vital to his patient's well-being and interest in life. The closest liaison with the family doctor is necessary in handling such discoveries. It is particularly important that the normal ethical procedures of the profession are followed, because there is nothing more demoralizing to a sports team or governing body than to lose confidence in its technical advisers because of mishandling of important issues.

A problem can often arise in the considerable difference of opinion between doctors involved in the management of, say, an athlete with a cardiac murmur in relation to the amount of activity to be permitted. On the one hand, a traditionally conservative profession tends all too easily to assume that all pathologies are bad pathologies, and to forbid exertion. On the other hand, a patient can usually find an opinion to support a firm defiance of any restriction of activity. As far as the governing body is concerned the final decision in such cases has to rest with its own medical adviser. His decision must be regarded as final by that governing body. It must therefore be based upon a properly appreciated balance of the risks operating in relation to the anticipated stresses in any particular case. It is good clinical conduct to offer the patient more than a mere prohibition of activity. The responsible physician might reasonably offer more detailed advice about alternative occupations and recreations in future.

Gynaecological problems
Gynaecological problems and menstruation, as well as problems of chromosomal sex-testing are covered in Chapter 10.

Clinical tests
In terms of routine monitoring of a squad of athletes, the number of tests to be performed will depend on the resources available as well as the research ideals aspired to! A simple full blood count is essential because many athletes are found to be anaemic, usually due to iron deficiency. A few male sportsmen become iron deficient under heavy training stress, especially if prolonged, and it is probably wise to regard all female athletes in the child-bearing age as iron deficient unless specifically proved otherwise. There are also, of course, the dietary faddists With mixed populations, sickle-cell anaemia may be detected which can occasionally give rise to unexpected clinical difficulties, especially at altitude (including air travel).[1] Routine urinalysis is essential, and if at all possible resting stan-

dard ECG recording should be performed. In cases of abnormality not associated with clinical symptoms, these should be complemented by exercise ECGs, and will serve as a valuable baseline for future reference. Because of the relatively recent recognition of the wide range of changes previously regarded as pathological in fit, high-performance sportsmen, a baseline ECG can be invaluable if subsequent changes are found (see Chapter 8). A routine chest X-ray at reasonable intervals is desirable, certainly in mixed urban populations.

Physiological testing

The particular physiological tests selected for routine examination of sportsmen will depend upon the facilities available and the specific requirements of the sport involved. There has in the past been a tendency to collect information without clear purpose, and on general principles the range of tests performed should be confined to those specifically relating to the athlete's present or potential requirements, including those yielding data which might be directly used in guiding the lines of future training programmes. These are fully covered in Chapters 2 and 4 (Physiology and Training).

Long-term studies of an athletic population are invaluable as indicators of the benefits of exercise, and it is unfortunate that Britain has for long lagged behind certain countries, especially those of Eastern Europe, in recording clinical and physiological data of athletes in longitudinal studies. Even now, little is known about the long-term sequelae of intensive exercise, and a number of the age and distance limits imposed by the rules seem to be a little artificial. If a marathon has been run by a 6-year-old in 4 h 27 m and by a 53-year-old woman in 4 h 45 min, perhaps there is considerable scope for further long-term studies of defined athletic populations![3]

Infections

Of paramount importance is the detection of infection in athletes. The time-honoured writings of past authorities pointing to focal sepsis as a cause for poor performance[3] may seem strange to many of today's medical graduates, but the finding of a chronic low grade tonsillitis or (often) of dental sepsis may explain poor form in a sportsman and be speedily rectified by appropriate treatment. As the dental health of the Western European nations is generally poor, there is clearly little chance of finding no need for active dentistry in an athletic population, and the reader is encouraged both to look for dental decay, and to read Chapter 20 for further guidance.

Of more immediate importance is the question of intensive exertion and competition during infection. Though overt bacterial infections and tuberculosis may be uncommon in Western Europe today, it is increasingly appreciated that viral illnesses give rise to considerable morbidity. While it may generally be regarded as safe to continue competition during a mild coryza it must be a golden rule that fever is an absolute contraindication to athletic exertion. This may be justified on two main grounds. Firstly in the case of bacterial infections, for instance tonsillitis or sinusitis, the athlete is not likely to perform adequately with an active septic condition, even if under correct treatment with the appropriate antibiotic. The possibility of venereal infections should here be remembered and extra-genital spread may give rise to gonococcal arthritis, pharyngitis, and endocarditis, one sports death being recorded from the last.[4] Also, Reiter's syndrome may cause diagnostic confusion if it presents with limited symptoms such as pubic symphysitis, rather than as the classic triad of urethritis (or dysentery), arthritis and conjunctivitis.

Secondly, if there is any doubt whatever about the diagnosis, it should be remembered that many of the viral illnesses include a myocarditis in their repertoire of infiltrations, and a number of deaths occur each year where there is clear post-mortem evidence of influenzal infection. There is evidence that exertion may actually be harmful in the incubation period of viral illness, for instance during the pre-icteric phase of acute infectious hepatitis,[5] although it has been suggested that exercise may not be harmful during the recovery phase of this condition.[6] Of particular importance is glandular fever (infectious mononucleosis) a condition particularly prevalent in the young and in communities such as students. It may be insidious in onset and because of its chronicity and the side-effect of depression it may give rise to particularly prolonged disability. Its low grade hepatitis may cause protracted alcohol and effort intolerance, and the myocarditis may cause considerable effort dyspnoea.

It should also be borne in mind that the depression so commonly found associated with viral infections will be especially undermining to an athlete with his constant restlessness to get back into heavy training.

There is, to date, no clear evidence of any adverse or advantageous effects of exercise on the body's immunological systems.[7] While there are many accounts of the epidemic spread of infections in sporting groups, these have not been accompanied by antibody studies, and may reflect simply the ease with which infections spread in closed community groups. While sportsmen as a group have no increased immunity to infection, it should be remembered that exercise may sometimes be harmful, for instance in the prodromal phase of poliomyelitis when it increases the risk of subsequent paralysis.[8]

Hazards of exercise

Having mentioned the dangers of exertion during viral infection, it is necessary to consider briefly the causes of death in sport. Most reported studies have shown that in all sports a high proportion of the deaths occurring are due to essentially preventable accidents.[4,9] Among the non-accidental causes, ischemic heart disease, unsuspected pre-existing cardiovascular anomalies such as aberrant cardiac vessels, and infections account for the vast majority of deaths.[4,9–12] While many deaths due to drowning and exposure are preventable by the simplest application of common sense, only a proportion of the cardiovascular deaths may be preventable because they frequently occur in previously fit young individuals. However, a number of these deaths occur in people who, in retrospect, are found to have had symptoms suggestive of myocardial insufficiency, cardiac arrhythmias, or infection. For instance, Prokop[13] has clearly described many of the non-traumatic dangers associated with skiing holidays, especially in the middle-aged and elderly. He points out that a storm at 2000 to 3000 m altitude may increase the resting pulse rate by 20 beats per minute, and the blood pressure by 30 to 40 mmHg. Many subjects arriving for a recreational holiday in the mountains may not be able to make the necessary physiological adjustments easily, especially where there is pre-existing disease. Here again adequate preliminary medical supervision might eliminate many of these illnesses and deaths, particularly those marked increases in disability and death occurring about the third day of altitude exposure.

Cardiovascular disorders

Sportsmen may be classified into three groups, namely: normals; 'normals', but with latent cardiovascular disease; and abnormals. In normal subjects there may be considerable variations from the standard descriptions of normal ECGs found in medical text books (see Chapter 8). In abnormal subjects there are, by definition, findings of abnormal heart sounds or rhythm, hypertension, or symptoms suggestive of cardiovascular disease. While at the present time the role of planned exercise programmes in cardiovascular disease is the subject of much study, there is universal agreement that any exercise programme in non-normals must be closely monitored by physician and physiologist alike. For those who have suffered myocardial infarction there are considerable possibilities for active graded rehabilitation following the pioneer studies of Kavanagh and Shephard[14] bringing post-coronary subjects through a training programme to the completion of the Boston marathon race.

However it is in the second group, the apparently normal with latent abnormality, that perhaps most danger lurks. It may be difficult to justify cardiac catheterization of a symptomless young athlete with an atypical murmur, and it may seem unjustifiably harsh to prohibit activity in a patient with symptoms perhaps suggestive of angina without absolute proof of cardiac abnormality on simple tests. It is here that the closest co-operation is necessary between the clinician immediately responsible for the patient and his sporting environment, and the back-up team of cardiologist and exercise physiologist. It should be possible by carefully monitored exercise testing to clarify most cases of doubt, but the practical reality remains that in many situations, such a resolution may be difficult to achieve for administrative or geographical reasons for all but the élite in sport. Nevertheless, a detailed clinical history and examination will often provide a safe basis for realistic advice in a given case. For instance, a female international sportswoman who at the height of her career complained of increasing fatigability in the absence of anaemia was found to have a battery of murmurs consistent with rheumatic valve disease. Her determination to continue her sport at all costs could be more confidently countered when she admitted to increasing nocturnal dyspnoea.

Diagnostic difficulties may arise with transient symptoms such as palpitations or blackout. One youthful sportsman complained only of palpitations at the end of each training session or race on final maximal effort. Clinical examination was normal, but ECG revealed changes of recent anterior myocardial infarction. Dizziness or blackout may suggest transient cardiac arrhythmias, Stokes–Adams attacks, or cerebrovascular insufficiency which may not be associated with positive clinical findings on examination, but the possibility of 'weight lifter's blackout' should be borne in mind in situations involving the Valsalva manœuvre.[15] Here the sudden release of greatly raised intrathoracic pressure causes transient delay in left ventricular refilling and hence a momentary drop in blood pressure and cardiac output. This is essentially a harmless condition, but may well be alarming!

Blood doping
Experimental re-transfusion of subjects with their own red cells after an interval of four weeks[16] was thought to give improved performance, but this has subsequently been denied by further studies.[17] In view of the dangers inherent in the whole process of blood transfusion, it is unlikely that further developments can be expected.

Respiratory system
Reference has been made to active infection and this includes bronchitis and respiratory tract infection from any cause. While active tuberculosis is a contra-indication to vigorous sporting activity, this condition, once fully treated, is consistent with normal life. Smoking constitutes a real hazard to health with very considerable evidence accumulating for a causal relationship between smoking and bronchitis, carcinoma of the bronchus, and atheromatous vascular degeneration. Of immediate practical importance to the athlete is that the products of cigarette combustion bind haemoglobin and therefore impair maximum potential ventilatory function.

Asthma
Many successful sportsmen suffer from asthma of varying degree, and it has been shown that while exercise can induce bronchospasm in some subjects, not all sports activities do so to an equal degree. Thus Fitch and Morton[18] showed that running and cycling produced exercise-induced asthma in twice as many asthmatic subjects as did swimming tests. This suggested that swimming might be a preferred exercise for asthmatics, but paradoxically a number of asthmatics gain *relief* from their bronchospasm by exercise, especially if running or cycling regularly! Disodium cromoglycate and salbutamol are effective in relieving bronchospasm in exercising subjects, but a major problem for the asthmatic high-performance sportsman is that many of the drugs usually used to control bronchospasm fall within the prohibited categories at international games. There is therefore considerable reason to identify asthmatic subjects early and manipulate possible changes of treatment well in advance of the acute and dramatic situations associated with major games. Unfortunately, some authorities, including the International Olympic Committee, have lacked a little imagination as well as charity in their attitude towards the disabled sportsman in their unduly rigid definitions of prohibited drugs.

Haemoptysis
Occasionally an athlete may cough up a little blood after hard exertion. Clinical and radiological findings are usually normal and the commonest cause is bronchiectasis, which may not otherwise be symptomatic. Any regular or profuse haemoptysis calls for full investigation including bronchoscopy or contrast radiography.

Dyspnoea

In non-asthmatic subjects, dyspnoea may be immediately related to effort, or may persist for some time afterwards. This often occurs after hard exercise in cold weather, and probably reflects bronchial oedema due to the direct effect of unwarmed air on the bronchial mucosa. Clinical examination is usually normal, the symptoms closely related to effort, and the athlete can be firmly reassured.

Alimentary system

Traveller's diarrhoea is discussed in Chapter 9. Many athletes are worried by constipation though this more often represents a preoccupation with their body systems and an ignorance of the range of normal bowel functions. The commonest cause in the active sportsman is simple dehydration and many sportsmen, having no idea of how much fluid they lose in their training environment, never compensate adequately with fluid intake.

'Stitch' is often ascribed to gastrointestinal causes, especially unwise eating habits such as taking a substantial meal shortly before vigorous exertion. This is certainly one cause, where the remedy is obvious. Some athletes suffer 'stitch-like' symptoms of abdominal discomfort which are relieved by any of the standard alimentary antispasmodics. However, the majority of cases of 'stitch' are not clearly defined, do not necessarily recur to any troublesome degree, and respond so well to determined abdominal muscle exercises as to suggest that in this group the cause is a functional weakness of the external abdominal musculature.

Diabetes mellitus need not stop activity, though clearly the disadvantages of a fluctuating blood sugar level, especially in an unstable diabetic, may suggest that some forms of activity are more suitable than others. Short duration events allow for more adequate pauses for adjustment of therapy or food intake as well as avoiding the risks of hypoglycaemia associated with prolonged activity. Adequate food intake should be secured before training or competitive activities to minimize the risk of sudden hypoglycaemia, and in any case sugar or chocolate should be readily available at the point of activity in case the athlete becomes hypoglycaemic. The symptoms will be well recognized by the experienced diabetic, but include difficulties in focusing, a feeling of hotness and tiredness, perhaps mental confusion or a lack of co-ordination in movement, and failing concentration. It is important that the sportsman's colleagues should be aware of his condition so that they may be able to come to his aid on occasion. They should also be aware that in any situation where the diabetic becomes acutely confused or even comatose the prompt application of sugar is required. In diabetic coma, no catastrophe will result from this, but in hypoglycaemia obvious improvement will be secured and further damage avoided. Fifteen or twenty minutes rest should be allowed for a diabetic on his recovery from a hypoglycaemic state. Headache may follow, which may further embarrass concentration and skill. While diabetes may be a serious and difficult impediment, the intelligent diabetic can, by fully understanding and controlling his own condition, lead a near-normal life.

Though diet is fully discussed in Chapter 11, brief mention may here be made of alcohol. While this has in the past been widely used as a sedative, e.g. in modern pentathlon pistol shooting events, it is not likely to be of much benefit to any endurance athlete prior to or during the event, because the peripheral vasodilatation may interfere with the sweat and heat loss mechanism. Further, any excess intake will clearly impair motivation and concentration over a prolonged period. Deliberate alcohol intake before aggressive team games could be regarded as doping by intent, and is probably unlikely to help skill.

The use of other dietary supplements is discussed elsewhere. It is, however, fair to say that although there are clear indications for dietary supplementation and for special arrangements during defined events such as marathon running and in hot climates, the doctor is more often consulted about quite extraordinary degrees of dietary faddism. The majority of dietary supplements taken in sport are totally unjustifiable, unnecessary, and expensive. There is little evidence that for the average sportsman more than an average diet is required.[19, 20]

Renal system

In normal high performance sport there are three major problems associated with renal function—dehydration, traumatic haemoglobinuria, and athletic pseudonephritis.

Dehydration

In a recent review, Costill[21] has described the considerable losses of up to 21 per cent of plasma water sustained in four hours' running. In a hot environment it is virtually impossible to replace sweat loss during a protracted competitive event. Even so, it is important to try to keep pace with fluid loss and 200 to 300 ml of fluid taken every fifteen minutes are recommended. Absorption of solutions containing more than 2·5 g glucose/100 ml of water was found by Costill to be delayed.

It is important to recognize that a small group of athletes may develop a state of chronic dehydration with symptoms of diminished endurance capacity due to increased fatigability, diminished sweating capacity, and an undue increase in body core temperature because of the lowered capacity for heat loss. It is most important to emphasize to these athletes that it is necessary to take several litres of fluid a day, despite a possible lack of thirst. Rough guides to the adequacy of hydration can be obtained by daily weighing or by estimation of urinary output.

Salt supplements

Associated with excessive fluid loss, especially in hot climates, is sodium depletion. While this is rarely a problem in temperate climates and normal exercise situations, this may become a problem of considerable magnitude either in outdoor sport in hot ambient temperatures or in indoor sport such as fencing, where restrictive clothing causes increased sweating. Sodium depletion usually accompanies dehydration and its symptoms consist of headache, thirst, anorexia and nausea, apathy, drowsiness, postural giddiness, and muscular cramps. Ultimately blood pressure falls and peripheral circulatory failure may ensue. Before the advent of slow release medication, the practical problems of avoiding nausea while consuming sufficient salt to combat depletion were almost insuperable, but Clarkson[22] described the successful use of a slow release product (Slow Sodium— Ciba Laboratories) in the English team in the World Cup Football Competition in Mexico in 1970. Ambient temperatures approached 38 °C (100 °F) and it was found that many of the players were unable to maintain fluid and electrolyte balance. Slow Sodium (sodium chloride 600 mg, equivalent to 10 mEq of Na and Cl) was administered in doses of up to 50 tablets in one day or 20 in 10 min without gastrointestinal side-effects. Absorption continued for up to three hours so that it was possible to anticipate sodium and sweat loss occurring during a game.

Haemoglobinuria

Haemoglobinuria following exertion has been ascribed to haemolysis due to direct trauma to circulating erythrocytes in otherwise healthy subjects. This is usually found in healthy young men after walking or running, is only very rarely found in women, and has also been described following the repeated hand trauma involved in karate.[23,24] In this condition there is haemoglobinuria with a red or brown discoloured urine, but there are no red cells present on urine microscopy. The condition tends to disappear if more adequate padding is used, or exertion takes place on softer surfaces.

Athletic 'pseudo-nephritis'

It has long been known that proteinuria occurs after physical exertion,[25] and that protein, casts, and red cells as well as frank haematuria occur in marathon runners.[26] It has been found[27] that under severe exercise conditions a urinary picture identical to that of acute nephritis may be found, and protein, red and white cells, as well as casts may appear. Gross haematuria following exertion may cause considerable alarm. The differential diagnosis from acute nephritis may be difficult but the absence of sepsis, anaemia, or hypertension, together with a normal WBC are helpful. In one of Gardner's[27] cases a sore throat was present, but the subsequent course of the illness, with a normal ASO titre, was felt to have excluded acute nephritis. Recovery in this condition is always rapid and spontaneous provided that effort is avoided. This does, however, raise the question of appropriate advice in the particular case in respect of further severe effort. This condition is not identical with the frank haematuria associated with direct renal trauma as found, for instance, in boxers or rugby forwards—the 'athlete's kidney' of Kleiman.[28] Caution is advised in allowing return to full sports activity after either renal trauma or 'pseudo-nephritis', and investigation is required to establish the diagnosis. Precipitate return to exertion after acute glomerulonephritis is also contraindicated.[29]

Sex

So rich is the mythology of sex in relation to sport that it is difficult to separate facts from some of the historically hallowed dogmas, mostly based on notions of morality and arbitrary discipline. On the assumption that sex is a normal human activity and is here to stay, the athlete and his coach may be counselled along certain common-sense simple lines. It is almost certainly true that more disability is caused by guilt, doubt, and ignorance about sexual functions than by sexual activity itself. It is important that the athlete should understand clearly that there is no evidence to suggest that masturbation, nocturnal emissions (wet dreams), or sexual intercourse have any consistent effect on athletic performance. Individuals, or couples, will determine a normal level of sexual activity for themselves and if this is a normally integrated part of their lives they will not find any difficulties in relation to training and competition. However it should be understood that intensive training may well cause enough fatigue to diminish libido and cause temporary impotence. There is also evidence that in the male tight underclothing, such as the 'jock-strap', depresses spermatogenesis by raising testicular temperature. Provided that all these factors are understood and acknowledged to be rapidly reversible, then no problem need arise in the minds of the individuals concerned. Practical details such as changing the timing of intercourse on occasion may help a couple to cope with particularly intensive spells of training.

There is no evidence whatever to suggest that a sportsman 'looses his edge' by indulging in sexual activity, and there is no logical reason for banning sexual activity before competitive events. On the basis that human beings are, after all, creatures of habit and that deprivation of normal activity may be more harmful than indulgence, the attitude of a team manager who seeks to deny normal behaviour to his team is more a source of wonder than is the attitude of the team wishing merely to indulge their normal way of life! Because the doctor interested in sport is in close contact with a young and sexually active group of people, he will be consulted frequently about matters of sexual technique, performance, contraception, venereal disease and so on. Needless to say, the doctor who applies his own censorious attitudes to such approaches will simply alienate his team. The normal sympathy and understanding given to patients is required in this field no less than in others concerned with sport.

Skin

Certain dermatological conditions come to the attention of the sports doctor. Acne and boils are frequently the source of embarrassment and anxiety, though they rarely indicate any deficiency disease. Attention should be paid to scrupulous bathing or showering, with washing and drying of the skin as well as to regular cleansing of athletic kit to minimize the risk of perpetuation and spread of bacterial skin infections. The merits of treating any particular case of acne will clearly be a case for individual judgement, but the side-effects of antibiotics should be borne in mind in the young athlete striving to exert himself fully.

Fungal infections occur commonly as Athlete's foot (*Tinea pedis*) and Dhobie itch (*Tinea cruris*). These conditions are rampant where there is poor hygiene in communal washing facilities, and particular attention should be paid to careful washing of feet and drying of the interdigital clefts. Athlete's foot may occur as an acute inflammatory condition with a vesicular or pustular eruption with considerable itching, or may present as a chronic condition with slight reddening and scaling of the skin with nail involvement causing undue friability. For the acute condition, withdrawal from sport may be necessary because of the painfully raw feet, and warm potassium permanganate (1 in 8000) foot baths thrice daily, may be given. Thereafter for both Athlete's foot and Dhobie itch Whitfield's ointment is usually satisfactory (salicylic acid, 1 g (3%); benzoic acid, 2 g (6%); and carbowax to 30 g (91%)). Alternative commercial products are available, such as Monphytol (boric acid, 2%; clorbutol, 2%; methyl undecylenate, 5% salicylic acid, 31%; propyl undecylenate, 1%). Many prefer a dusting powder such as Mycil (Chlorphenesin, 1%) powder. A dusting powder may be a useful prophylactic measure for a spell after an acute attack as it should be borne in mind that the fungal infection may persist in the footwear.

Warts may occur as simple warts on any part of the body or as more troublesome plantar warts (verrucae) on pressure areas on the foot. While silver nitrate or podophyllin application may often be successful with these conditions, they may each be particularly persistent and require several attempts at treatment including electrocautery and surgical removal. As these conditions tend to be spread in communal areas such as wet floored changing rooms and swimming baths, it is important that someone with these conditions should not expose untreated skin to such flooring. A firm waterproof dressing over a treated lesion would seem to be the minimum reasonable measure to adopt; further restriction will probably be ignored by the sportsman in any case.

Heat rashes and blisters are common in sport. There is a considerable tendency for the sportsmen under hot and sweaty conditions to form blisters on pressure areas (such as the fingers involved in the gripping of fencing weapons or rackets or the feet in sports shoes). It should be borne in mind that many athletes go straight out to compete or train in brand-new shoes and pay the inevitable penalty of friction blistering. There is no particular reason for or against the wearing of socks in running shoes, and this must be left to individual preference but it would seem wise for the athlete to wear-in new footwear in the normal way. As a prophylactic measure, the direct application of zinc oxide or similar plaster without lint to pressure areas under the shoe may often prevent the appearance of blisters, and the same applies to other sites on the body.

In the event of frank blistering, a most effective way of minimizing the time lost from training and competition is for the blister to be thoroughly cleaned and then de-roofed in sterile manner and left to dry either in the open air, or with the, albeit painful, application of spirit. Zinc oxide or similar plaster without lint is then applied direct to the whole blister area. While this may seem unduly painful, it is a highly effective way of returning rapidly to training, and there is no logic in applying layers of lint, etc. which simply allow the persistence of rubbing between the skin layers and adjacent dressings and shoes. The prophylactic application of surgical spirit to feet is a time-honoured habit which may often be helpful in the prevention of blisters.

Drug rashes and contact dermatitis may occur in sport. Drug rashes may be seen after almost any powerful drug, including Streptotriad tablets taken prophylactically for Travellers' diarrhoea. Prompt withdrawal of any offending drug together with soothing applications such as calamine lotion and an antihistamine to minimise itching may be required.

Pruritis ani is often seen in sportsmen. The irritation and discomfort in the anal region may be exacerbated by scratching and secondary infection. This lesion is usually due to the wearing of tight clothes, and is often associated with a change in training conditions, e.g. hot weather causing an increase in sweating. Treatment consists of scrupulous toilet hygiene, with careful washing and drying of the affected parts followed by the application of one of the hydrocortisone creams or lotions. Rarely, general sedation may be required.

Fig. 7.1 Sports medicine medical examination pro-forma.

Name in full			Date / /
Address			
Date of birth / /		Occupation	
Events			
Best performances			
Marital status S. M. D. W. Ch:			
Name and address of own GP			

Part 1 Outline of training

Number of sessions per week
Type

Runs	Miles per week	Summer	Winter
	Intervals	Summer	Winter
Circuits			
Callisthenics			
Weights	Type of session	Sessions per week	
Other games	Type	Number per week	

Part 2 Past medical history

(a) General

Any previous history of:

Epilepsy	Allergy
Asthma	Migraine
Bronchitis	Anaemia
Hay fever	Glandular fever

Sleep (hours per night)	
Travel	

Acclimatization to:

Heat	Altitude
Any regular medication	

Protective innoculations

Smallpox	19	Cholera	19
DPT	19	YF	19
Polio	19	Others	19

(b) Injuries

A brief history of injury, treatment, time off training, etc.

Part 3 Medical examination

CVS

Pulse (resting)	BP (Lying)	/	
Heart sounds: (i)	Systole	(ii)	Diastole
Arterial walls	Varicose veins		
Fundi. Rt	Fundi Lt		

RS

Auscultation	
Clear	Added sounds (specify)

Abdomen

Liver	Spleen	Kidneys
Scars	Hernial orifices	
Genitalia	Epidermophytosis	

Breasts

Glands

ENT

Teeth: Upper	Lower	Mucosa	Pole/well
Throat	Tonsils removed/clear/inflamed		
Ears	Right	Left	
Wax			
Drums			
Valsalva			

CNS

Reflexes:	Right	Left
B		
S		
T		
K		
A		

Special investigations
Urine. Sugar (Clinistix)   Albumen (Albustix)

If albumen is positive use sulphosalicylic acid test, if still positive full MSU test in laboratory.

Blood. Hb:..........G %. if under 13G% male or 12G% female, send blood for full blood count.

Vitalograph. FVC Litres. FEV 1 sec: Litres.
FEV, 1 sec/FVC%
ECG attach trace.
Chest x-ray. Report:

Part 4 Locomotor system

(a) General

Height.............cm   Weight............kg.

Circumference of chest at nipple level:

Inspiration............................... cm

Expiration .... cm

Expansion .... cm

(b) Joint mobility

Indicate full (F) or limited (L); note particularly difference in range of paired joints.

		Right	Left		
Foot	Hallux MTP				
	Toenails				
	Epidermophytosis				
	Blisters/Corns				
Ankle	Flexion				
	Extension				
	Inversion				
	Eversion				
Knee	Flexion				
	Extension				
Hip	Flexion				
	Extension				
	Abduction				
	Adduction				
	Int: Rotation				
	Ext: Rotation				
Wrist	Flexion				
	Extension				
	Pronation				
	Supination				
	Abduction				
	Adduction				
Elbow	Flexion				
	Extension				
Shoulder	Flexion				
	Extension				
	Abduction				
	Adduction				
	Rotation				
Spine	Flexion	Lumbar	Dorsal	Cervical	
	Extension				
	Lat: Flexion (R)				
	Lat: Flexion (L)				
	Rotation (R)				
	Rotation (L)				

(c) Event specific examination (e.g. TA's in runners. Arm in throwers).

Part 5 Conclusions of medical examination

(a) Certification

FIT
UNFIT TEMPORARILY ⎱ FOR INTERNATIONAL COMPETITION
UNFIT PERMANENTLY ⎰

In the event of TEMPORARY UNFITNESS state here the date when full fitness is regained:

Signature of Medical Examiner
(Name in Block Capitals)

(b) Notification
To Athlete's own GP Date   /   /   Initials

To Governing Body   Date   /   /   Initials

(c) Follow up endorsements
19. Certificate of fitness received   Date   /   /   Initials
     Notified to Governing Body   Date   /   /   Initials
19. Certificate of fitness received   Date   /   /   Initials
     Notified to Governing Body   Date   /   /   Initials
19. Certificate of fitness received   Date   /   /   Initials
     Notified to Governing Body   Date   /   /   Initials

Hygiene

It will be noted that questions of personal as well as corporate hygiene are of considerable importance in sport. It is, after all, in the athlete's own interests to keep himself healthy and free from preventable diseases. It cannot help an athlete to impair his respiratory capacity by smoking. Attention to personal hygiene with adequate washing and drying are important in the prevention of skin disorders which can spread rapidly through communal changing facilities, and associated with this should be scrupulous attention to athletic clothing. A further responsibility rests on the shoulders of organizers of sports facilities to ensure that the maximum available precautions are taken in the arrangement of changing facilities with ample provision for washing and showering as well as regular attention to the cleaning of floor surfaces with regular disinfection.

P.N.S.

References

1. Green, R. L., Huntsman, E. G. and Serjeant, G. R. (1971) The sickle cell and altitude. *Br. Med. J.*, **iv**, 593.
2. Temple, C. (1973) In *Athletics Weekly*,, Feb. 3.
3. Abrahams, A. (1961) *The Disabilities and Injuries of Sport*. London: Elek.
4. Izeki, T. (1973) Statistical observation on sudden deaths in sport. In Proceedings XVIII world congress of sports medicine. *Br. J. sports Med.*, **7**, 172.
5. Krikler, D. M. and Zilberg, B. (1966) Activity and Hepatitis, *Lancet*, **ii**, 1046.
6. Repsher, L. H. and Freebern, R. K. (1969) Effects of early and vigorous exercise on recovery from infectious hepatitis. *New Eng. J. Med.*, **281**, 1383.
7. Jokl, E. (1974) The immunological status of athletes. *J. sports Med. phys. Fitness*, **14**, 165.
8. Russell, W. R. (1947) Poliomyelitis, the preparalytic state, and the effect of physical activity on the severity of the paralysis. *Br. med. J.*, **2**, 1023.
9. Moncur, J. A. (1973) A study of fatalities during sport in Scotland. In Proceedings XVIII World Congress of Sports Medicine, *Br. J. sports Med.*, **7**, 162.
10. Jokl, E. (1971) *Exercise and Cardiac Death*. London: University Park Press.
11. Jokl, E. (1958) *The Clinical Physiology of Physical Fitness and Rehabilitation*. Springfield, Ill.: Charles C Thomas.
12. Opie, L. H. (1975) Sudden death and sport. *Lancet*, **i**, 263.
13. Prokop, L. (1972) Non-traumatic incidents during Skiing *In Proceedings International Congress of Winter Sports Medicine*. Sapporo: Organising Committee of International Congress of Winter Sports Medicine.
14. Kavanagh, T. and Shephard, R. J. (1973) The importance of physical activity in post-coronary rehabilitation—a special review. *Ann. phys. Med.*, **52**, 304.
15. Compton, D., Hill, P. M. and Sinclair, P. D. (1973) Weight-lifters' blackout. *Lancet*, **ii**, 1237.
16. Ekblom, B., Goldberg, A. N. and Gallbring, B. (1972) Response to exercise after blood loss and infusion. *J. appl. Physiol.*, **33**, 175.
17. Williams, M. H., Goodwin, A. R., Perkins, R. and Bocrie, J. (1973) Effect of reinjection upon endurance capacity and heart rate. *Med. Sci. Sports*, **5**, 181.
18. Fitch, K. D. and Morton, A. R. (1971) Specificity of exercise in exercise-induced asthma. *Br. med. J.*, **iv**, 577.
19. Anonymous (1970) Diet and athletics. *Br. med. J.*, **iii**, 361.
20. Williams, J. G. P. (1968) Nutrition and sport. *Practitioner*, **201**, 324.
21. Costill, D. (1974) Muscular exhaustion during distance running. *Physn and Sports-Med*. 2:36
22. Clarkson, E. M., Curtis, J. R., Jewkes, R. J., Jones, B. E., Luck, V. A., de Warderer, H. E. and Phillips, N. (1971) Slow Sodium: an oral slowly released sodium chloride preparation. *Br. med. J.*, **iii**, 604.
23. Spicer, A. J. (1970) Studies on march haemoglobinuria. *Br. med. J.*, **i**, 155.
24. Streeton, J. A. (1967) Traumatic haemaglobinuria caused by karate exercises. *Lancet*, **ii**, 191.
25. Collier, W. (1907) Functional albuminuria in athletes. *Br. med. J.*, **i**, 4.
26. Barach, J. H. (1910) Physiological and pathological effects of severe exertion (marathon race) on circulatory and renal systems. *Archs. Intern. Med.*, **5**, 382.
27. Gardner, K. D. (1955) Athletic pseudo-nephritis. *J. Am. med. Ass.*, **161**, 1613.
28. Kleiman, A. H. (1960) Athlete's kidney. *J. Urol.*, **83**, 321.
29. Alyea, E. P. and Parish, H. H., Jnr. (1958) Renal response to exercise—urinary findings. *J. Am. med Ass.*, **167**, 807

8

Sports cardiology

Introduction

This chapter sets out to describe briefly the physiological adaptation of the heart to exercise associated with sport, the peculiarities of the 'athlete's heart' in particular the ECG and then discusses the physician's involvement in screening for competition, cardiovascular symptoms in athletes, and then finally the long term effects of sport on the heart in terms of the possible benefits of sporting activity in prolonging life.

Physiological aspects

The transport of the metabolic substrates to, and the products of metabolism from, the active tissue is carried out by the cardiovascular system. The transportation rate is dependent on the cardiovascular response to exercise to meet the increased demands.

The cardiac response to exercise is complex and involves the interaction of changes in heart rate, ventricular end diastolic volume, ventricular end systolic volume, and the heart's neurohumoral background. The relative roles of each of these variables in the adaptation of the heart to the demands of exercise have been the subjects of investigation for many years.

The regulation of the circulation in exercise is probably guided primarily by factors sensitive to an adequate cardiac output. Heart rate and stroke volume are the variables, stroke volume being more likely to be directly influenced by such factors as venous return or peripheral vascular resistance. Green[1] in 1970 stated: 'In man an alteration in heart rate may or may not alter the cardiac output. It is unwise to assume that it does unless it is known that the stroke volume is unaffected. But in exercise, up to quite high levels of work, the increase in heart rate may account for practically all the increase in cardiac output with stroke volume remaining constant.'

Then, using the data of Asmussen and Neilson[2] he stated that, 'In severe exercise with cardiac outputs of 40 l/min an increase in stroke volume must occur, since such outputs require a stroke volume of 200 ml, with a heart rate of 200 beats/min.'

Under laboratory exercise conditions, athletes have sustained heart rates in excess of 200 beats/min for short periods of time. Åstrand[3] concluded from a measure of the oxygen transport/heart beat, that (in subjects above eight years of age), 'There are no findings indicating a decrease in stroke volume with increasing heart rate, not even at the highest rates,' Åstrand[4] and Saltin[5] using cardiac catheterization, stated that at heart rates above 110 beats/min almost maximal stroke volume was reached.

Glick and co-workers[6] suggested that, although a simple increase in heart rate in a resting individual improves the contractile state of the myocardium, the shift of the myocardial force velocity curves that occur during exercise can be attributed only in part to this change in rate. During maximal exercise, the acceleration of the heart rate alone is not sufficient to allow the achievement of a cardiac output large enough to satisfy the requirements of the peripheral tissues, unless stroke volume also rises substantially. Although the increase in cardiac output that occurs during moderate exercise is accomplished almost exclusively through an increase in heart rate after an initial increase in stroke volume, if the former is held constant, the heart is still capable of elevating its output to an appropriate level by raising the stroke volume.

Ross, Linnhart and Braunwald[7] stated that in the resting state, the cardiac output is not altered by large changes in the heart rate alone. It is clear that, in the absence of augmented metabolic requirements, homeostatic mechanisms keep cardiac output constant despite wide variations of heart rate.

Braunwald and co-workers[8] concluded that: 'The normal cardiac response to exercise involves the integrated effects on the myocardium of simple tachycardia, sympathetic stimulation and the operation of the Frank–Starling mechanism. During sub-maximal levels of exertion, cardiac output can rise even when one or two of these influences are blocked. However, during maximal levels of muscular exercise, the ventricular myocardium requires all three influences to sustain a level of activity sufficient to satisfy the greatly augmented oxygen requirements of the exercising skeletal muscle'.

Linden[9] reviewed the problem of upright exercising man and gave sample values of cardiac performance at rest and maximal exercise (Table 8.1). These are values taken from a fit, normal man. Athletes can and do demonstrate higher

Table 8.1 Sample values of cardiac performance at rest and maximal exercise in a fit normal man.[9]

	Resting	Exercising
Oxygen uptake (ml/min)	400	3000–3500
Cardiac output (l/min)	5	25
Heart rate (beats/min)	70	180
Stroke volume (ml)	70	140
Residual (end-systolic) volume (ml)	75	40
End-diastolic volume (ml)	145	180
Cycle time (sec)	0·85	0·33
Ventricular systole (sec)	0·3	0·2
Ventricular diastole (sec)	0·55	0·13

values, i.e. cardiac outputs of 35–40 l/min have been reported.[4] Mean maximum heart rates of 192 ± 5 beats/min are regularly recorded from cyclists exercising on a laboratory ergometer.

It is therefore obvious that interrelationships exist between various physiological factors that will influence the performance of the cardiovascular system and hence the man performing exercise. In addition, if athletes and non-athletes are studied it is possible to see differences in these relationships which can be attributed to conditioning and consequently increased performance.

Cardiac output is dependent on the product of heart rate and stroke volume, and increases to meet the increased demands of the active tissues. This can be seen in Table 8.2. Heart rate response to increasing work in laboratory tests has

Table 8.2 Circulatory parameters of increased O_2 transport in a normal sedentary young man capable of a 12-fold increase in $\dot{V}o_2$.[10]

Base line posture	$\dot{V}o_2$	=	H-R	×	S.V.	×	a - $\dot{V}o_2$ difference
Supine	↑12	=	↑(3.5x)	×	↑(1x)	×	↑(3.5x)
Upright	↑12	=	↑(2.3x)	×	↑(2x)	×	↑(2.6x)

shown this relationship to be linear at sub-maximal work levels.[11] There is a widening of the arteriovenous oxygen difference as more oxygen is transferred from haemoglobin to myoglobin and to the mitochondria in the working muscles to accommodate increased metabolism.

Brooke, Hamley and Thomason[12,13] demonstrated a non-linear response of heart rate to steadily increasing work load on a cycle ergometer for highly proficient male cyclists habituated to the task. After an initial linear response (Bowen effect removed), curvilinearity was noted at between 60–80 per cent work task. Thomason[15] noted that those subjects who did most work showed an earlier curvilinear response. In the other studies no correlation was found between maximum heart rate and total work capacity, and numerous other workers have reported a similar lack of correlation.

Shephard[16] suggests that endurance fitness can best be described by the pulse response at sub-maximal work: these measurements during exercise are better than ventilatory measurements in showing dependence with total work capacity. Work by Thomason[15] demonstrated high correlation between sub-maximal heart rates and total work capacity in skilled cyclists.

Wasserman and co-workers[17] noted that the interdependence of work, heart rate and ventilation suggests that control mechanisms during exercise are closely related to cellular metabolism and to changes in the internal chemical environment, and it is on this interdependence and on the characteristics of the cellular metabolism that a complete test of exhausting physical work capacity needs to be based. However, measurement of these parameters needs both accuracy and precision.

Measurement of cardiac output by any technique is difficult and outputs over 30 l/min must be treated with some circumspection as accuracy at these outputs is probably no greater than ± 20 per cent.

A summary of the response of the cardio-respiratory system to exercise can be seen in Tables 8.3–8.5. These data are compiled from several sources and can only be an estimate of what actually happens.[18] A review of the subject in detail, with the effects of temperature, is given by Rowell.[19] That differences do exist between sedentary and well conditioned men in their response to exercise is well documented as can be seen from Tables 8.6 and Fig. 8.1 which summarize these differences.[18,20]

From these tables it can be seen that differences in capacity and performance

Table 8.3 Distribution of blood flow (ml/min).

	Basal	Exercise
Heart	250	1 000
Muscle	1 200	22 000
Brain	750	750
Splanchnic	1 400	300
Kidney	1 100	250
Skin	500	600
Other	600	100
Total flow	5 800	25 000
O_2 uptake (ml)	240	2 000

Table 8.4 Contributions made by various components of the oxygen transport system to working muscle: increase during transition from rest to maximal exercise.

Oxygen uptake $\overset{\circ}{V}_{O_2}$)	12	fold increase.
Cardiac output (Q)	4	fold increase.
Heart rate (H-R)	2.7	fold increase.
Stroke volume (SV)	1.4	fold increase.
Arterio-venous difference (a-vO_2)	1.3	fold increase.

Table 8.5 Changes in haemodynamic values—transition from rest to maximal exercise as increase or decrease.

Systolic blood pressure	$+1\cdot6x$	Systemic resistance	$-2\cdot7x$
Diastolic blood pressure	$+1\cdot1x$	Pulmonary resistance	$-2x$
Mean blood pressure	$+1\cdot4x$		

Table 8.6 Average cardiovascular values for sedentary men and male endurance athletes compiled from various sources.[21]

	Heart volume*		Blood volume (ml) (l)		Total haemoglobin (g)	
Sedentary men		769		5.3		805
	n = 342		n = 174		n = 174	
Endurance athletes		986		7·5		1130
	n = 124		n = 27		n = 27	
△Difference		+217		+2·2		+325

* Resting presystolic estimated from PA and lateral X-rays of the chest.
(Authors note—These are absolute values and have not been normalized for body surface area but endurance athletes tend to have a normal or low surface area.)

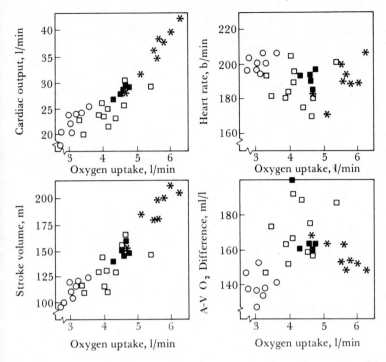

Fig. 8.1 Individual data obtained during maximal exercise: male subjects. Showing cardiac output, heart rate, stroke volume and arteriovenous oxygen difference during maximal exercise in relation to maximal oxygen uptake in top athletes who were very successful in endurance events ★, well-trained but successful athletes ■, 20–30 year old men well-trained □ and 25 year old habitually sedentary subjects ○. From Ekblom[22] adapted by Åstrand & Rodahl.[11]

do exist between conditioned and non-conditioned men. It is obvious from the literature that much more detailed investigation of the circulatory changes occurring during exercise, and chronically as a result of long term training, needs to be carried out. The major question is whether differences between the superior athlete and the normal man are innate or can be acquired by intensive training.

Adaptation of the cardiovascular system is most dramatic in the endurance athlete, so much of the data in this chapter is orientated towards these sportsmen. Many other sportsmen will be able to participate at a high level in their sport with relatively poor cardiovascular function. However it is self evident that a high maximum cardiac output, and thus oxygen uptake and sustainable maximum work rate, is of considerable value in nearly all sports which do not rely completely on skill. A tennis player who can run for every ball for example will have a decided advantage.

Long distance cycling, endurance running, cross-country skiing, rowing, canoeing, and high altitude mountaineering all put the cardiovascular system at a premium and at the highest levels select those with a combination of natural cardiovascular endowment and the quality of 'compliance to conditioning' (i.e. the ability to benefit from training by further enhancing their physiological attributes). The heart is not the sole determinant of performance and some athletes appear to compensate for deficiencies in maximum cardiac output by greater desaturation of mixed venous blood during exercise.[23] Obviously motivation plays an overwhelming part in determining performance. However, because of the selective effect of endurance athletics and the physiological consequences of prolonged heavy exertion, many athletes have evidence of enlargement of the heart beyond normally accepted limits. This condition is called 'athlete's heart' and will now be discussed. It is important to realize, however, that this condition may be found as an occupational 'disease'. One of the authors has seen a young man of 20 with many of the attributes of the athlete's heart described below. He took part in no active recreation at all but had worked for the previous three years in a carpet warehouses moving rolls of carpet weighing between 50 and 200 lb (22·5 to 90 kg).

Athlete's heart

In Samson-Wright[10] an attempt is made to explain the 'athlete's heart'. Maximal performances, i.e. 35–40 l/min cardiac output, are only achieved by international-class athletes. Such trained athletes have much larger end-systolic reserves than do ordinarily fit young adults—professional cyclists for instance, who probably call upon their end-systolic reserve in a sprint to a greater extent than any other performers, have end-systolic volumes of the order of 180 ml and their estimated heart weight is 500 g, instead of the normal 300 g. Characteristic of these highly trained individuals is a heart rate at rest which is far slower (i.e. 40 beats/min) than those of the untrained but moderately fit young adult: thus Kilby, a 1964 Olympic marathon runner, had a resting rate of 38 beats/min. Training, then, invariably lowers the heart rate, but the reason for this is obscure. The maximal steady heart rate which can be achieved in exercise by trained or untrained individuals is the same, approximately 180–190 beats/min. However, instances of heart contractions equivalent to over 200 beats/min (i.e. heart contraction rates measured on ECG by the R–R intervals of 0·25 sec) have been recorded. The trained man's ability to reach a cardiac output of say, 36 l/min depends upon his ability to eject a stroke volume of 200 ml—a 'tidal' volume which exceeds the total end-diastolic volume (180 ml) of the man who can summon up a cardiac output of only 25 l/min (Fig. 8.2). The professional cyclist has drawn upon his huge end-systolic reserve and his more muscular left ventricle can eject 200 ml of blood in 0·2 sec.

The ejection fraction, i.e. stroke volume/end-diastolic volume is as low at rest in athletes as it is in normal subjects, therefore a larger total reserve volume exists.

Moderate exercise can be achieved by the trained athlete with quite trivial increases of heart rate—the untrained man with much less end-systolic reserve begins to encroach upon his heart rate reserve much sooner and may show little evidence of an increased stroke volume in moderate exercise.

Frequent reports of X-rays taken amongst groups of sportsmen and control groups of non-participating subjects state that there is a significant difference in cardiac size between sporting and non-sporting subjects (Table 8.6). 'In trained athletes the resting pulse is often slow and there may even be mild hypertrophy and dilation of the heart as a consequence of the chronic increased work

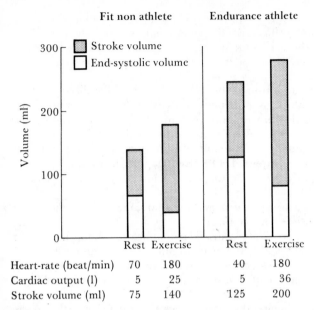

Fit non athlete   Endurance athlete

	Rest	Exercise	Rest	Exercise
Heart-rate (beat/min)	70	180	40	180
Cardiac output (l)	5	25	5	36
Stroke volume (ml)	75	140	125	200

Fig. 8.2 Cardiac reserve of endurance athlete. This comparison is between a fit young man and a world-class endurance athlete. The average sedentary male would be incapable of raising his cardiac output to 25 l, and incapable of doubling his resting stroke volume. The figures for end-systolic volume in the endurance athlete would depend on the circumstances under which the measurements are made.

requirements upon the heart. There is no evidence that this (physiological) hypertrophy is detrimental to the individual.'[24]

The endurance athlete thus has a large capacity heart with a slow 'tick over'. There are probably other adaptations that allow him not only to achieve a high maximum cardiac output but to maintain a high value for prolonged periods of time.

The increase in chamber size of the heart may well be complemented by an increase in blood vessel size and the diameter of the valve orifices. There are virtually no data available on this feature of the athlete's heart. However, the autopsy on De Mar, the legendary American marathon runner, apparently showed that the cardiac chambers were large and also that the great vessels and coronary arteries were larger than in comparable subjects.[25] Dilatation of these vessels would seem to be a necessary adaptation to the high flows that have been demonstrated.

A cardiac output of 40 l/min through an aortic root of 2·7 cm diameter (Feigenbaum's figure[26] for the average aortic root diameter) would generate a mean blood velocity of 260 cm/sec and a mean Reynolds number of 18 000. These figures would be reduced to a mean aortic blood velocity of 117 cm/sec and mean Reynolds number of 12 000 by an aortic root diameter of 4 cm, which would reduce somewhat the very large energy losses involved in accelerating the blood up to such high velocities and also reduce the dissipative energy losses resulting from the turbulence in the aortic flow that would seem inevitable with such high mean blood velocities and Reynolds numbers.[27] Similar reasoning applied to the mitral valve orifice would suggest that the limit to maximum cardiac output could be the size of the mitral valve orifice, since the left atrial pressure is limited to levels below that at which pulmonary oedema would develop.

Thus sustained high cardiac output would seem to require generalized enlargement of the heart and great vessels and, since cardiac output appears to be the limiting factor in defining the maximum oxygen uptake,[19] it could well be the development of large pressure losses across the mitral valve and in the aortic root which acts as the ultimate determinant of performance. This hypothesis is supported by personal observations (DTP) using Doppler ultrasound to study flow patterns in the subclavian arteries. On severe exercise the flow appears to become highly turbulent.

The slow resting heart rate of the athlete and the anatomical and physiological increase in cardiac dimensions and volumes may not be the sole ways that the heart adapts to prolonged exertion. It seems likely that at the cellular level there are biochemical changes that enable the heart to function at high levels of output for prolonged periods. These changes are suggested from analogy with skeletal muscle and the experimental work in animals still gives contradictory evidence.[28,9]

One of the most obvious changes that can be seen in 'athlete's heart' is in the electrocardiogram (ECG). The ECG in the athlete and the changes seen with training will now be discussed.

Electrocardiography

Electrocardiography, the art of recording the electrical activity associated with the heart's action, has progressed from an empirical basis to a much more scientific one since A. D. Waller first coined the word in a paper read before the Royal Society in 1890.[30] It has always been a tool of the clinician; changes in wave patterns have been regarded as significant when taken in the light of other information available and the results of autopsies. This has resulted in the construction of compendia correlating various patterns with specific diagnoses, in addition to inference of information on the periodicity and conductivity of the cardiac muscle.

Simonson[31], discussing the concept and definition of normality of ECG recordings, stated that a satisfactory description of normality in valid statistical terms can be given only for functions or properties that can be quantitatively measured, and Schaeffer[32] argued that: 'The ECG is the record of a superimposition of the electromotive forces which originate during the activation process in the individual heart muscle fibres. An ECG is not an indication of the function of the heart—this can only be determined by the analysis of stroke volumes ejected at known pressures. The very purpose of an ECG is to give information about the direction and velocity of the excitation wave and subsequent repolarization. Observations, theories and derivations which do not lead to information of this kind are useless.'

Sources of biological variability such as age, sex, relative body weight, and chest configuration, are interdependent. Therefore, their individual effect on the ECG is complex and analytical separation is sometimes difficult.

A review of the effect of these variables leads to the conclusion that information of ECGs reported without consideration of them is of little value.[33]

Errors in recording procedures can be many. Attempts have been made to standardize equipment and improve its performance by the American Heart Association Technical Committee recommendations of 1967.[34]

An abundance of literature on ECGs of athletes, before and after exercise (and now, due to technical advances, during exercise), have attempted to demonstrate differences in the ECGs of sportsmen from those of the normal population. It must be remembered that unless these changes can be measured quantitatively and analysed, then the results must be regarded with some reserve, for a clinically abnormal population is not being studied but rather the part of the normal population which are placed at the upper end of the spectrum with regard to physical ability.

A 'once only' ECG might show some abnormality, which could be due to a multiplicity of factors and, therefore, may not be due to the athletic prowess of the subject. It seems that the value of the ECG in detecting early or minor departures from normal may be enhanced greatly by making serial observations under standardized conditions and comparing the changes observed with the listed maximal permissible day-to-day differences.[35] Abnormalities can thus be detected by comparing tracings even though individual recordings are within normal limits.

Blackburn and others in 1967 reported[36] on the standardization of the exercise electrocardiograms and stated that: 'Despite many limitations, empirical interpretation of the electrocardiographic response to exercise is a useful clinical tool which is inadequately exploited. It was concluded that a first step towards standardization of the exercise ECG method should be recording with the same lead system before, during and after the stress.'

Michaels[35] on day-to-day variability of the ECG from 36 males and 22 females (age range 30–70), found 5 per cent with some abnormality, and 12 per cent with occasional atrial or ventricular ectopic beats, while 'normal' standards for ECG wave amplitudes and time intervals for males and females at various age groups have been given.[37]

The idea that the ECG response may be affected by physical work has long been held. Bloch,[38] Delachaux,[39] and Cureton[40] have all reported T wave inversion in athletes who were training hard, and Lepeschkin[41] reported greater amplitudes of T waves in athletes than non-athletes. Carlile[42] found that severe physical effort causes, in some subjects, a progressive flattening of the T wave in the resting ECG, while Plas[43] found four stages of wave changes in cyclists during the Tour de France:

1 S–T segment elevation;
2 T wave becoming biphasic;
3 S–T segment and T wave tend to combine;
4 S–T segment becomes curved and elevated, T wave is negative

These changes persisted for several weeks but after 2 months, disappeared in the reverse order.

Rosnowski[44] stated that an increase in QRS amplitude after prolonged exercise was usual, while Sesenbach[45] reported that excessive exercise in normal individuals will produce depression of the S–T segment and flattening and inversion of the T wave.

Wasserburger and colleagues reported that RS–T elevation occurs in approximately 1 per cent of the normal population.[46] When exercising 48 subjects with RS–T elevation, they did not find it lowered during the cycle tests.

Beckner and Winsor[47] reporting on findings from ECGs of 40 non-runners and 155 male runners with at least 5 years' training, found large QRS complexes and tall T and U waves, while Beswick and Jordan using ECGs of 60 male athletes reported similar findings.[48]

Karvonen[49] noted bradycardia, slow conduction at atrial and ventricular level, high voltages, and cardiac enlargement, confirmed by Smith, Cullen and Thorburn in reports of bradycardia, high voltage QRS complexes and tall T and U waves.[50] In some subjects, but not all, P and T waves increased in amplitude directly after an endurance race. Partial right bundle branch block is demonstrated with increasing frequency, the greater the distance run. Åstrand[51] reporting on resting ECGs of 12 Swedish champion girl swimmers, found, at rest, pronounced sinus arrhythmia, abnormal P waves, and in 4 cases a tendency to high voltage of the QRS complexes, as well as tall T waves, and stated that these T waves may have been an indication of left ventricular enlargement.

Thomason, Hamley and Brooke[52] studied resting supine ECGs of young females, including physical education specialists, British international swimmers, and a control group. From resting ECG recordings taken at 6-monthly intervals for the 3 years of their course, they found the QRS amplitude in lead II was greater statistically in those subjects who undertook a lot of physical activity. A linear regression of this QRS amplitude in those subjects who stopped or markedly decreased their yearly physical work was demonstrated. The non-PE student's R2 wave amplitude did not differ from that of the normal population as reported by Simonson for that age group. Measurement of the P, QRS and T wave amplitudes for standard leads I, II, III in this study, and subsequent analysis of them, did not demonstrate any further significant statistical correlations.

Hunt[53] reporting on ECGs from swimmers before and after a hard race found sinus arrhythmia in 40 per cent of them before and after the race—45 per cent had inverted T waves in lead III.

Many athletes have marked sinus arrhythmia during the recovery phase of exercise and at rest. Treffene[57] has investigated this phenomenon in a group of swimmers and cross-country runners. Many of them had an exaggerated sinus arrhythmia during their recovery from exercise, especially the élite swimmers. The arrhythmia commenced at a specific heart rate for each individual varying from 150 to 100 beats per minute during return from a peak of 180 to 200 beats/ min. The arrhythmia could start within 40 seconds of the termination of exercise and measurement of the R–R interval could show oscillation between values as wide as 0·5 sec and 1·2 sec (equivalent to heart rates of 150 and 50 beats/min respectively) within 3 or 4 cardiac cycles. The sudden slowing from normal recovery heart rate occurred inconsistently with each respiratory cycle but always at the same phase of respiration when it did occur.

Beckner and Winsor,[47] and Thomason and Hamley[52] demonstrated larger heart shadow size and R2 wave amplitudes in athletes than non-athletes. Barach[54] Gordon and co-workers[55] and Bramwell and Ellis[56] have all pointed out that cardiac enlargement is a usual finding among marathon runners and is not indicative of cardiac disease.

The usual types of abnormal tracings found in athletes are associated with arrhythmicity. Studies carried out in recent years by the authors, using athletes, bear this out. The following are case histories of various athletes and groups of athletes. It must be remembered that most athletes do not demonstrate any abnormality of wave patterns.

Sample cases

Case 1: 1964 British olympic swimmer, female

She swam within 10 per cent of her fastest time to date and then was connected to the ECG in the resting supine position at the bath side: Standard Lead II.

This trace shows a marked sinus arrhythmia with varying P wave configuration, and complete failure to conduct on one occasion in the 1 minute strip. Varying R–R P–R and P wave configurations are also seen in the 1 min 15 sec strip (Fig. 8.3).

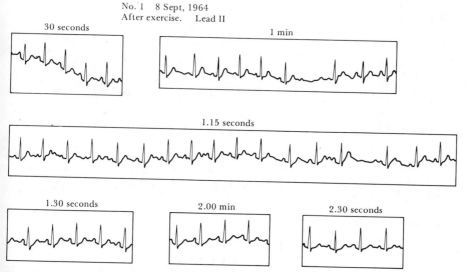

Fig. 8.3 ECG tracings, case 1.

Case 2: Marathon runner pre-exercise testing on treadmill standing prior to experiment: Lead V5

This record shows ventricular ectopic beats superimposed on a sinus bradycardia (heart rate, 48). Normally there is a compensatory pause after a ventricular

ectopic beat, because retrograde conduction from the ventricles renders the conduction pathway to the next sinus beat refractory. Because of the slow sinus
rate, the AV node in this case is only relatively refractory, and so although

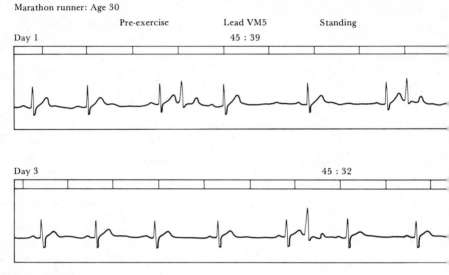

Marathon runner: Age 30

	Pre-exercise	Lead VM5	Standing
Day 1		45 : 39	

Day 3   45 : 32

Fig. 8.4 ECG tracings, case 2.

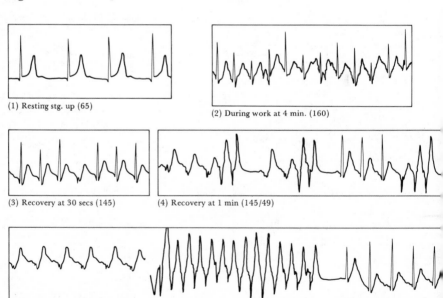

(1) Resting stg. up (65)

(2) During work at 4 min. (160)

(3) Recovery at 30 secs (145)

(4) Recovery at 1 min (145/49)

(5) Recovery at 1.30 mins (113)?

Recovery at - 2 mins (122)   2.30 mins (102)   3 mins (105)   4 mins (105)   5 mins (113)   10 mins (105)

Fig. 8.5 ECG tracings, case 3.

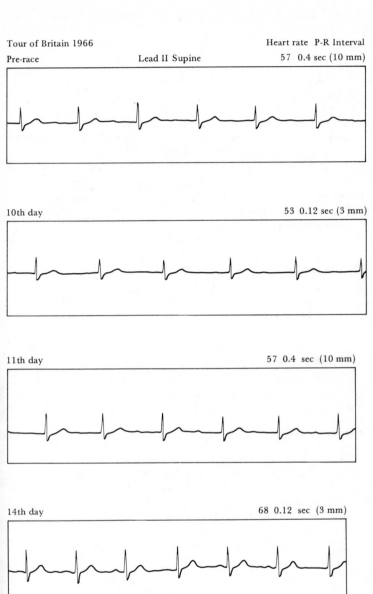

Tour of Britain 1966
Pre-race   Lead II Supine

Heart rate P-R Interval
57 0.4 sec (10 mm)

10th day

53 0.12 sec (3 mm)

11th day

57 0.4 sec (10 mm)

14th day

68 0.12 sec (3 mm)

Fig. 8.6 ECG tracings, case 4.

there is a slight increase in P–R interval in the post-ectopic beat, there is no real post-ectopic (Fig. 8.4).

Case 3: British cycling champion

Had complained of tightness in his chest when he slowed down during a race. This tightness sometimes persisted for half hour spells.

In exercise test on cycle ergometer, maximum work load achieved 350 watts at 90 rev/min, while ECG was continuously monitored throughout.

This record appears to illustrate a very rapid ventricular tachycardia, starting with coupled ectopics after 1 min and then persisting for 3 seconds. The alternative diagnosis is a supraventricular tachycardia with aberrant conduction. This illustrates the fact that dysrhythmias are more likely to occur in subjects without ischaemic heart disease during the recovery phase. This tachycardia with a rate of 200 beats/min may well account for this cyclist's symptoms, which only occurred after prolonged severe exertion.

To elucidate an athlete's symptoms it is obviously necessary to stress him to his limits.

This case is quite unique and is not to be taken as an example of the dangers of exercise (Fig. 8.5).

Case 4: British cyclist in Tour of Britain 14-day cycle race, 1966

Lead II supine at the same time each evening always at least 2 hours after the end of the day's racing. Abnormal P–R interval on certain days.

This example of variation in the P–R interval independently of the heart rate suggests that the vagal influence on the AV node can be quite independent of the vagal influence on the SA node, since it seems most likely that the large variations in P–R interval are produced by variations in vagal tone (Fig. 8.6).

Case 5: British cyclist in Tour of Britain 14-day cycle race, 1966

Lead II supine at least 2 hours after the end of the day's racing—complete omission of QRS complex. This phenomenon was not present before the start of the race. Occurred after the 4th day and persisted for the next 10 days. Coach stated that subject was not performing well from day 4 until day 14. Subsequent laboratory investigation failed to demonstrate this phenomenon in recovery after exhaustive exercise testing.

Another example of AV block occurring intermittently. It is doubtful whether this could have had anything to do with his poor performance (Fig. 8.7).

Tour of Britain 1966

Subject 1:   Age 22   60 : 29   Lead II Supine

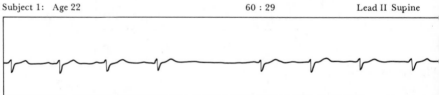

Fig. 8.7 ECG tracings, case 5.

Case 6: British cyclist in Tour of Britain Cycle Race, 1965

This phenomenon occurred on the 6th day of the race and persisted throughout the rest of the race. ECG taken at least 2 hours after completion of race prior to eating, Lead II supine.

Another example of intermittent AV block, this time with classical Wenckebach periods of progressive lengthening of the P–R interval before the dropped beat (Fig. 8.8).

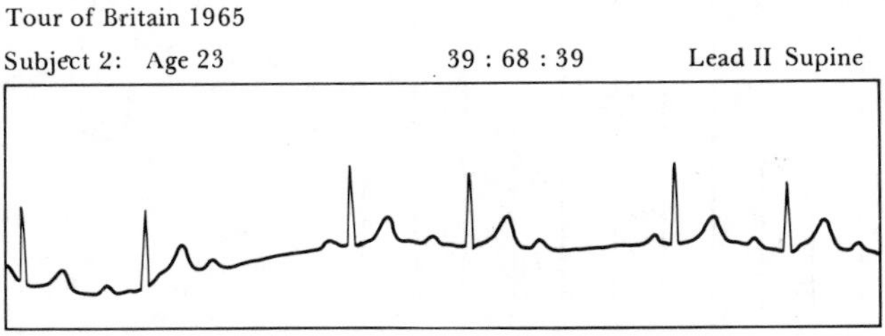

Tour of Britain 1965

Subject 2: Age 23   39 : 68 : 39   Lead II Supine

Fig. 8.8 ECG tracings, case 6.

The following graphs are results from various studies of the ECGs of sportsmen and women.

Graphs 1, 2, 3 (Figs 8.9–8.11)

Resting supine standard Lead I, II, and III were taken from: (1) 100 female PE students, (2) 40 female PE students who were also International and area

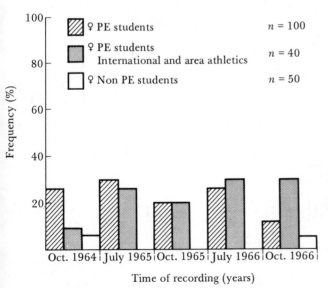

Fig. 8.9 Demonstrates the percentage frequency of S–T elevation Lead II > 1 mm against time into 3-year course.

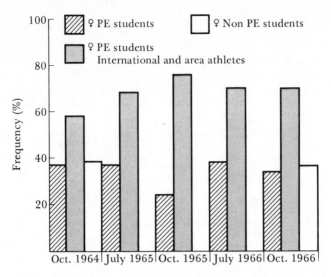

Fig. 8.10 Demonstrates percentage frequency of inverted T waves in Lead III against time into 3-year course. Age range 18–21 years.

athletes, and (3) 50 non-PE students of the same age range (18–21 years). Recordings were taken at the start of a 3-year course and at intervals throughout.

It is of interest to note that in Group 1 the weekly level of physical activity dropped throughout the 3-year course. The weekly level in Group 2 remained

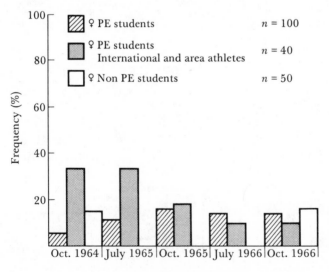

Fig. 8.11 Demonstrates percentage frequency of sinus arrhythmia against time into 3-year course. Age range 18–21 years.

constant or increased, while that of Group 3 was similar to the normal population for that age range.

The cases reported are from practicing 'athletes' and not clinical problems. That there are differences between the normal population and some athletes in respect of certain aspects of the ECG is apparent. However, one cannot, using electrocardiography alone, determine why there are these differences, only that they exist. It should be noted that some top-class athletes demonstrate what may be regarded as clinically abnormal tracings.[58, 59] The most dramatic abnormalities are those of the T wave,[59] since T wave flattening or inversion may be taken by the clinician as an indication of ischaemia or pericarditis if the athlete complains of chest pain. These T wave abnormalities will in many cases disappear on stress testing.

The presence of these 'abnormalities' of the ECG in athletes reinforces the imperative that an ECG should never be interpreted without full knowledge of the subject. In addition to the usual details of race, body build, medication, blood pressure, etc., it seems that information is needed on the subject's level of physical activity if this is of sufficient intensity and duration.

Finally, the plan of Smith and others for a long term prospective study of athletes on an international basis, in order to assess the significance of the electrocardiogram and other changes,[50] must be reiterated.

Fit for competition?—screening of athletes

One of the most difficult problems that can face a doctor is to decide whether a particular subject is normal and fit for competitive sport or whether some minor abnormality found on routine examination indicates that there will be definite risks associated with participation. For example a systolic murmur may indicate severe heart valve disease or a cardiomyopathy, or merely a minor haemo-dynamic disturbance related to the shape of the chest. Similarly an electrocardiographic abnormality may be a benign variant of normal, or the clue to disease of the coronary arteries. It therefore seems appropriate to discuss the screening or routine examination of athletes prior to competition.

Routine screening of athletes is not widespread in the United Kingdom, but in the U.S.A. there is increasing demand for medical certification of fitness to compete in certain sports and recreations. Judging from the literature, routine screening with exercise ECG is uncommon and is usually undertaken following a totally unexpected death in University athletes.[60, 61]

Screening, if it is undertaken, should have the objective of finding abnormalities likely to present risk of sudden death or injury to the subject or the detection of any condition that would be aggravated seriously by participation in the relevant sport.

As far as the heart is concerned the question is not whether there is any minor abnormality, but whether that abnormality under the stress of competition could lead to sudden death, or whether the cardiac lesion would be made worse by participation.

Exclusion of athletes from the sport of their choice on the grounds of a minor abnormality of the heart would be both unscientific and counterproductive in that it would inhibit athletes from submitting to this type of routine screening. Fortunately sudden death from cardiac causes in young athletes is uncommon and is probably dwarfed by the mortality from trauma in body contact sports.

Where an athlete has commercial value, another question has to be asked: This is whether any abnormality that is found indicates a lesion that will limit performance, either at the time, or in the future. This problem was dramatized a few years ago in Britain when a football player, who was being transferred from one club to another for a very large fee, was found to have a congenital abnormality of the heart, and the transfer was stopped. Presumably the physician involved thought him a bad investment.

Before discussing the physical examination of athletes or other potential sportsmen it would seem appropriate to discuss the cardiac symptoms of which an athlete may complain.

Cardiac symptoms

Athletes or sportsmen are likely to seek the opinion of a doctor (or be sent to see him) on the basis of several symptoms.

Syncope

Fainting or syncope on exercise is a classical warning of severe heart disease, since it may indicate a low fixed cardiac output which cannot increase to compensate adequately for the increased vascular bed which opens up on exercise. It may also indicate a dysrhythmia precipitated by exercise, or even coronary insufficiency.[62]

The more common causes of syncope on exertion are aortic and pulmonary stenosis, and hypertrophic obstructive cardiomyopathy, all of which have definite physical signs and can cause sudden death on exertion. Syncope during exertion therefore is a serious symptom and in the absence of physical signs must still be investigated with an ECG and cardiologist's opinion. It should therefore be considered an absolute contraindication to further severe exertion until it has been investigated.

Syncope can, however, occur in normal fit athletes AFTER exertion. Luckily this is appreciated by many of them and is one of the reasons why cyclists and runners keep moving at the end of a race. This prevents the pooling of blood in the legs which can result in cerebral ischaemia and thus syncope. Syncope at the end of a race, particularly at the end of an endurance race on a hot day when the blood volume may be depleted, should therefore not be treated with the same seriousness as syncope occurring during exertion. The postural hypotension that may occur at the end of a marathon for example rapidly recovers with replacement of some of the fluid loss.

Syncope unassociated with exertion or after exertion is more frequent during recovery from, or incubation of, an infection or in a state of severe fatigue when the cardiovascular reflexes may be more sluggish. Alcohol has the same effect

Palpitations

Palpitations or consciousness of the heart beat may become evident during training following illness when the heart rate response to exertion will be temporarily
greater than normal. Pounding of the heart during severe exertion is not usually
noticed by the fit athlete, but irregularity of the pulse during recovery or at rest
may be sufficiently noticeable to worry the athlete.

Irregularity of the heart rate may be caused by strong vagal tone with sinus

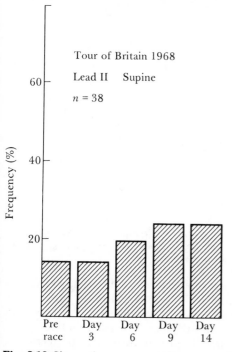

Fig. 8.12 Shows the percentage frequency of sinus arrhythmia throughout the 14-day
Tour of Britain cycle race, 1968. n = 38 British riders. From Lead II supine recorded at
least 2 hours after the end of the day's racing and prior to the evening meal.

arrhythmia or even a 'wandering pacemaker' in which the sinus node is inhibited
and atrial or nodal pacemakers take over. Even second degree heart block with
Wenckebach phenomena can result from this strong vagal tone[63] (Fig. 8.8) causing
missed beats followed by a large jolt. The most frequent cause of this symptom
is ventricular ectopic beats which are surprisingly common in athletes.

Ventricular ectopic beats
These may occur at rest or only during recovery from exercise and are then often
associated with a sinus arrhythmia. In the vast majority of cases they are of no
significance and usually are not noticed, but the jolting post-ectopic beat may
reach the athlete's consciousness.

Ectopic beats have obtained a sinister reputation through their association with

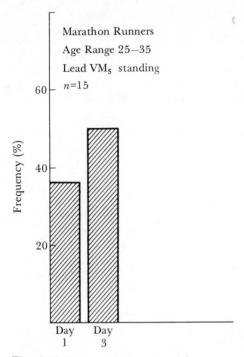

Fig. 8.13 Shows the percentage frequency of S–T elevation—Lead VM_5 standing, in 15 male marathon runners, age range 25–35, n=15, prior to starting an exercise test on a laboratory treadmill. All subjects rested on Day 2.

ischaemic heart disease in the post-myocardial infarction situation where they may herald ventricular fibrillation. No such risk is attached to the subject with an otherwise normal heart and the vast majority of athletes with ventricular ectopic beats can be strongly reassured that these are a normal finding.

Frequent ventricular ectopic beats have been seen in the resting records of a racing cyclist, an ultra-long distance runner (100 miles) and a young female sprinter, only one of whom (the long distance runner) was conscious of them.

Ventricular ectopic beats occurring on exercise and increasing in frequency with the severity of the exercise, or varying in configuration (i.e. from more than one focus), or associated with symptoms of dizziness are, however, of sinister significance and merit an expert opinion.

Consciousness of the heart beat while anticipating a race is so common as not to merit further discussion.

Lethargy and fatigue

Athletes tend to be obsessional introverts and occasionally may complain of lethargy and fatigue, symptoms which may still be ascribed by some of the older generation to a 'strained heart'. These symptoms are common after a really maximal effort, especially if the athlete was not fully conditioned, and can be made worse by excessive efforts of the athlete to prove his fitness.

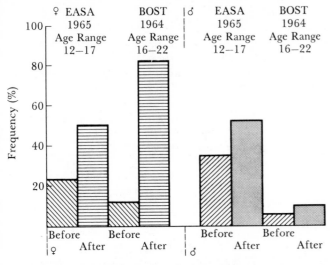

Fig. 8.14 Shows the percentage frequency of sinus arrhythmia before and after swimming. All recordings were Lead II supine. Each subject rested prior to the 'before' recording, they then swam within 10 per cent of their best time for their distance. Immediately, they left the pool and the 'after' recording was taken, usually within 1 min of the end of the swim. Sinus arrhythmia in this context was taken as arrhythmia which persisted for some little time. It was interesting to note that this arrhythmicity did not occur, until at least 1 min–1 min 30 sec after the swim. This is similar to results seen by Treffene.[57] E.A.S.A. ♀ and ♂ n = 20 were the participants on the Amateur Swimming Association Easter Swimming School, 1965. They are among the best non-international swimmers in the country. B.O.S.T. ♀ and ♂ n = 18 members of the British Olympic Swimming Team for the 1964 Olympics, Tokyo.

There is absolutely no evidence that the normal heart can be 'strained' by exertion even to the point of complete exhaustion, and most of these symptoms arise from peripheral muscle.

However these symptoms arising after a viral infection must raise the possibility of a viral myocarditis, and competition or even training at the time of, or very shortly after, a pyrexial illness is probably unwise because of this. Exercise associated with an attack of myocarditis (which is often associated with myalgia) can precipitate heart failure and is certainly unlikely to be beneficial.

Unaccustomed breathlessness

This is an unlikely symptom for an athlete, but like palpitations and lethargy may occur during convalescence from an illness. In the fit athlete, it is probable that many systems limit performance at the same level. Illness can make the cardiovascular or respiratory system limit activity when the peripheral circulatory and muscular systems are unaffected, which may give rise to this feeling which will also occur with exercise induced asthma; the latter can easily be detected with a Peak Flow meter. If not asthmatic in origin this symptom usually improves spontaneously with reassurance.

Chest pain

Chest pain on exertion need not be angina and many runners suffer transient chest pain. A burning retrosternal raw pain after severe exertion in cold weather is presumably due to a tracheitis, and for some reason, despite similar ventilation rates, tends not to occur with increasing fitness and presumably adaptation to the low relative humidity of the cold air.

A spontaneous pneumothorax may occur on exertion and will produce a sudden pleuritic pain associated with breathlessness, the degree of breathlessness depending on the size of the pneumothorax. A pneumothorax may occur with sudden trauma to the chest.

Angina is unlikely to occur but would tend to appear at repeatable levels of exertion.

Physical examination

Routine physical examination of amateur athletes is not yet widespread except in particular sports such as boxing. However, in the litigious U.S.A. it is becoming increasingly common for the organizers of races (particularly those for the 'joggers') to demand medical certification of fitness to compete.

It is sometimes difficult to know what real purpose this serves since normal physical examination does not exclude ischaemic heart disease, aneurysm of the arteries of the circle of Willis in the brain, or other causes of imminent sudden death. However, a doctor may restrain a particularly misguided individual such as a hypertensive 55-year-old man who has taken no exercise for 35 years and who has a sudden yen to take up parachuting (which requires a medical certificate).

Luckily sudden death during athletic competition is uncommon so the risks run by the certifying doctor are small.

The findings that may worry the doctor on physical examination may be those of organic heart disease, benign variants of normal, or manifestations of the 'athlete's heart syndrome'.

Heart-rate

A slow resting heart rate, which is often slightly irregular, is very common in endurance athletes. It may be as slow as 30 beats/min. If it is very slow, the effect of vigorous exercise should be to remove the vagal tone and increase the heart rate to well over 100 beats/min. If the bradycardia is caused by congenital complete heart block, the heart rate may rise to 90 beats/min or even slightly more, but a normal pulse rate response to exercise will not be possible.

Congenital complete heart block would have to be confirmed by an ECG recording but itself may not preclude competitive sport, since maximum oxygen uptake levels in these people may fall within the range of normal for non-endurance athletes.[23]

Irregularity of the heart beat at rest should be abolished by exercise and if this is the case, an ECG in an asymptomatic subject is not justified. A marked bradycardia will be accompanied by compensatory increase in the heart size.

Blood pressure

Regular exercise tends to lower resting systolic blood pressure slightly and the hypertensive response to moderate exercise lessens with training. It is difficult to give any hard and fast rules as to what levels of blood pressure might be considered dangerous for participation in any particular sport. Mild elevation of blood pressure (say up to 110 diastolic) has been shown statistically to increase the chances of myocardial infarction and strokes by a factor of 2 or 3. These increased risks are operative all the time and may be accentuated by some forms of exercise. Any sport in which there is powerful prolonged isometric exercise, such as weight-lifting and perhaps wrestling, produces marked rises in blood pressure, which, if the pressure is already raised, may be undesirable.

Sports in which a temporary loss of mental faculties or physical control could be lethal, such as underwater diving or parachuting, would obviously need to be stricter in their criteria than others.

If a raised blood pressure is found on routine screening it should obviously be checked on 2 or 3 occasions before further action is taken. If it is markedly raised and requires treatment, highly competitive sport is probably unwise, but regular exercise and sociable sport are not.

Cardiac enlargement

Some degree of cardiac enlargement, with displacement of the apex beat of the heart beyond the midclavicular line, is common in athletes and is a result of physiological hypertrophy. It is common to feel a 'left ventricular impulse' consistent with the large stroke volume consequent on a slow heart rate. However, anything more than moderate hypertrophy, and certainly any evidence of right ventricular hypertrophy would need a specialist opinion. Cardiac enlargement would need to be verified by X-ray and ECG.

Murmurs

The assessment of heart murmurs is difficult and if there is any doubt specialist advice should be sought. However if there is a soft systolic ejection murmur with normal splitting of the second heart sound, a normal carotid pulse, little if any cardiac hypertrophy, and no symptoms, the murmur is likely to be of no significance, and may just reflect an increased stroke volume. Murmurs can be heard in virtually every athlete after severe exertion and are then 'physiological'.[27]

Individual conditions that may produce heart murmurs will now be briefly discussed.

Systolic murmurs

Aortic stenosis may be present as a congenital abnormality besides the more common type of degenerative stenosis that develops in late middle age. Minor abnormality of the aortic valve (a bicuspid valve) is present in about 2 per cent of the male population, often gives rise to a systolic murmur, and may later proceed to stenosis or incompetence of the valve. Significant stenosis will manifest itself by a prolonged weak carotid pulse, but there may be no increase in heart size or hypertrophy on the ECG with the congenital variety. Sudden death may occur with tight aortic stenosis on exertion so specialist advice should be sought if there is any doubt.

Pulmonary murmurs
A pulmonary systolic murmur may be found with pulmonary stenosis, atrial septal defect or depressed sternum, and again specialist advice with chest X-ray and ECG may be required.

Hypertrophic obstructive cardiomyopathy
This is a cause of sudden death in young people and may be associated with exertion or excitement. There is a rather jerky carotid pulse and a late systolic murmur and sometimes a family history of sudden death.

Again specialist advice should be sought as the diagnosis can be established with echocardiography, and the presence of this condition would be an absolute contraindication to strenuous competitive sport.

Pan-systolic murmurs
These occur with ventricular septal defects and mitral regurgitation, neither of which may be a contraindication to participation in sport, provided the lesion is not severe. Again specialist advice should be sought.

Diastolic murmurs
These are all of pathological significance and require further specialist investigation.

Abnormalities of the heart on investigation

Many physicians still tend to regard the changes of athlete's heart as pathological. For example an Olympic sculler was failed on his medical for the RAF on the basis that he had a very slow heart, an abnormal ECG (partial right bundle branch block with a wandering pacemaker and large voltages), and an enlarged heart on chest X-ray. Specialist advice overruled this decision but the physiological consequences of prolonged athletic training are generally too little appreciated. Moderate cardiac enlargement on chest X-ray and a wide variety of ECG changes must therefore be accepted as normal for the athlete.

Exercise testing for ischaemic heart disease

Exercise testing is a widely used screening procedure to look for evidence of ischaemic heart disease in the middle-aged population and is not usually used for athletes.[60, 61]

The scope of this type of testing is beyond this chapter and is well reviewed.[64–67] However, in discussion of the contraindications to active participation in sport, the results of exercise testing are sometimes quoted, so the merits of this sort of testing must be considered.

Exercise testing consists of the search for an abnormal ECG response to exercise, an ischaemic resting trace being a contraindication to such a search.

The diagnostic criteria for ischaemia can be set at various levels of selectivity which will give a varying proportion of correct, false positive, and false negative results. The incidence of false positive results (excessive ST segment depression in normals with no symptoms and no evidence of heart disease) is particularly high in young women.

The technique of testing varies. A constant load may be given for a varying length of time (Master's test), or the work load may be increased as a stepwise function with time, or, with special equipment, at a continuous rate.

Where fit young athletes are being tested, a test to exhaustion without standby resuscitation equipment is probably justifiable. Where a middle-aged or even unfit young population is being studied there is a small but definite risk of exercise-induced cardiac dysrhythmias or even ventricular fibrillation. The test should therefore not be made without continuous monitoring of the ECG and a defibrillator should be immediately available.

Exercise testing is of considerable value in population studies of the incidence of ischaemic heart disease and is of some prognostic value, but because of the high incidence of false positive and false negative results, the results of such a test should not be taken in isolation. Gross ST segment depression obviously merits further study. Unfortunately even severe coronary artery disease may not give a positive result, and impending myocardial infarction can be silent in this respect.[68] A 46-year-old man with atypical chest pain unrelated to exercise, with a normal resting ECG and normal cardiac enzymes, was exercised to a heart rate of 160 beats/min with no chest pain and no ischaemic changes on ECG. Thirty hours after the test, with no intervening attacks of pain, he sustained a full thickness anteroseptal myocardial infarct with pathological Q waves from V1 to V5. (DTP personal observation).

Although this chapter is hardly concerned with the specific problems of diagnosis of ischaemic heart disease, the subject has been raised because of its relevance to the prevention of sudden death in sport, since it has been suggested that routine exercise testing with ECG control would reduce this risk.[60, 61]

Although some of these unfortunate but very rare fatalities might be prevented by this type of screening, the procedure is not without its problems, both logistic and diagnostic.

Action to be taken if abnormalities are found on routine screening

Sudden death in sport for medical reasons is fortunately very rare: examples will be discussed below. It is therefore only justified to advise non-participation in sport where there are symptoms or signs strongly indicating the likelihood of a potentially lethal condition such as aortic stenosis, hypertrophic cardiomyopathy, or ischaemic heart disease.

Where there is a possibility of an abnormality such as an atrial septal defect, or other non-lethal cardiac condition, it would be quite wrong to forbid athletic activity whilst further investigation is awaited, if the athlete has no symptoms and regards himself as normal. This happened in the case of a swimmer who was stopped from training and competition, on the basis that his physical signs and chest X-ray were consistent with a small atrial septal defect (ASD) thought not big enough to justify catheterization or operation.

Before stopping a sportsman's chief interest in this way every attempt should be made to define the severity of the problem and whether or not the lesion will be aggravated by exercise, or pose a threat to health. In this example it is difficult to see how an ASD, if it were small, would do either. If it was thought that it would, then the swimmer should have had a cardiac catheterization to define the severity of the lesion. On the other hand, left heart catheterization in athletes must be fully justifiable as there is always the small risk of arterial damage which may limit the athlete's subsequent activities.

Screening and sudden death

Unfortunately, normal or even excellent levels of athletic endeavour are quite consistent with severe cardiac disease, and normal or super normal exercise tolerance may be found immediately before sudden death. This enigma has been a particular interest of Jokl.[69]

The incidence of sudden death in young athletes is small. Apart from the cases of aortic stenosis, hypertrophic cardiomyopathy, and myocarditis, there have been reports of anomalies of the coronary circulation[62, 69, 71] and the conduction system of the heart in young people dying during exertion.[70]

Many of these cases might well be impossible to diagnose without hindsight but some could have been anticipated if it had been appreciated that:

1 Young people can get angina, if they have anomalies of the coronary circulation.
2 Exertional syncope is a very serious symptom and requires urgent investigation.
3 Routine physical examination and, if warranted, ECG for athletes complaining of chest pain or dizziness during exertion should be followed by specialist referral if there are doubts.

Severe exertion during or immediately after any pyrexial illness is potentially hazardous because of the risks of myocarditis: it is not heroic, it is foolhardy.

There is no evidence that athletic training or severe exertion make sudden death from the Wolff–Parkinson–White syndrome more likely[60] or that it necessarily makes attacks of tachycardia more frequent.

The presence of conduction abnormalities is more difficult. Complete right bundle branch block can be of no significance, but left bundle branch block always indicates heart disease and so does right bundle branch block with a left axis. If these abnormalities are seen to develop, the possibility of underlying ischaemic heart disease must be considered and severe exertion is probably best avoided.

Exercise and risk factors in ischaemic heart disease

The prevention of ischaemic heart disease has become one of the primary objectives of health care and for this purpose exercise is being widely advocated.[72]

Ischaemic heart disease has been found to be associated with certain characteristics which are known as risk factors. Thus of large groups of people who have been studied by epidemiologists, those with high blood pressure, those who smoke, those who are excessively overweight or have excess fat in their blood, and those who lead a sedentary existence are found to have a higher chance than average of suffering from the clinical manifestations of ischaemic heart disease. These factors are cumulative, and predict a statistical risk rather than a certainty. Many subjects with multiple risk factors will not suffer from ischaemic heart disease, and the converse is also true. None of the factors is exclusively causative and some individuals with no risk factors will nevertheless defy the statistical probabilities and suffer from ischaemic heart disease despite being non-smoking, normotensive, normolipaemic, thin manual workers.

Because there are many risk factors ischaemic heart disease appears to be a multifactorial system where manipulation of one risk factor does not always have a very marked effect. Indeed not all the risk factors are amenable to manipulation. For example excess fat in the blood may not be significantly changed by diet so the risk factor may not have been changed. Adequate control of a raised blood pressure has little effect on the subsequent risk of myocardial infarction which continues to be higher than normal in those who have been hypertensive. Here reversal of a risk factor may not nullify its cumulative effect, if it has been active for a sufficient time. Smoking on the other hand is a risk factor that is effectively reversed. If a heavy smoker stops smoking his chances of having a myocardial infarct drop gradually to those of a non-smoker.

Where does lack of exercise fit into this scheme of things? The position here is being studied but so far there are few definite answers. The method of approach has been the study of:

1 The longevity of former athletes as opposed to non-athletes.[73–76]
2 Comparative groups of matched newly exercising and non-exercising middle-aged men who have previously been physically inactive.
3 Comparison of ischaemic heart disease incidence in subjects with a similar occupation (e.g. Civil Servants) with leisure activities demanding varying levels of physical activity.[77]
4 Comparison of ischaemic heart disease incidence in different occupations, comparing those involving a considerable amount of physical activity with sedentary jobs.[78]
5 Studies of cultures where ischaemic heart disease is almost unknown and there is a very high level of physical activity, e.g. the Takumara Indians[79] compared with Western society and the levels of physical activity found there.[80]

Studies of the longevity of sportsmen show that the college athlete has a life expectancy slightly greater than average, but in Rook's Cambridge study less than that of students with 1st Class Honours.[73] Studies of the longevity of sportsmen have all been retrospective and there is no information available on the length of time after leaving University or top class competition that the chosen sport was followed. It is a fair assumption that following marriage and the demands of parenthood, most of these athletes gave up their sport if they had not done so on leaving University. Few of them would have pursued a vigorous training schedule for more than perhaps 10 years. The other information which is lacking in these studies is the incidence of other risk factors in the athletes, such as smoking and obesity.

The few studies of 'chronic' athletes suggest that vigorous physical exertion pursued into middle age is associated with a considerable increase in life

expectancy[75, 81] and with various indices of cardiac performance more characteristic of athletic young men than middle-aged normals.[82]

Unfortunately, even these studies are open to question. It could be argued
that the middle-aged Finnish cross-country skier who has ischaemic heart disease,
having had his coronary in a snow drift 10 kilometres from the nearest doctor,
is not going to survive to form part of a group of athletes against whom to match
the less enterprising controls. However, the mortality among 'chronic' athletes
is not high and more of them drop out because of musculoskeletal problems than
ischaemic heart disease. However, a prospective study is obviously needed.

Even a prospective study in which a group of club athletes is followed for
50 to 60 years is open to the objection that athleticism is a way of life associated
with certain other factors which may be beneficial apart from the exercise. These
might include moderation in smoking, and a tendency to select a more 'natural'
diet. Even if the other risk factors are evenly distributed, the tendency to take
up sport may be associated with an innate physiological or psychological factor
which in itself is protective rather than the exercise.

For these reasons studies of highly 'self selected' groups such as Finnish skiers
or German long distance runners are of value in suggesting that exercise is unlikely to be dangerous in the 'chronic athlete', but are of limited value in predicting the effects of exercise programmes on previously inactive middle-aged men.

Studies of exercise programmes in middle-aged men who have not previously
taken regular exercise have often been started after the subjects have already
shown some evidence of ischaemic heart disease. Claims have been made of
reduced mortality from ischaemic heart disease in many of these studies[83–85] when
compared with predicted values for comparable groups. However, in most of
these studies there is a relatively high drop out rate from the exercising groups,
and matching of the exercising and non-exercising groups for other risk factors
requires a huge prospective study, which has not yet been reported.

Morris has shown that occupations associated with heavy physical exertion have a lower incidence of ischaemic heart disease than more sedentary jobs,
and the relative lack of coronary artery disease has been confirmed at *post
mortem*.[77]

Studies of Takumara Indians[79] and other studies of primitive societies with
documented very long average life expectancy all show a very high level of general
physical activity, and usually a 'subsistence' level of nutrition, principally of vege-
tarian origin.

Possible beneficial effects of regular exercise on the cardio-vascular system

Since the statistical data on the effects of exercise programmes is still controversial, it is reasonable to mention briefly the possible ways in which regular
exercise can benefit the cardiovascular system. This topic is discussed in more
detail by Fox[86] and the influence of exercise on coronary risk factors is discussed
by Bonanno and Lies.[87]

Regular exercise involving rhythmic contraction of large muscle groups such
as swimming, running or jogging, and cycling has been shown in a large number
of studies to increase the maximum rate of oxygen transport. This enables tasks

to be undertaken with a smaller fraction of the total aerobic capacity than they previously required.

On theoretical grounds exercise would be expected to increase the size of the coronary arteries which would make the effects of atheromatous deposits less critical, but as yet there is no evidence for exercise increasing the size of the arteries or increasing collateral flow around a stenosis. Such evidence would be very difficult to obtain, and the arteries may only be responsive to exercise before degenerative changes have occurred.

In experimental animals exercise has been shown to make the myocardium relatively resistant to hypoxia[88] but the exercise consisted of twice daily swimming for 75 minutes.

Exercise boosts the fibrinolytic activity of the blood[89,90] and it is perhaps not unreasonable to hope that this helps to prevent the arterial system 'silting up'. Sedentary subjects have an abnormal response to sudden severe exertion, with a subsequent lowering of fibrinolytic activity which is not found in active subjects.

As far as coronary risk factors are concerned,[86,87] regular exercise appears to have a beneficial effect in lowering resting systolic blood pressure. It has little effect on blood lipids and body fat unless several hours a week of exercise are taken, but the triglycerides are reduced within 96 hours of exercise.

Recent work suggesting the aetiology of carbon monoxide in ischaemic heart disease[91] has shown that smokers have a significant fraction of their blood haemoglobin fixed to carbon monoxide in the form of carboxyhaemoglobin. The normal half-life of breakdown of this substance (which may be of great aetiological importance in the genesis of atheroma) is considerably shortened by physical activity and exercise would have a significant effect in lowering the level of carboxyhaemoglobin in the blood.[92,93] Thus smokers would benefit from exercise in another way.

The psychological effects of exercise may well be beneficial in terms of relieving tension and so overactivity of the sympathetic nervous system. Most participants in physical activity claim they feel benefit from it.

There are, therefore, many unanswered questions in this field. The type of exercise showing the greatest benefit in terms of oxygen uptake[94] may not be that which gives the greatest protective effect to the heart, although they are likely to be the same.

On balance the small risk of cardiac complications from strenuous exercise seems to be far outweighed by the benefits, provided that regular exercise becomes a way of life at an early age. Strenuous exercise programmes started in middle age carry significant risks, especially in those who have had previous episodes of ischaemic damage to the heart, or who have a large number of risk factors.[95]

Ideally, regular exercise involving oxygen uptakes of over 70 per cent of maximum should be taken at least 3 times weekly, and if started early in adult life would not require the sort of medical supervision that makes exercise programmes of the American style logistically and financially daunting. It is a sad form of exercise or sport that can only take place within reach of a cardiac defibrillator.

D.T.P.
H.T.

References

1. Green, J. H. (1970) *An Introduction of Human Physiology*, 2nd Edn. London: Oxford University Press.
2. Asmussen, E. and Nielson, M. (1955) Cardiac output during muscular work and its regulation. *Physiol. Rev.*, **35**, 778.
3. Åstrand, I. (1960) Aerobic work capacity in men and women with special reference to age. *Acta physiol. scand.*, **49**, Suppl. 169.
4. Åstrand, P. O., Cuddy, T. E., Saltin, B. and Steinberg, J. (1964) Cardiac output during submaximal and maximal work. *J. appl. physiol.*, **19**, 263.
5. Saltin, B. (1964) Circulatory response to submaximal and maximal exercise after dehydration. *J. appl. physiol.*, **19**, 1125.
6. Glick, G., Sonneblick, E. H. and Braunwald, E. (1965) Myocardial force–velocity relations studied in intact unanesthetized man. *J. clin. Invest.*, **44**, 978.
7. Ross, J., Linhart, J. W. and Braunwald, E. (1965) Effects of changing heart rate in man by electrical stimulation of right atrium: studies at rest and during exercise and with isoproterenol. *Circulation*, **32**, 549.
8. Braunwald, E., Ross, J. and Sonneblick, E. H. (1967) *Mechanisms of Contraction of the Normal and Failing Heart*, London: Churchill.
9. Linden, R. J. (1965) In *Scientific Basis of Medicine, Annual Review*. London: Athlone Press, 164.
10. Keele, C. A. and Neil, E. (1971) Samson-Wright's Applied Physiology, 12th Edn. London: Oxford University Press.
11. Åstrand, P. O. and Rodahl, K. (1970) *Text Book of Work Physiology*. New York: McGraw-Hill.
12. Brooke, J. D., Hamley, E. J. and Thomason, H. (1968) Response of heart rate to physiological work. *J. Physiol.*, **197**, 61.
13. Brooke, J. D., Hamley, E. J. and Thomason, H. (1969) Normal and strain heart rate responses to workload increasing continuously and by steps. *J. Physiol.*, **201**, 33.
14. Brooke, J. D., Hamley, E. J. and Thomason, H. (1968) The Multiple regression of heart, lung and physique measures on work capacity in subjects trained to withstand fatigue. *International Symposium on Stress & Fatigue*. Per. Comm. & Int. Ass. for Occup. Health, Paris.
15. Thomason, H. (1972) The use of the electrocardiogram for the analysis of tolerance to work and the measurement of work capacity. *Unpublished Ph.D. Thesis*. University of Loughborough.
16. Shephard, R. J. (1969) *Endurance Fitness*. Toronto: University of Toronto Press.
17. Wasserman, K., Van Kessel, A. L. and Burton, G. G. (1967) Interaction of physiological mechanisms during exercise. *J. appl. Physiol.*, **22**, 71.
18. Buskirk, E. R. (1973) Cardiovascular adaptation to physical effort. In *Exercise Testing and Exercise Training in Cardiovascular Heart Disease*, ed. Naughton, J. P. and Hellerstein, H. K., New York: Academic Press.
19. Rowell, L. B. (1970) Human cardiovascular adjustments to exercise and thermal stress. *Physical. Rev.*, **54**, 75.
20. Bar-Or, O. and Buskirk, E. (1974) In *Science and Medicine of Exercise and Sport*, 2nd Edn, ed. Johnson, W. R. and Buskirk, E. R., New York: Harper & Row.
21. Grande, F. and Taylor, H. (1965) in *Handbook of Physiology Circulation*—III. Washington D.C.: American Physiology Society.
22. Ekblom, B. (1969) Effect of physical training on oxygen transport system in man. *Acta physiol. scand.*, Suppl. 328.
23. Ikkos, D. and Hanson, J. S. (1960) Response to exercise in congenital complete atrioventricular block. *Circulation*, **22**, 583.

24. Schlant, R. C. (1966) In *The Heart*, ed. Hurst, W. J. and Logue, R. B., New York: McGraw-Hill.
25. Currens, J. A. and White, P. D. (1961) Half a century of running. *New Engl. J. Med.*, **265**, 988.
26. Feigenbaum, H. (1972) *Echocardiography.* New York: Lea and Febiger.
27. Tunstall-Pedoe, D. S. (1970) Velocity distribution of blood flow in major arteries of animals and man. *D. Phil. Thesis.* Oxford University.
28. Opie, L. H. (1974) Exercise training, the myocardium and ischaemic heart disease. *Am. Heart J.*, **88**, 539.
29. Naughton, J. P. and Hellerstein, H. K. (1973) In *Exercise Testing and Exercise Training in Cardiovascular Heart Disease.* New York: Academic Press.
30. Waller, A. D. (1889) On the electromotive changes connected with the beat of the mammalian heart, and of the human heart in particular. *Phil. Trans. Roy. Soc.*, B. **80**, 169.
31. Simonson, E. (1966) The concept and definition of normality. *Ann. N.Y. Acad. Sci.* **134**, 541.
32. Schaeffer, H. and Haas, H. G. (1962) Electrocardiography. *Handbook of Physiology*, *Section 2*, Circulation 1. Washington D.C.: American Physiological Society.
33. Thomason, H. (1968) The comparative study of some physiological changes occurring in women students during the three years of a physical education course. *Unpublished M.Sc. Thesis.* University of Salford.
34. American Heart Association Committee (1967) Recommendations for standardisation of leads and of specifications of instruments in electrocardiography and vectocardiography. *Circulation*, **35**, 3.
35. Michaels, L. and Cadoret, R. J. (1967) Day to day variability in the normal E.C.G. *Br. Heart J.*, **29**, 913.
36. Blackburn, H., Taylor, H. L., Okamato, N. Rantaharju, P., Mitchell, P. L. and Kerhof, A. C. (1967) In *Physical Activity and the Heart*, ed. Karvonen, M. J. and Barry, A. J., Springfield, Ill.: Charles C Thomas.
37. Simonson, E. and Blackburn, H. (1960) Comparison of age differences in the E.C.G. of men and women. *Malatt. cardiovasc.* **1**, 311.
38. Bloch, C. (1935). *Wein Arch. inn. Med.*, **28**, 55: Ibid, **28**, 229.
39. Delachaux, A. and Rivier, J. (1948) Electrocardiogrammes anormaux chez des athletes. *Helv. med. Acta.* **15**, 424.
40. Cureton, T. K. (1951) *Physical Fitness of Champion Athletes.* Urbana: University of Illinois Press.
41. Lepeschkin, E. (1951) *Modern Electrocardiography.* Boston: Williams & Wilkins Co.
42. Carlile, F. and Carlile, U. (1959) T wave changes in the electrocardiogram associated with prolonged periods of strenuous exercise in sportsmen with special reference to application in training swimmers. *Communication to a meeting of the New South Wales Sports Medicine Association.*
43. Plas, F. (1963) Electrocardiographic changes during work and prolonged effort, *J. sports Med. phys. Fitness*, **3**, 131.
44. Rosnowski, M. (1937) Influence de l'effort corporal sur le coeur chez les sportifs; etude electrocardiographique. *Archs Mal. Coeur*, **30**, 133.
45. Sesenbach, W. (1946) Some common conditions not due to primary heart disease but which may be associated with changes in electrocardiogram. *Ann. intern. Med.*, **25**, 632.
46. Wasserburger, R. H., Siebecker, K. L., Jr and Lewis, W. C. (1956) The effect of hyperventilation on the normal adult E.C.G. *Circulation*, **13**, 850.
47. Beckner, G. L. and Winsor, T. (1954) Cardiovascular adaptations to prolonged physical effort. *Circulation*, **9**, 835.

48. Beswick, F. W. and Jordan, R. C. (1964) Cardiological observations of the 6th British Empire and Commonwealth Games. *Br. Heart J.*, **23**, 113.
49. Karvonen, M. J. (1959) Effects of vigorous exercise on the heart. In *Work and Heart*, ed. Rosenbaum, F. F. and Balknap, E. L., New York: Hoeber.
50. Smith, W. G., Cullen, K. J. and Thorburn, I. O. (1964) Electrocardiograms of marathon runners in the 1962 Commonwealth Games. *Br. Heart J.*, **23**, 469.
51. Åstrand, P. O., Engstrom, L., Erikson, B., Karlberg, P., Nylander, I., Saltin, B. and Thoren, C. (1963) Girl swimmers. *Acta paediat. scand.*, Suppl. 147.
52. Thomason, H., Hamley, E. J. and Brooke, J. D. (1968) Modifications electrocardiographiques liées a la change annuelle de travail physique chez de jeunes adulte de sexe feminine. *Travail hum.*, **31**, 344.
53. Hunt, E. A. (1963) E.C.G. study of 20 champion swimmers before and after 110 yard sprint swimming competition. *Can. med. Ass. J.*, **88**, 1251.
54. Barach, J. H. (1910) Physiological and pathological effects of severe exertion, marathon race, on circulatory and renal system. *Archs intern. Med.*, **5**, 382.
55. Gordon, B., Levine, S. A. and Welmaers, A. (1924) A group of marathon runners with special reference to circulation. *Archs intern. Med.*, **33**, 425.
56. Bramwell, C. and Ellis, R. (1931) Circulatory mechanisms in marathon runners. *Q. Jl Med.*, **24**, 329.
57. Treffene, R. J. (1974) Personal communication.
58. Lichtman, J., O'Rourke, R. A., Klein, A. and Karliner, J. S. (1973) Electrocardiogram of the athlete, alterations simulating those of organic heart disease. *Archs. intern. Med.*, **132**, 763.
59. Hanne-Paparo, N., Wendkos, M. H. and Brunner, D. (1971) T wave abnormalities in the E.C.G.s of top ranking athletes without demonstrable heart disease. *Am. Heart J.*, **81**, 743.
60. Rose, K. D. (1969) Relationship of cardiac problems to athletic participation. *J. Am. med. Ass.*, **208**, 2319.
61. Storstein, L. and Opie, H. (1973) Latent coronary insufficiency in young athletes. *Acta med. scand.*, **193**, 525.
62. Usher, B. W. and McGranahan, G. M. (1972) Syndrome of exertional syncope functional coronary insufficiency and death in young males. *Circulation*, **46**, Supp. 11, 231.
63. Cullen, K. J. and Collin, R. (1964) Daily running causing Wenckebach heart block *Lancet*, **ii**, 729.
64. Bruce, R. A. (1973) Principles of exercise testing. In *Exercise Testing and Exercise Training in Coronary Disease*, ed., Naughton, J. and Hellerstein, H. K., New York: Academic Press.
65. Naughton, J. and Haider, R. (1973) Methods of exercise training. In *Exercise Testing and Exercise Training in Coronary Heart Disease*, ed. Naughton, J. and Hellerstein, H. K., New York, Academic Press.
66. Gorman, P. A., Byers, W. S. and Haider, R. (1973) Exercise electrocardiography. In *Exercise Testing and Exercise Training in Coronary Heart Disease*, ed. Naughton, J. and Hellerstein, H. K., New York: Academic Press.
67. Amsterdam, E. A. (1974) Ed. Symposium on exercise in cardiovascular health and disease. *Am. J. Cardiol.*, **33**, 713.
68. Bruce, R. A., Hornstein, T. R. and Blackmon, J. R. (1968) Myocardial infarction after normal response to maximal exercise. *Circulation*, **38**, 552.
69. Jokl, E. and McLellan, J. T. (1971) *Exercise and Cardiac Death*. Basle: Karger.
70. James, T. N., Froggat, P. and Marshall, T. K. (1967) Sudden death in young athletes. *Ann. intern. Med.*, **67**, 1013.

71. McLellan, J. T. and Jokl, E. (1968) Congenital anomalies of coronary arteries as cause of sudden death associated with physical exertion. *Am. J. clin. Path.*, **50,** 229.

72. Semple, T. *et a¹* (1973) Myocardial infarction. How to prevent. How to rehabilitate. International Society of Cardiology.

73. Rook, A. (1954) An investigation into the longevity of Cambridge sportsmen. *Br. med. J.*, **i,** 773.

74. Polednak, A. P. (1972) Longevity and cardiovascular mortality among former college athletes. *Circulation*, **46,** 649.

75. Pomeroy, W. and White, P. D. (1958) Coronary heart disease in former football players. *J. Am. med. Ass.*, **167,** 711.

76. Pyorala, K. (1965) Cardiovascular studies on former endurance runners. Report from Institute of Occupational Health of Finland, No. 19.

77. Morris, J. N., Chave, S. P. W., Adam, C., Sirey, C., Epstein, L. and Shuhan, D. J. (1973) Vigorous exercise in leisure time and the incidence of coronary heart disease. *Lancet*, **i,** 333.

78. Morris, J. N., Heady, J. A., Raffle, P. A. B., Roberts, C. G. and Parks, J. W. (1953) Coronary heart disease and physical activity of work. *Lancet*, **ii,** 1053 and 1111.

79. Groom, D. (1971) Cardiovascular observations on the Tarakumara Indian runners—the modern Spartans. *Am. H. rt J.*, **81,** 304.

80. Durnin, J. V. G. A. (1967) Activity patterns in the community. *Can. med. Ass. J.*, **96,** 882.

81. Karvonen, M. J., quoted by Jokl, E. (1964) In *Heart and Sport*, American Lectures in Sports Medicine series. Springfield Ill.: Charles C Thomas.

82. Lang, E. (1970) Cardiovascular system of elderly long-distance runners. Preliminary report on 100 elderly long-distance runners. *Z. Kreislaufforsch*, **59,** 139.

83. Hellerstein, H. K. (1968) Exercise therapy in coronary disease. *Bull. N.Y. Acad. Med.*, **44,** 1028.

84. Gottheimer, V. (1968) Long range strenuous sport training for cardiac reconditioning and rehabilitation. *Am. J. Cardiol.*, **22,** 426.

85. Rechnitzer, P. A., Pickard, H. A., Paivio, A. V., Yuhasz, M. S. and Cunningham, D. (1972) Long term follow up study of survival and recurrence rates following myocardial infarction in exercising and control subjects. *Circulation*, **45,** 853.

86. Fox, S. M. (1973) Relationship of activity habits to coronary heart disease. In *Exercise Testing and Exercise Training in Coronary Disease*, ed. Naughton, J. and Hellerstein, H. K., New York: Academic Press.

87. Bonanno, J. A. and Lies, J. E. (1974) Effects of physical training on coronary risk factors. *Am. J. Cardiol.*, **33,** 761.

88. Scheur, J., Penpargkul, S. and Bhan, A. K. (1974) Experimental observations on the effects of physical training on intrinsic cardiac physiology and biochemistry. *Am. J. Cardiol.*, **33,** 744.

89. Cash, J. D. (1966) Effect of moderate exercise on the fibrinolytic system in normal young men and women. *Br. med. J.*, **ii,** 502.

90. Menon, I. S., Burke, F. and Durar, H. A. (1966) Effect of strenuous and graded exercise on fibrinolytic activity. *Lancet*, **ii,** 700.

91. Wald, N., Howard, S., Smith, P G. and Kjeldsen, K. (1973) Association between atherosclerotic diseases and carboxyhaemoglobin levels in tobacco smokers. *Br. med. J.*, **i,** 761.

92. Castleden, C. M. and Cole, P. V. (1975) Carboxyhaemoglobin levels of smokers and non-smokers working in the city of London. *Br. J. ind. Med.*, **32,** 115.

93. Wald, N., Howard, S., Smith, P. G. and Bailey, A. (1975) Use of carboxyhaemoglobin levels to predict the development of diseases associated with cigarette smoking. *Thorax*, **30,** 133.

94. Roskamm, H. (1967) Optimum patterns of exercise for healthy adults. *Can med Ass. J.*, **96,** 895.
95. Cantwell, J. D. and Fletcher, G. F. (1969) Cardiac complications while jogging. *J Am. med. Assoc.*, **210,** 130.

9

Team medical care

Introduction

For doctors associated with a sporting team or governing body of sport, the main point to emphasize is that the major championship occasion is the exceptional highlight in what should be a continuing programme of medical care for a team or squad. The various general medical aspects have been described in Chapter 7 and it is emphasized that the routine medical checks and fitness tests applied over the seasons should form the basis of mutual trust between the doctor and sportsman, and between both parties and the team management and coaches. All too often, teams meet a doctor for the first time at the point of departure for a major event, and it is then not possible at such short notice for many avoidable medical problems to be prevented. Often there is the bitter complaint by a team doctor that he is simply presented with a group of assorted mental, medical, and locomotor cripples about whose medical backgrounds he is totally uninformed. The governing bodies of sports have a responsibility in this respect; various degrees of supervision exist within the different sports and National Olympic Associations.

Why a team doctor? While it may seem an unnecessary luxury, indeed a pandering to a spoilt élite, to provide a doctor for travelling sportsmen, many teams have learnt from bitter past experience that it is often simpler, cheaper, and far more effective to take a doctor to a distant venue than to rely on the vagaries of fortune and the sort of *ad hoc* 'middle-of-the-night' multilingual arrangements that may sometimes have to occur in case of emergency. It is hoped that the provision of a competent team physician may lift a considerable burden of worry from the team management on the one hand and reassure the sportsmen on the other.

The team physician's role in relation to a specific championship event starts with his assessment of the competitive venue with its associated problems. The various components such as altitude, temperature, and humidity will be taken into account and he will be required to advise on appropriate clothing, diets and supplements, inoculation procedures, and travel and acclimatization arrangements. Most major events, in fact, provide full medical cover in the form of highly competent clinics. What problems do arise relate mainly to the scale of major games and the language problems involved. It may take a considerable time to secure simple treatment for a simple complaint in a major games environment, whereas the team's physician may reduce this inconvenience to an absolute minimum by being on the spot to deal with it.

The question of the team physician's medical bag will be a fairly individual one. Clearly there are basic essential drugs which will be broadly similar to those required in the average general practice situation. Additional medications may be required because of particular circumstances applying locally, e.g. salt tablets for hot climates. Further equipment such as simple surgical and suturing kit will depend largely on the practitioner's own wishes and competence: it is useful to be able to offer simple surgical emergency treatment of minor wounds. Most doctors will find that a timely approach to the pharmaceutical industry will be sympathetically met by the donation of drugs and equipment. The regular team physician will wish to keep his own personal team trunk, perhaps with a small portable first aid and travel kit separately.

On arrival at a competition venue the team physician will seek an early contact with his local opposite numbers and should have little difficulty in establishing a good rapport and access to both diagnostic and treatment facilities.

The question of supporting ancillary medical staff for teams is often raised. This is partly because many of today's sports teams become accustomed to passive massage as part of their psychological preparation for competition. This is in contradistinction to the role of the properly qualified physiotherapist whose treatments will be specifically related to diagnosed lesions. If a registered physiotherapist accompanies a team then it is reasonable for him or her to be provided with those items of equipment found to be most useful. On the other hand, there is no reason why a masseur should not be welcomed as a useful member of a team, and in many team situations it is the masseur who acts as general factotum-cum-father confessor and unofficial personnel manager. Provided that he does not overstep his limits of competence and enter the slippery realms of diagnosis, then no harm should be done and there is no reason why a medical practitioner should not be able to co-operate happily with a good masseur.

Travel problems

Departure times are usually dictated by the general management's charter arrangements but it is importan, for team and management alike to understand the physiological adjustments required when moving across time zones. Hauty and Adams[1] shifting volunteer populations, established some useful guidelines. With direct north-south transportations there were no undue disturbances in circadian rhythms, though obviously the fatigue associated with travel was disruptive. With a 10-hour journey westwards it took roughly four days to realign the normal diurnal temperature variation to normal, with some eight days being required for adjustment of sweating mechanisms, and two days for reaction times to speed up to normal levels. By contrast a 10-hour journey eastwards showed longer adjustment times by factors of about 50 per cent over westward shifts.

These figures are given simply to indicate that there are problems of circadian readjustment involved in team travel, and that a wise management will make good allowance for them in shifting sportsmen. Just as the executive is strongly advised against going into conference directly from the aeroplane, so is it also asking almost the impossible of an athlete to perform at his best directly after a long journey. Having said this, it should be pointed out that there is considerable individual variation and that the general excitement associated with travel and the team situation often helps to produce surprisingly good performances in spite of inadequate acclimatization. It must be stressed that two or three days are necessary for most people to adjust adequately to any new environment in terms of living conditions, sleep, and diet. The team should be told that if the journey itself is not broken at frequent intervals then a habit should be made of walking about fairly frequently on the train or aeroplane in order to prevent undue vascular stasis in the legs. Travel sickness is fairly unusual and is simply dealt with by any of the standard remedies. Very rarely there may occur an acute claustrophobic crisis in transit which may have fairly alarming repercussions on the team. One such situation was resolved by the application of gentle psychotherapy on one side of the unfortunate victim and the positioning of a very large manager on the other!

Traveller's diarrhoea

Travellers' diarrhoea is notoriously crippling if a team's dietary and hygiene environment is poor. After much mystery and study[2-6] and years of eponymous description (Delhi belly, G.I. trots, Montezuma's revenge, etc.) the mundane truth is that travellers' diarrhoea usually occurs shortly after arrival in a new environment and is caused by exposure to an unaccustomed strain of *Escherichia coli*.[7] This causes a self-limiting attack of diarrhoea. Its significance to the athlete with his other problems of adjustment and his need to continue high quality training and competition is obvious. As so often, prevention is better than cure and scrupulous attention to hygiene, starting with supervision of the team's diet and drinking water, and extending through deliberate instruction to avoid exposure to uncertified drinking water, unpeeled fruit and salad, as well as ice-cream, should virtually prevent the occurrence of this problem.[8]

It has been a time-honoured custom to take prophylactic medicines against travellers' diarrhoea. Both Streptotriad and similar sulpha drugs have been widely advocated with evidence of success.[5] Entero-Vioform (iodochlorhydroxyquinoline) has also been used with effect.[9,10] However, dietary indiscretions, especially when associated with alcoholic excess, will cause diarrhoea whether these prophylactics are taken or not. Also changes in diet or methods of food preparation can by a purely chemical effect alter the nature and consistency of the stool to cause looseness (or constipation!). The stress of competition may itself cause anxiety-induced diarrhoea, often confused with travellers' diarrhoea.

Bacterial dysenteries are largely preventable diseases if simple hygiene precautions are applied. One has therefore to ask whether prophylactic treatments are necessary at all. In this context the widely documented side-effects of streptomycin and the sulphonomides[11] need no further recording, and recently documented evidence of neurological disease following admittedly very high doses of Entero-vioform[12,13] suggest that these therapies are not without risk. This is especially important when it is remembered that today's top athletes may travel the world frequently and thus be exposed to repeated small doses of these drugs— the classical way of producing subsequent sensitivity. Cases of typical drug rash have been seen following the first doses of Streptotriad in a team previously exposed to this drug.[14] The blunt chemical approach should therefore be discarded in favour of the more reasoned application of dietary and hygiene advice. In the event of the occurrence of travellers' diarrhoea there is usually a prompt response to kaolin mixtures or simple codeine phosphate. The latter, in 30 mg tablet form, has the advantage of compactness and convenience, and is highly effective. It should, however, be noted that codeine metabolites may interfere with dope tests and that whatever the physician's personal feelings, non-opiate derivatives should be used within twelve hours of competition. Acute gastrointestinal illnesses should be dealt with by bed rest in addition to any necessary antiemetic or bowel sedating measures, and particular care should be taken over hygiene as in most team situations there may be room sharing to the point of frank over-crowding.

Sunburn

Sunburn may cause prickly heat or frank burning. Prickly heat (miliaria) is due to blocking of the sweat glands in a hot atmosphere, so that efficient sweating is prevented. This may be a most disabling condition and if someone is known to be sensitive to prickly heat, particular attention should be paid when he moves to a sunnier sports environment so that carefully conditioned exposure to sun is planned and the risk of acute exposure avoided.

   Sunburn itself is often unexpectedly severe, for instance at altitude or where there is sufficient wind present for the immediate burning effect not to be noted. Ideally, sunburn should be avoided in a team by the careful instruction of individuals in the technique of dosed exposure day by day. However, despite precautions, one usually meets one or two individuals with severe sunburn in any given team. While claims have been made for the prophylactic effect of vitamin A preparations[15] such as Sylvasun, it would be wise to publicize the use of mechanical barrier creams such as Uvistat (mexenone 4%, Ward Blenkinsop) if athletes are to be exposed to strong sunlight.

Insect bites

Insect bites are often a problem, perhaps more frequently when a team is exposed to a foreign environment containing insects such as mosquitoes to which the transferred population has no resistance. This may call for the provision of insect repellent creams and lotions beforehand and antihistamine tablets and soothing applications, such as calamine, for subsequent treatment.

General

The doctor has a further role to play in respect of prevention of foreseeable medical problems such as those arising from footwear. The usual problems are the provision of new shoes to teams so that the chances of blistering are high during competition and, in hot situations, the popularity of 'flip-flops' which leads to a high incidence of stubbing of toes that may seriously impede competitive chances.

   The team physician should be fully familiar with regulations regarding doping and sex testing where applicable, and even this may not be as simple as it sounds. The doping regulations applied at major games are not based upon drugs therapeutically useful but on drugs thought possibly to be able to help performance. There may well be occasions when the physician is in some difficulty when he wishes to select one of the 'prohibited' drugs for legitimate medical treatment. It can also be extremely embarrassing for a competitor on a major occasion to be found to have been cheating his own team physician in respect of the taking of stimulant drugs detected on dope tests!

At the present time the major problems concern the control of asthma and allergic conditions. The situation is far from finalized, though it is fair to say that the International Olympic Committee and its Medical Commission, as well as the medical committees of the major sports, do try to keep therapeutic and doping situations under constant surveillance in order to be fair to the individual patient as well as to prevent cheating.

The question of anabolic steroids has recently been prominent and now that there are adequate radio-immunoassay methods available for screening tests it is hoped that these drugs will no longer be a source of difficulty in sport[16] (see also Chapter 12).

In some sports, notably athletics, a female is required to produce evidence of her femininity in order to be eligible for international competition. While the application of 'sex tests' may seem amusing for normal women, embarrassments have arisen in the past with the disqualification of chromosomally abnormal women. Even though in such cases full karyotyping and a full gynaecological examination take place before any disqualification, the real point is that no such situation should be allowed to happen under the full glare of publicity associated with major international competition. It follows, therefore, that all female athletes should be properly tested, classified, and certified at an early stage in their careers (see also Chapter 10).

The role of the team doctor is potentially important in that while no credit belongs to the idle, the prompt and cool management of potentially disastrous situations can be of inestimable value to team morale and performance. If the physician can command the respect and confidence of competitors and officials alike, he may then play an important part in helping to produce the best performance from his team. He is uniquely placed to see the interplay of personalities between team members and the team and its managers, and perhaps to influence matters, hopefully for the better. It should be emphasized that the place of the team doctor is with his team and that the acceptance of the privilege of accompanying a team constitutes a full-time commitment to that team. While it may be impossible to cover all the sports venues and training areas at once in a team comprising several different sports the physician should nonetheless make every effort to be available on a regular basis for informal surgery consultations, and try and make a point of spreading his attentions to all factions within the team.

There will inevitably be situations where the physician finds himself offering considerable support to some members of the team who may have difficulty coping with the stress of competition and the emotional demands involved, and there is considerable scope for helping athletes with their own personality problems in this context. As Carstairs[17] so eloquently put it, 'athletes may be as delicately tuned as race horses ... the highly trained athlete can easily become hypochondriac and excessively concerned about minor physical discomforts or trivial ailments. It seems that the very act of training makes one abnormally aware of one's physical functioning, and when this happens, athletes paradoxically find themselves in danger of joining the ranks of the psychoneurotics'. It is thus easy to see how important can be the role of the team doctor especially in the very high stress situations of major championships. The teams will often contain young novices who need considerable support and there are often characters present who seem fated to drag the whole team's morale down to their own poor level.

The behaviour of coaches or officials may at times add to a competitor's personal uncertainties, and in this respect tactful adjustment of the situation by the physician may be possible. It is also true to say that a number of athletes are, by definition, selfish and difficult characters who thrive on the antagonisms found in team situations, and who urgently require conflict with the authority figures of the team management. Adding the conflicts engendered by those physically magnificent athletes who seem to have to fail on the big day itself, it is possible to see the rich scope available for the physician interested in human behaviour. While the psychological aspects of sport are well covered in Chapter 3, the team physician may perhaps best function at the level of general purpose confidant and physician/psychiatrist because he may in fact be dealing with major or minor degrees of psychiatric stress to the point of illness. It is probably generally agreed now that staleness is a form of depression which may call for considerable psychotherapeutic support, perhaps from the doctor, or perhaps from the doctor together with the coach or manager. On rare occasions it may require specific antidepressant drug therapy. There is much scope for the use of sympathetic discussion, reassurance, and occasionally the use of placebo medication to tide the athlete over his or her crisis.

Bearing in mind that the team situation involves repercussions of individual problems through a team, it is particularly important that the physician should try to keep a constant control of the variables leading to personal psychological stress and breakdown. The borderline between success and failure in modern terms is so fine as to be virtually non-existent. Bearing in mind the need to balance perfectly the degree of arousal against the level of performance, the deliberate manipulation of morale becomes an important variable in team management. Too often, the team's officials are remote from the team, and the lack of elementary psychological knowledge in team management can add considerable stress to a team. Thus a potentially good team may perform badly under ideal circumstances, and an indifferent team may rise above itself in competition against all odds. Poor conditions such as unpleasant accommodation and bad diet may actually act as very powerful stimulants to good team morale if the management can cope with the situation. By contrast ideal arrangements may be completely sabotaged by unsympathetic and out-of-touch management. Considering the tension that must be generated when a young sportsman, (perhaps only a teenager) faces major competition in front of an audience of perhaps one-hundred thousand spectators, it requires little imagination to realize that a number of these sportsmen will not be able to cope successfully with this stress. The repercussions may well involve aggressive behaviour towards team mates and officials. Here the role of the team doctor is potentially one of considerable importance as he is in the privileged position of sitting on the invisible fence between team and management while being privy to the secrets of both. A consequent danger is that, by the close identification necessary with his team in order to help contain their problems, he may fall foul of the management and be regarded as yet another potentially hostile element. The opposite danger is equally unfortunate, especially if the doctor makes little attempt to identify with his team—he is regarded by the team as yet another manager and therefore by them also as another potentially hostile element! The successful team doctor has ideally to be 'all things to all men'.

In conclusion, it will be seen that there is much in favour of the integrated role of the team physician in the team structure of spor*sman, coach, and manager. Only in this way is it likely that the team will be nelped to achieve its optimum results under stress, and only in this way is the long-term mutual confidence engendered which can develop a squad's performance gradually and happily over a period of years. From this and the preceding chapters it will be clear that there is no one sort of doctor who makes the perfect team physician. Sound knowledge of general medicine and a healthy dose of common sense are pre-requisites. The ability to identify with the conflicting elements present in any team is essential, and a close understanding of the particular techniques and injuries related to the sports involved can on occasion play a decisive role.

P.N.S.

References

1. Hauty, G. T. and Adams, J. (1966) Phase shifts of the human circadian system and performance deficit during periods of transition. *Aerospace Med.*, **37**, 7, 10, 12.
2. Kean, B. H. and Waters, S. (1958) The diarrhoea of travellers. *A.M.A. Archs ind. Hlth*, **18**, 148.
3 Kean, B. H. and Waters, S. (1959) The Diarrhoea of travellers. *New Engl. J. Med.*, **261**, 71.
4. Kean, B. H., Schaffner, W., Brennan, R. W. and Waters, S. (1962) The Diarrhoea of travellers. *J. Am. med. Ass.*, **180**, 367.
5. Turner, A. C. (1967) Traveller's diarrhoea: a survey of symptoms, occurrence and possible prophylaxis. *Br. med. J.*, **iv**, 653.
6. Sperryn, P. N. (1968) The prophylaxis of traveller's diarrhoea in athletes. *Br. Ass. Sports Med. Bull.*, **3**, 124.
7. Rowe, B., Taylor, J. and Bettelheim, K. A. (1970) An investigation of travellers' diarrhoea. *Lancet*, **i**, 1.
8. Woodruff, A. W. (1965) Personal communication.
9. Anonymous (1957) Queries and minor notes. *J. Am. med. Ass.*, **164**, 505.
10. Richards, D. A. (1970) A controlled trial in traveller's diarrhoea. *Practitioner*, **204**, 822.
11. Anonymous (1972) Martindale: The Extra Pharmacopoeia, 26th edition, ed. Blacow, N. W., London: The Pharmaceutical Press.
12. Nakac, K., Yamamoto, S., Shigematsu, I. and Kono, R. (1973) Relationship between subacute myelo-optic neuropathy (S.M.O.N.) and Clioquinol: nationwide survey. *Lancet*, **i**, 171.
13. (a) Spillane, J. D. (1971) Correspondence. *Lancet*, **ii**, 1371.
    (b) Spillane, J. D. (1972) Correspondence. *Lancet*, **i**, 154.
14. Sperryn, P. N. (1967) Medical Report, Universiade 1967. British Universities Sports Federation.
15. Turner, A. C., Barnes, R. M. and Green, R. L. (1971) The effect of a preparation of vitamin A and calcium carbonate on sunburn. *Practitioner*, **206**, 662.
16. Sperryn, P. N. (Ed.) (1975) Proceedings of International Symposium on anabolic steroids in sport. *Br. J. sports Med.*, **9**, 2.
17. Carstairs, G. M. (1970) Psychology of athletic performance. Second Adolphe Abrahams Memorial Lecture. *Br. J. sports Med.*, **2**, 73.

10

Women in sport

In childhood, there is very little difference between boys and girls as regards capacity for physical activity and what difference there is would seem slightly to favour the girls, who in development are a little in advance of boys up to puberty. From late adolescence onwards, the boys rapidly outstrip the girls in physical development. They are capable of more prolonged and strenuous activity although it seems that there remains little difference in the capacity to develop motor skill. With puberty, the male and female bodies take on their typical forms expressing the secondary sexual characteristics.

Body form and sex

It is because of the characteristic differences in body form and function that physiological performance capacity in many activities shows such marked difference between the sexes. This, in turn, has necessitated the separation of men from women for fair sporting competition in certain events, particularly since historically so many sports evolved from activities specifically developed to foster and bring out martial or virile characteristics involving feats of strength and endurance. In the past, female participation in sport and physical recreation was discouraged mainly for aesthetic and cultural reasons. Whatever the argument of the Women's Lib movement, it remains true that even today female competitors in many sports are unable to take on men on equal terms. The answer to the argument that prizes for female tennis players in international tournaments should be as great as those given for men is that the women should show the same level of performance capacity. In fact, the women are probably better off as they are since it is unlikely that a woman tennis player, however good, could play sufficiently well in open world tennis to gain from open tournaments the same financial rewards that she can presently gain from closed tennis tournaments for women only.

Women therefore by virtue of their sex are at a disadvantage in a very large number of sports. The nature of the characteristic differences in body form is variable. Certainly there are some women who are relatively manly in physique, as there are some men who are relatively feminine but, as there is wide variation in body type within a given height and weight range, a degree of overlap must be expected.[1] Even so there are certain physical characteristics, as also physiological characteristics, which tend to be more prominent in women than men. The ratio of lean body mass to adipose tissue is one of the most obvious[2] as is the presence of the breasts.

Skeletal differences include a greater bone strength and density in the male,[3] and a greater degree of pelvic tilt and obliquity in the female associated with oblique femoral axes.[4] At the same time, women also have a greater carrying angle and tendency to cubitus valgus at the elbow.[5] All of these characteristics tend to militate against high quality performance in most sports. Where women do, however, score, is in flexibility, since mean joint range is greater, on average, in women than men.[6] Furthermore, relative differences in stature may be of advantage to women in certain activities such as equitation.

Differentiation of sex

In order to make for fair competition for women, some means have to be found to exclude men. This makes for immediate difficulties since it is impossible to define precisely what is meant by 'woman'.[7] Most people have a clear subjective idea of femininity and the vast majority of women share definable characteristics with their sisters, characteristics which are not apparent in those who are clearly of the male sex. The borderline between the presence and absence of individual characteristics may be quite clear cut, but these borderlines may not coincide when the characteristics are assembled in a given individual.[8] It is with the small number of cases in which there is overlap of the borderlines that problems arise, since in such situations, an individual may be variously classified as male or female according to the particular characteristics utilized as criteria for defining sex. The number of available characteristics for such definition is quite large.

The sex of the individual is essentially determined by the chromosomes which in development must give rise to an individual with the correct gonad. This in turn must produce the appropriate hormones to induce correct development and form in the genitalia and of the secondary sexual characteristics. Such hormonal control must be maintained through puberty while the individual must have developed an outlook appropriate to his or her actual sex.

Problems relating to chromosomes readily arise. The male is essentially XY and female XX. Absence or a duplication of certain chromosomes produces peculiar patterns, for example, the XXY of the male Klinefelter syndrome or the XO of the female Turner's syndrome (to say nothing of the mixed chromosomal patterns seen in mosaics). Differentiation between male and female using the chromosome pattern has hitherto depended upon the presence and number of X chromosomes; in subjects with the XX configuration, nuclear chromatin material can be demonstrated in a significant percentage of cells. In the majority of cases this would serve to indicate female origin of the cellular material, but in Klinefelter syndrome, although the presence of chromatins suggests femininity, the individual having a Y chromosome in addition to the two X's is clearly male. By a similar process, the patient with Turner's syndrome having only one X chromosome although female, presents as male on nuclear chromatin testing. Even more confusion may occur in cases of mosaics. Lest male chauvinists feel unduly complacent, the significance of certain male chromosmal abnormalities is still under review following the discovery that the XYY configuration was associated with an increase in the rate of admission to maximum security hospitals. While the social and psychological characteristics of these individuals are still being defined, they tend to be taller than average males, and possibly more aggressive. As these may conceivably offer athletic advantage, a day may be foreseen when male athletes could also be required to display normal XY chromosomal configuration.[9,10]

Normally, under the influence of the appropriate chromosome, the individual develops a testis or an ovary. In some rare situations, as in some cases of mosaic, both ovary and testis may be present in the same person. Such an individual may well be brought up as a female and exhibit many of the characteristics of a female, and yet, from the point of view of differentiation by gonad, must be defined in one sense as male as having a testis.

The developing gonads produce appropriate hormones to stimulate development of genitalia, and (in puberty) the secondary sexual characteristics. Occasionally, however, the hormone balance becomes disturbed as a result of which the individual is modified in development. Relatively the commonest example is adrenal virilism in which the suprarenal gland produces male hormones in a female, thus giving rise to considerable masculinization.

In testicular feminization, which is rare, but which produces grave difficulties, the patient has XY chromosomes and has testes, but the hormonal response is female and the individual presents in all respects as a female, although infertile. Such an individual is by virtually all definitions female, but, having a testis and an XY chromosome, must be capable of definition as male on chromosomal and gonadal grounds.

Even where there is no genetic gonadal or biochemical disorder, anatomical development may still be impaired and, in extreme cases, the sex of the individual thereby concealed and the individual in consequence brought up on the wrong side of the line; specifically, males appear to be females due to failure of development of the genitalia.

Finally, the sex of an individual can be disturbed psychologically. In this context, homosexuality is of little relevance but transvestitism may complicate the issue. It must therefore be understood that although in the vast majority of cases, the definition of sex as far as the demands of sporting activity are concerned is a relatively simple matter, there remain a small proportion of individuals in the intersex zone who need immensely delicate and sympathetic handling. Fortunately, at the present time, it is accepted that one test is not sufficient to determine the functional sex of an individual in these difficult cases. In general, female athletes requiring to prove their femininity before admission to athletic competition who fail to establish their femininity in the first instance, are permitted to go through a series of examinations of progressive thoroughness. Much further study needs to be completed, however, before a perfectly effective means of determining the sex of an individual for purposes of sports competition has been finally achieved.

Physical activity in females

The woman by virtue of her special role in the process of reproduction exhibits not only changes in degree in the distribution or character of the general body tissues but also peculiarities of form and function strictly her own which are relevant to the context of sport and physical recreation. The periodic cycle of ovulation and menstruation produces not only local changes in the gonads but also general physiological disturbances which may be quite profound. The development of the embryo following conception alters not merely the woman's general physiological behaviour but also drastically modifies, if only temporarily, body structure particularly that of the abdomen. After parturition, during the puerperium and later, involutional changes are taking place, while lactation may increase the particular problems posed in respect of certain types of physical activity by the presence of the female breast.

Menstruation

The effects of menstruation on the individual subject vary enormously. In some individuals, the cycle progresses throughout its entirety without any apparent disturbance. In others, the changes are quite profound and may indeed be sufficient to give rise to regular periods of significant incapacity. In the majority of cases, the cycle gives rise to little apparent disability, though the physiological changes which take place may significantly affect human physical performance. For example, the weight gain associated with water retention during the premenstrual period will clearly be disadvantageous as will the feeling of dragging in the abdomen as well as the fullness if not discomfort felt in the breasts. Psychological changes are also demonstrable during the cycle, showing considerable fluctuation in the level of intellectual and psychological performance capacity.[11]

Physical activity has frequently been shown to improve the woman's capacity to cope with the physiological changes in menstruation, and indeed it has in some series been shown that physical training is a valuable means in the treatment of dysmenorrhoea.[12] The effects of menstrual periodicity on physical performance have also been studied.[13] Although there is some individual variation, the majority of women do tend to perform less well during the premenstruum, and most female athletes are able by observation over a significant number of cycles to pinpoint the time phases of each cycle during which they are at their best and at their worst. Those who are disadvantaged by the physiological function of menstruation can have their menstrual cycles adjusted so that their competitive events occur at the optimum time of their cycle. Oestrogens, progestogens or progesterone can be used alone or in combination. Each group has its own indications and applications.

Menstrual control

Sportswomen tend to be young, healthy, nulliparous females, who must be able to maintain a steady, consistent performance of high quality in which even slight variations spell defeat. Their best performances are frequently achieved in those years during which sexual development is occurring, for once full development is complete the peak may be passed. Undoubtedly the menstrual hormones play an important part in any sportswoman's career, but it is not possible to generalize about their influence. It is just as erroneous to say that all sportswomen are affected by menstruation as it is to say that none are affected. For each woman the influence of menstruation is a personal and very individual effect, and the old adage 'know thyself' is vital to success. The only way in which this essential knowledge can be obtained is by meticulous recording on a personal menstrual chart of every variation in performance together with the dates of menstruation. It is then possible to discover whether performance is related to a particular phase of the menstrual cycle, and which hormone levels are most advantageous. Many sportswomen are mesomorphs, and therefore not so markedly influenced by menstrual hormones.

Menstrual hormones

A full understanding of the menstrual hormones entails an appreciation of the various organs involved together with the feedback mechanisms. The hormones are: the hypothalamic releasing factors which act on the pituitary; the follicle stimulating hormone (FSH), and the luteinising hormone (LH) which are pro-

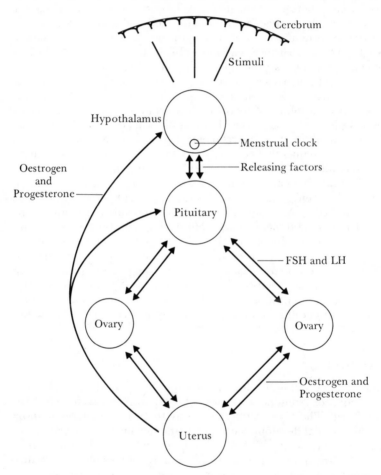

Fig. 10.1 Menstrual hormones.

duced by the pituitary and act on the ovaries; and oestrogen and progesterone produced in the ovaries and which act on the endometrium (Fig. 10.1). At each and all levels there is a feedback mechanism controlling the entire system. The menstrual regulating centre, or menstrual clock, is situated in the hypothalamus where it is easily influenced by cerebral stimuli.

Menarche

In the United Kingdom the average age for the first menstruation has been found to be between 13·1 and 13·4 years[14,15] with a range from 11 to 16 years. The exact timing of the menarche is influenced by genetic, racial, socio-economic, and climatic factors.[16] Pubertal development begins with a gradual increase in breast size and the sprouting of pubic and axillary hair, which proceeds slowly for some two years before the first menstrual loss, and these changes continue for a further two years after the menarche. At the same time secondary skeletal changes are taking place with broadening of the female pelvis and an increase in the carrying angle of the arms.

Normally, menstruation will have commenced by the age of 17 years. If it has not, a physical examination should be made to ascertain the presence or absence of pubertal development. Where there are signs of breast growth and pubic hair it may be assumed that there is merely a delay in development, and menstruation may be expected to occur naturally. In the absence of breast and secondary hair development, endocrinological investigations should be undertaken to discover the cause of this primary amenorrhoea.

Normal menstruation

At the menarche the duration of loss may be 2 to 9 days, but it is usually scanty. This duration gradually decreases so that by the age of 16 years it lasts for an average of 6 days, which is nevertheless longer than it will be in adult life when the duration averages 4 days with a range from 2 to 7 days.[17]

The normal adult menstrual cycle varies from 21 to 35 days, and is rarely that precise 28 days suggested in biology text books, except when controlled artificially by hormone therapy. It is important to appreciate that among normal healthy 16-year-olds as many as 20 per cent still have cycles exceeding 40 days. Often in adolescence the cycle may become shorter when a regular boy friend is on the scene, but if the attachment is broken off the girl may revert to her long irregular cycle.

Both the length of the cycle and the duration of loss may be affected by stress. This was well demonstrated among 91 boarding school girls sitting their 'O' level examinations[18] (Fig. 10.2). The number of girls menstruating each day during examination week is compared with the preceding weeks. The increase in menstruations occurred during this period of stress, because some girls had a shortened cycle, others a lengthened cycle; some found the duration of loss prolonged into examination week, and yet others missed menstruation entirely during this critical week. The effect of stress on menstruation is variable, although the pattern of each individual tends to remain the same throughout life, either in the alteration of the cycle or the duration of loss. The stress may be of the positive happy variety, e.g. weddings, promotion, etc., or of the negative type such as failure, bereavement or jilting.[19] It is interesting that when women live together in dormitories or on the college campus their menstrual cycles tend gradually to synchronize so that after some months there is a tendency for them all to menstruate at the same time.

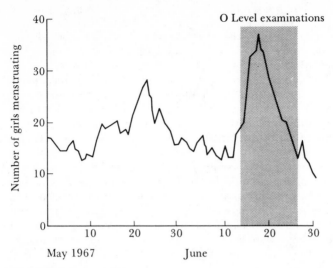

Fig. 10.2 Effect of 'O' level examinations on 91 menstruating schoolgirls. (From Dalton, K.[18] by permission of the publishers.)

Dysmenorrhoea

Two distinct types of primary dysmenorrhoea have been distinguished, and as the treatment is different it is important to differentiate the types, spasmodic and congestive.[20]

Spasmodic dysmenorrhoea
This only occurs in ovular cycles, so its onset is about two years after the menarche and it ends after a full term pregnancy. The pain presents suddenly on the first day of menstrual loss with a colicky, lower abdominal spasmodic pain occurring at intervals of 5 to 20 minutes. The girl may appear pale and shocked and is eased by lying down curled around a hot water bottle. The pain is limited to the perineum, but there may be reflex vomiting or fainting. The pain subsides by the second or third day of menstruation. Gynaecological examination is invariably normal. During the acute phase analgesics and antispasmo⁴ᵢcs are indicated. The specific treatment is oestrogen therapy, which needs to be started on day 5 and continued for 21 days. Ethinyloestradiol (10–100 µg daily) or an oestrogen-progestogen contraceptive preparation may be used. It should be continued for at least six months and then gradually reducing doses used. If only partial relief is obtained, the dose of oestrogen should be increased in subsequent months, while if there is no menstruation on stopping the course the dose should be lowered.

Congestive dysmenorrhoea
This may begin with the menarche and increase in severity after each pregnancy. It has a gradual onset some days before menstruation with a lower abdominal, heavy, continuous, dragging pain increasing with the onset of menstruation. Usually there are accompanying symptoms of the premenstrual syndrome with ten-

sion, abdominal bloatedness, weight gain, nausea, headaches, joint pains, acne, and oedema. In mild cases diuretics may be helpful, but the specific treatment is progesterone as discussed under treatment of the premenstrual syndrome.

Premenstrual syndrome
This covers any symptoms which recur regularly at the same phase of the menstrual cycle: usually they occur just before and at the beginning of menstruation but occasionally also at ovulation. The commonest symptoms are tension (with depression, irritability and lethargy), headache, asthma, weight gain, bloatedness, rhinitis, joint pains, and acne. The symptoms usually abate quite suddenly with the onset of the full menstrual flow. The premenstrual syndrome tends to increase in severity with age and parity, especially if the pregnancies have been complicated by toxaemia or puerperal depression. It is therefore unlikely that severe cases of the premenstrual syndrome will occur in competing sportswomen. The treatment of this syndrome is the administration of progesterone by suppositories or pessaries in an initial dose of 200 or 400 mg daily from midcycle until the onset of menstruation. If symptoms occur at ovulation then treatment may be commenced on day 12 and continued until menstruation. If the initial dose regime is successful an attempt may be made gradually to shorten the course or reduce the dosage to a level compatible with full relief of symptoms. If the initial dose does not completely relieve symptoms then the dose may be increased to 400 mg thrice daily by suppositories or pessaries. Diuretics are helpful if there is bloatedness or weight gain, but they do not affect the psychological symptoms of depression, irritability, or lethargy.

Variations with menstruations
In studies of large populations of women between 15 and 55 years of varying parity, it has been shown that during the 8 days of the paramenstruum (4 days before and the first 4 days of menstruation) there is an increase in accident proneness,[21] lowering of mental ability,[18,22] lowered resistance to infection,[23] increased suicide attempts,[24 26] and increased hospitalization. Nevertheless it is important to appreciate that for each individual there are rarely more than 2 or 3 days when she is at greatest risk. It is up to each individual, by careful recording, to appreciate her own specific pattern. Those showing variations in sporting performances are advised to record on their menstrual chart the dates on which they are off peak[27,28] (Fig. 10.3). While some of the common variants are normally detrimental to sporting performance as well as in everyday life, at least one of them could result in improved performance, namely the increase in aggression which occurs in premenstrual tension. Detrimental variants to sportswomen include the temporary and minor rise in intra–ocular pressure, which assumes importance in those sports requiring high visual acuity. A rise in weight occurs at ovulation in some women, and in others during the premenstruum, and may be reflected in lowered performance. Hand and arm steadiness vary during the cycle with the greatest unsteadiness occurring during menstruation and then during the premenstruum.[29] Simple reaction time does not appear to differ during the menstrual cycle in normal healthy individuals,[13,30] suggesting that it is the judgement and mental ability which are decreased, resulting in increased accident proneness during the premenstruum. Even a slight degree of premenstrual

	Jan.	Feb.	Mar.	Apr.
1				
2		✓		✓
3				
4				
5	✓			
6		✓		
7		✓		
8				
9			✓	
10				
11				
12			✓	
13			✓	
14	*			
15	*			✓
16	M *			✓
17	M			
18	M			
19	M	*		
20	M	*		
21		M		
22		M		
23		M	*M	*
24	✓	M	M	*
25	✓		M	M
26			M	M
27			M	M
28			M	M
29				M
30			✓	
31				
Total				

Fig. 10.3 Performance and menstruation. M, menstruation; ✓, good performance; *, poor performance.

dyspnoea due to engorgement of the bronchial or nasal mucosa may prove a handicap in many sports.

In a survey of female university students in Finland[31] it was found that those studying physical education and those who were actively engaged in sports had significantly less premenstrual tension and headaches, although the incidence of students between 19 and 22 years, as many as 22 were found by cytological smears and 17-ketosteroid estimations to have monophasic, anovular cycles, and in these students there were no differences in performance during the various phases of the menstrual cycle. Both these studies suggest that with sportswomen there is a self-selective process, in that only those women who find themselves little affected or completely unaffected by their menstrual hormonal pattern participate in competitive sports, which tends to debar those with the premenstrual syndrome and marked swings in performance, mood, and physical well-being.

Menstrual adjustment

For those sportswomen who are able to demonstrate consistent fluctuations at the same phase of each menstrual cycle, it is justifiable to adjust the time of menstruation so that the competition dates coincide with the time of maximum efficiency. Although the time of optimal performance is highly individual, it is frequently in the preovulation (days 9–12) or postovulation (days 17–20) phases, but there are also a few who perform best during menstruation. There are three groups of hormones which are available for this adjustment, which will usually bring on menstruation, or withdrawal bleeding, within 48 hours of stopping medication. If it is desired to shorten the cycle by only 2 or 3 days, or if the cycle is already overdue, then medication need only be given for 3 days, while if it is desired to shorten the cycle to 16 days then medication needs to be given continuously from day 5 until day 14.

Oestrogens
These are of value in those who tend to have immature sexual development or spasmodic dysmenorrhoea. The side-effects are nausea, headaches, weight gain and depression. They may be given as ethinyloestradiol ($10–50\,\mu$g daily) or may be administered as an oral contraceptive with a progestogen.

Progesterone
Progesterone is used in those with congestive dysmenorrhoea, premenstrual tension, bloatedness, cyclical weight swings, headaches, and mood swings. Unfortunately, it cannot be administered orally but can be absorbed per rectum or per vagina in doses of 200 to 400 mg daily.

Progestogens
Progestogens are useful for those with irregular or anovular menstruation. They can be administered orally either as norethisterone (5 mg) or as the progestogen-only pill. Progestogens cause proliferation of the endometrium but lower the blood progesterone level,[33] and so may cause or exacerbate premenstrual symptoms. Where there is no special indication for one particular group of hormones, then a contraceptive pill may be used containing $50\,\mu$g of oestrogen and some progestogen.

Single event
If help is sought to adjust the cycle some two or three months before a vital competition, then it is best to adjust it in the earliest available month so that the

	Jan.	Feb.	Mar.	Apr.	May	Jun.	Jul.
1					⋮		M
2					⋮		M
3					⋮		M	M
4					↓	M	
5						M	
6					M	M	
7					M		
8					M		
9						C	
10							
11							
12			M				
13			M				
14			M				
15			M	M			
16		M	M	↑			
17		M	M	⋮			
18	M	M		⋮			
19	M	M		⋮			
20	M			⋮			
21	M			⋮			
22				⋮			
23				⋮			
24				⋮			
25				⋮			
26				⋮			
27				⋮			
28				⋮			
29				⋮			
30				⋮			
31							
Total							

Fig. 10.4 Adjusting menstruation in a woman with regular cycles. The menstrual cycle in May was shortened. Normal menstruation occurred in June and July. M, menstruation; C, competition; ↑, treatment started; ⋮, treatment stopped.

sportswoman can compete during the critical cycle without medication. For example, in Fig. 10.4 poor performances were noted by the candidate in the late premenstruum and early menstruation in February to April. The menstrual cycle in May was shortened to 21 days by giving medication from day 5 to 19, and next two menstruations occurred at their normal interval, allowing the candidate to perform during her optimum phase of the postmenstruum. In Fig. 10.5 the time of the poor performances were again in the premenstruum, but the candidate had irregular menstruation with a cycle varying from 26 to 35 days. The men-

	Jan.	Feb.	Mar.	Apr.	May	Jun.	Jul.
1					:	↑	M
2					:	:	M
3					:	↓	M
4					:		M
5					:	M	
6					↓	M	
7						M	
8					M	M	
9						M	C
10						M	
11						M	
12							
13		M					
14		M					
15	M	M					
16	M	M					
17		M		M			
18	M			M			
19	M			M			
20	M			M			
21	M				↑		
22					:		
23					:		
24					:		
25					:		
26					:		
27					:		
28					:	↑	
29					:	:	
30					:	↓	
31							
Total							

Fig. 10.5 Adjusting menstruation in a woman with irregular cycles. Cycle length varies from 26 to 35 days. The menstrual cycle in May was shortened to 21 days. The June and July cycles were regularized with short 3-day courses of treatment. M, menstruation; C, competition; ↑, treatment stated; ⁝↓, treatment stopped.

strual cycle in May was again shortened to 21 days, but to avoid the possibility of a long cycle occurring in June or July 3-day courses of medication were given on days 24 to 26 of the cycle. In Fig. 10.6 the candidate only sought help nine days before the competition, which would leave insufficient time to shorten the cycle. She was therefore given progesterone suppositories to use each night until after the event. Although progestogens would also delay menstruation they would

	Jan.	Feb.	Mar.	Apr.	May	Jun.	Jul.
1							↑
2							:
3							:
4							:
5							:
6							:
7					M		:
8		M		M	M		:
9		M	M	M	M	C	:
10		M	M	M	M		↓
11		M	M	M	M		
12		M	M	M	M	M	
13		M	M	M	M	M	
14		M	M	M	M	M	
15			M			M	
16						M	
17						M	
18						M	
19							
20							
21							
22							
23							
24							
25							
26							
27							
28							
29							
30							
31							
Total							

Fig. 10.6 Late adjustment of menstruation. Late consultation only 9 days before event, treated with progesterone. Although progestogens will delay menstruation they will not prevent premenstrual deterioration of performance. M, menstruation; C, competition; ↑, treatment started; ↓, treatment stopped.

not have prevented the deterioration of performance which she experienced during the premenstruum, and may well have made it worse.

Continuous programme
For those sportswomen whose performances are affected by menstruation and who have a continuous programme of events, menstruation may be completely suppressed for a few months. The occasional withdrawal bleeding which may

occur during such a regime is usually scanty, free from symptoms, and does not affect performance. Oestrogen, progestogen or progesterone may be used alone or in combination, as in the contraceptive pill, with continual daily administration and with the dose lowered at monthly intervals compatible with complete suppression. Sufferers from spasmodic dysmenorrhoea in particular, benefit from a few months absence of menstruation and may well be free from dysmenorrhoea when it is resumed.

Following continuous suppression by hormones, normal menstruation usually restarts within a couple of months. However if menstruation is delayed longer than three months, a 5-day course of clomiphene will stimulate the hypothalamus and restart the menstrual cycle so that menstruation may be expected after a 3-weeks' intervals. Those who stop hormone therapy and are anxious to conceive should be advised to start recording their early morning temperatures to discover whether they have ovular or anovular cycles; if the latter then clomiphene is again indicated even though their menstruation may be regular. One complication of long-term hormone therapy, particularly with progestogens, is the gradual development of a loss of libido, but fortunately this improves on stopping treatment.

It might be mentioned here that progestogens are testosterone analogues, and while at present there is no objection to their use either alone or in the contraceptive pill in competitive sport, it is possible that at some future date testosterone and its derivatives may be added to the list of drugs banned to competing sportswomen.

Menstrual regulation by endometrial aspiration is being tested in the United Kingdom and elsewhere.[34,35] The products of menstruation are evacuated through a soft plastic 4 mm cannula, a process which takes only a minute or two. However, this sudden endometrial change from the premenstrual to postmenstrual phase is not necesarily followed by the same rapid alteration in the hormone levels of the hypothalamic–pituitary–ovarian axis, and there is no certainty that it will result in a rise in sporting performance. Further studies are needed to investigate the short-term and long-term effect of this method of menstrual regulation on the physical and psychological variants of the menstrual cycle.

The possibility of prostaglandins or their analogues being developed as safe, effective menstrual regulators is still in the realms of speculation.

Pregnancy

There is no evidence that a normally established pregnancy in a fit woman is threatened by exercise at any particular level. In some women with poor obstetric histories or with impaired health, however, the obstetrician may prescribe rest at various stages of pregnancy.

There is little doubt that physical fitness during pregnancy contributes to ease of parturition. Certainly what evidence has been accumulated suggests that childbirth is generally easier if individuals are of an athletic disposition.[36,37] Of all the forms of sporting activity available, swimming is perhaps the most satisfactory and is much to be encouraged for mothers-to-be.

Following delivery, a certain amount of physical activity will assist the process of involution but such activity should be relatively light; intense competitive activity is generally contraindicated for several months. This is particularly the case if the mother is nursing the child herself, since the lactating breast is relatively larger and more cumbersome than its normal counterpart, and is therefore to some extent liable to injury, quite apart from producing mechanical problems. Lactation too is physically demanding so that the nursing mother is best advised not to engage in strenuous physical exertion until lactation is over. Following satisfactory completion of pregnancy, delivery, and subsequent involution, there is no physical reason why sporting activity should not be taken up again and indeed there are many famous women champions who have gained their titles after childbirth.

Injuries and other conditions

Injuries to the vulva, perineum and pelvic viscera are covered in Chapter 23. The management of other gynaecological conditions such as salpingitis, moniliasis, or ovarian cyst in sportswomen does not differ significantly from that in the normal active population.

K.D.

J.G.P.W.

References

1. Croney, J. (1971) *Anthropometrics for Designers*. London: Batsford.
2. Edwards, D. A. (1951) Differences in the distribution of subcutaneous fat with sex and maturity. *Clin. Sci.*, **10**, 305.
3. Bradbury, C. E. (1949) *Anatomy and Construction of the Human Figure*. New York: McGraw-Hill.
4. Caffey, J., Ames, R., Silverman, W. A., Ryder, C. T. and Hough, G. (1956) Contradiction of congenital dysphasia—predislocation hypothesis of congenital dislocation of the hip through study of normal variation in acetabular angles at successive periods in infancy. *Paediatrics*, **17**, 632.
5. Atkinson, W. B. and Elftman, H. (1945) Carrying angle of the human arm as a secondary sex characteristic. *Anat. Rec.*, **91**, 49.
6. Hupprich, F. and Sigerseth, P. O. (1950) The specificity of flexibility in girls. *Res. Q. Am. Ass. Hlth phys. Fitness*, **21**, 25.
7. Lennox, B. (1968) Some observations on the difficulty of determining sex. *Bull. Br. Ass. sports Med.*, **3**, 80.
8. Francois, J. and Matton-Van Leuven, M. T. (1973) Sexual evaluation of 'female' athletes. *J. Sports Med.*, **1**, 3, 5.
9. Jacobs, P. A., Brunton, M., Melville, M. M., Brittain, R. P. and McLemont, W. F. (1965) Aggressive behaviour, mental subnormality and the XYY male. *Nature*, **208**, 1351.
10. Leading Article (1974) What becomes of the XYY male? *Lancet*, **ii**, 1297.
11. Redgrove, J. A. (1971) Menstrual cycles. In *Biological Rhythms and Human Performance*, ed. Colquhoun, W. P., London: Academic Press.
12. Erdelyi, G. J. (1962) Gynaecological survey of female athletes. *J. sports Med. phys. Fitness*, **2**, 174.
13. Pierson, W. R. and Lockhart, A. (1963) Effect of menstruation on simple movement and reaction time. *Br. med. J.*, **i**, 796.
14. Scott, J. T. (1961) Report on the Heights and Weights (and other Measurements) of School Pupils in the County of London, 1959. London County Council, London.

15. Roberts, D. F., Rozner, L. M. and Swan, A. W. (1971) Age at menarche, physique and development in industrial N.E. England. *Acta paediat. scand.*, **60**, 158.

16. Tanner, J. M. (1962) *Growth at Adolescence*, 2nd Edn. Oxford: Blackwell Scientific Publications.

17. Dalton, K. (1973) *The Menstrual Cycle and Missing Menstruation*. Geneva: International Health Foundation.

18. Dalton, K. (1968) Menstruation and examinations. *Lancet*, **ii**, 1386.

19. Dalton, K. (1970) *The Menstrual Cycle*. Harmondsworth, Middlesex: Penguin Books.

20. Dalton, K. (1964) *The Premenstrual Syndrome*. London: Heinemann.

21. Dalton, K. (1960) Menstruation and accidents. *Br. med. J.*, **ii**, 1425.

22. Dalton, K. (1960) Effect of menstruation on schoolgirls' weekly work. *Br. med. J.*, **i**, 326.

23. Dalton, K. (1964) The influence of menstruation on health and disease. *Proc. R. Soc. Med.*, **57**, 262.

24. Dalton, K. (1958) Menstruation and acute psychiatric illnesses. *Br. med. J.*, **i**, 148.

25. Mandell, A. and Mandell, M. (1967) Suicide and the menstrual cycle. *J. Am. med. Ass.*, **200**, 792.

26. Tonks, C. M., Rack, P. H. and Rose, M. J. (1967) Attempted suicide and the menstrual cycle. *J. Psychosom. Res.*, **11**, 319.

27. Zaharieva, E. J. (1965) Survey of sportswomen at the Tokyo Olympics. *J. sports Med. phys. Fitness*, **5**, 215.

28. Wearing, M. P., Yohosz, M. D., Campbell, R. and Love, E. J. (1972) The effects of the menstrual cycle on tests of physical fitness. *J. sports Med. phys. Fitness*, **12**, 38.

29. Zimmerman, E. and Parlee, M. B. (1972) Behavioural changes associated with the menstrual cycle; an experimental investigation. *J. Appl. Soc. Psychol.*, **3**, 4, 335.

30. Loucks, J. and Thompson, H. (1968) Effect of menstruation on reaction time. *Res. Q. Am. Ass. Hlth phys. Fitness*, **39**, 2, 407.

31. Timonen, S. and Precope, B. J. (1971) Premenstrual syndrome and physical exercise. *Acta obstet. gynec. scand.* **50**, 331.

32. Papierowski, Z., Wyznikiewicz, Z. and Surma, H. (1972) Selected parameters of physical fitness in young women interested actively in sports training, in the course of their menstrual cycle. *Ginek. pol.*, **43**, 1205.

33. Nilluis, S. J. and Johansson, E. D. B. (1971) Plasma levels of progesterone after vaginal, rectal or intramuscular administration of progesterone. *Am. J. Obstet. Gynec.*, **110**, 4.

34. Davis, G. (1972) Menstrual Regulations. *Family Planning*, **21**, 57.

35. Davis, G. and Potts, M. (1972) Menstrual regulation, a review of a new technique with promise of providing effective fertility control on a world scale. *Soc. Study Fertility*, Symposium. Reading, U.K.

36. Erdelyi, G. J. (1961) Women in Athletics. In *Medical Aspects of Sport*, 2. Chicago: American Medical Association.

37. Zaharieva, E. (1972) Olympic participation by women: effects on pregnancy and childbirth. *J. Am. med. Ass.*, **221**, 992.

11

Nutrition in sport

Introduction

The contribution that nutrition can make to the general health of any individual, whilst usually accepted, has generally not been given the attention it deserves. However, in the field of sport it is axiomatic that the athlete is given an adequate and suitable diet not only to keep himself fit but also to provide the additional energy that he requires for his physical exertions.

Historically the role of nutrition in athletic performance has been recognized for a very long time. Thus, during the period of the first Olympic Games in Ancient Greece, history records how the athlete was concerned with what he ate.[1] Charmis of Sparta who was victor at the Games held in 668 B.C. is reported to have trained on a diet of dried figs. Tradition suggests that as a sprinter he found the extra sugar in the fruit helpful to his performance.[2] Since those early times a wide variety of substances have been proposed as helpful to the sportsman: one of the more original suggestsions was that royal jelly—the nutritive substance of the queen bee—would be beneficial to the athlete if added to his diet.[3] Such suggestions have, in the main, been based on the fads and fancies or the experience of coaches and trainers. With the development of nutrition as a science it has been possible to investigate the many claims that have been made and, in general, to refute their use as ergogenic aids. Nevertheless, it may well be the case that athletes do require some additional nutrients and that their provision either in the diet, or as dietary supplements, will make an increment in performance. It is important to realize, however, that any resulting increment is likely to be small but that such a small increase could make all the difference between winning and loosing.

Basic requirements

Like any other person the sportsman needs the normal amounts of the basic nutrients, viz. protein, carbohydrate, fats, vitamins, and minerals. Information as to the recommended daily intake of each of these nutrients has been provided by the Department of Health and Social Security[4] in the U.K. (For a more detailed consideration of the recommended intakes of vitamins in the normal subject see Kodicek[5].) The sportsman will need a diet which will supply him with all the recommended quantities of nutrients to keep him in good health, and will also require additional foods to supply him with the extra energy needed to make good the extensive expenditure resulting from his training. Athletes may consume a diet providing up to 5000 kcal (21·1 MJ) per day, although somewhat lower intakes are more usual.

The main nutrients should be presented in the proportion of four parts of carbohydrate to one part of protein and one part of fat. It is important that adequate amounts of protein are provided, and this will be ensured if 10 per cent of the total energy is provided by protein. It used to be thought that greater proportions of protein would be useful to the athlete and encourage muscle growth but there is in fact no evidence to support the view that any extra is beneficial.[6] Nevertheless, it is probably true that many athletes do consume larger amounts than are really necessary. Apart from the increased cost of such a diet, it can be pointed out that it is in no way harmful. It may be recalled, however, that many first-class sportsmen have been vegetarians: as long as sufficient protein is contained in the diet there should be no disadvantage in not consuming animal foods.

Provided, then, that the requirement of the basic nutrients is met and that adequate vitamins and minerals are given, the diet of the sportsman will differ little from an ordinary well-balanced diet except that it must include extra sources of energy. Meals should be as palatable as is practically possible. The actual amount of food necessary can generally be assessed by the natural appetite of each individual. When a subject who has recently taken little physical exercise commences a period of training he may lose a little weight consequent upon the using up of excess fat. But later there may well be a gain in weight resulting from hypertrophy of the muscles.

The question whether any additional nutrient can be helpful to the athlete in his performance is one which, as indicated in the introduction, has occupied the mind of the athletic competitor and his trainer for centuries.

Are additional vitamins beneficial?

It has been seen that the sportsman requires vitamins in amounts at least as much as the normal individual, and some authors have suggested that athletes should receive higher intakes on the grounds that their requirements may be appreciably raised in strenuous exertion. But are such proposals justifiable? Are they perhaps just the whims of coaches and trainers? When such questions are examined scientifically there is found, in general, little evidence to indicate that the need for vitamins is increased during prolonged muscular exercise. Nevertheless there are some instances when there is justification for believing that an increased demand may be made. This may best be illustrated by considering the case of vitamin E.

In various species of animal, deficiency of vitamin E causes the muscles to become dystrophic. It is reasonable, therefore, to consider that when muscles are under severe stress, as in an athletic contest, their demands for the vitamin may be raised to such an extent that these will not be met by the amounts available in an ordinary diet. A case could, therefore, be made for supplementation. Furthermore, evidence exists to demonstrate that the resistance of experimental animals to hypoxia and to hyperoxia is influenced by the vitamin E status. Because vitamin E can act as an antioxidant it is possible that additional amounts of this vitamin could protect against the stresses involved in vigorous muscular exercise. These, and other reasons for believing that vitamin E could aid performance, have been reviewed by Sharman, Down, and Sen.[7]

Several claims have been made that vitamin E can in fact improve performance,[8, 9] but Thomas[10] could find no significant differences between dosed and undosed subjects in a series of cardiorespiratory and motor fitness tests. Detailed observations, carried out on schoolboy swimmers given either 400 mg vitamin E daily or identical placebo tablets, showed that whereas training significantly improved physiological function and performance, vitamin E did not.[7] The possibility remained that had fully trained swimmers been investigated, so as to override any training effect, an improvement in performance with vitamin E might have resulted. In 1974, Sharman, Down and Norgan[11] reported carrying out such a trial with trained swimmers from an élite group in the United Kingdom which included amongst its members a number of Olympic competitors. However, no increments in performance from vitamin E were found. A similar result has since been reported by separate groups of workers in the United States.[12-14] From these observations, therefore, it seems fair to conclude that vitamin E has no ergogenic or work-producing properties.

Turning now to a consideration of the effects of vitamin C on performance, it would appear that extra quantities of this vitamin also do not have any beneficial property. In a trial involving nearly 300 subjects ascorbic acid (1 g) was given daily for 12 weeks, but no significant difference in performance was found between dosed and undosed groups.[15] It should be pointed out, however, that a large proportion of sportsmen probably obtain part, if not all, of their dietary intake from institutional sources, e.g. college refectory or works canteen, and that meals from such sources may be low in this vitamin. Because of the importance of the vitamin in adrenal metabolism it may well be desirable to supplement the athletes' diet. Fresh fruit, particularly the citrus fruits (oranges and lemons), black currants when in season, and fruit essences (e.g. Ribena) are all good sources of the vitamin.

Finally in this section it is necessary to consider the vitamins of the B group. The best known, namely thiamine, riboflavin, and nicotinic acid, are concerned with carbohydrate metabolism. As Scandinavian investigators have advocated the building up of glycogen stores, as an aid to endurance athletes, by consuming a high carbohydrate diet (see section below) it may well be asked 'Do increases in the amounts of carbohydrates metabolized result in higher demands for the B vitamins?'

Experiments with animals have shown that the rate of thiamine utilization depends on the amount of carbohydrate metabolized, and epidemiological studies in man also suggest that thiamine requirements are closely allied to carbohydrate intake. However, little accuracy is lost if they are related to the total energy intake, and it is now general practice to express requirements for thiamine per 1000 kcal (4·2 MJ) ingested. Increased physical activity increases thiamine requirements because of the greater energy involved; but when expressed per 1000 kcal (4·2 MJ) the requirement for the vitamin is constant and does not vary. The level required to saturate the tissues is 0·3 to 0·35 mg thiamine/1000 kcal (4·2 MJ), and any excess will be excreted. To allow for individual variations an intake of 0·4 mg per 1000 kcal (4·2 MJ) has been recommended.[4] Any excess will, as already stated, be excreted, so no benefit can be expected by providing larger quantities. This means that the vitamin is ruled out as an ergogenic aid, so long as needs are met for carbohydrate metabolism.

A similar conclusion is reached when riboflavin and nicotinic acid are considered. Daily intakes of 0·44 mg riboflavin/1000 kcal (4·2 MJ) and 6·6 mg nicotinic acid equivalents/1000 kcal (4·2 MJ) have been recommended.[4] No further increases have been considered necessary for physical activity apart from the related increase resulting from the larger number of calories needed in energetic exercise.

Vitamins are needed for general good health but the amounts are usually small. Quantities in excess of normal requirements[4] do not, in general, appear to provide any beneficial effects as far as physical performance is concerned. Care, however, must be taken to provide the athlete with the recommended daily intakes though the provision of further quantities seems unnecessary.

How muscles obtain their energy

'Living organisms, like machines, conform to the law of conservation of energy, and must pay for all their activities in the currency of metabolism'.[16]

E. Baldwin

The energy necessary for every muscle contraction comes ultimately from dietary sources, i.e. by the combustion of food. However, the immediate source is ATP (adenosine triphosphate). This compound is capable of splitting into ADP (adenosine diphosphate) and phosphoric acid and when it does it provides the actual power for muscle contractions. As muscles contain only small quantities of ATP it is important that the compound is continuously resynthesized. This is achieved by the recombination of its breakdown products, the necessary energy being provided by another energy-yielding reaction in the cell, viz. the splitting of creatine phosphate. This additional 'phosphagen', as it has been called, also has to be constantly replaced as it is present only in small quantities. There are two primary sources of energy for the resynthesis of the phosphagens: the combustion of food, and the process known as glycolysis, that is the breakdown of glycogen with the formation of lactic acid. As the latter process is reversible an input of energy from food combustion will cause a resynthesis of glycogen. Five biochemical reactions in all have therefore to be considered. Three of them: phosphagen splitting, food combustion, and glycolysis are energy providing; the other two: phosphagen resynthesis and glycogen reconstitution are energy absorbing.[17]

The relative amounts of fat and carbohydrate used during physical exercise will depend on the composition of the diet, the work intensity, the duration of the exercise, and upon the fitness of the subject concerned.[18] Because studies have shown that fat is mobilized from the body's reserve depots and that it is transported to the muscles and combusted in the cell during exercise, the alleged importance of carbohydrates for prolonged exercise has been challenged. However, Scandinavian workers have shown conclusively that carbohydrates play an essential role in building up glycogen stores. By developing the needle biopsy technique it has been possible to collect muscle specimens for direct determination of glycogen. The technique consists of making an incision in the skin, under local anaesthesia, and then inserting the needle into the deeper part of the vastus lateralis of the quadriceps femoris muscle. By using subjects on a bicycle ergometer modified so that only one leg is exercised it has been possible to investigate specimens both from exercised and resting legs. From these studies it has been shown that with prolonged heavy exercise the glycogen content of the working muscle is reduced from an average normal value of 15 g/kg of muscle to nearly zero when the subject is exhausted.[19] During prolonged exercise, when the relative work load is over 75 per cent of the subject's maximal oxygen uptake, there is a high and constant rate of carbohydrate combustion and this applies whether the muscle glycogen concentration is high or low. The importance of carbohydrate as a fuel during heavy exercise is therefore confirmed. In another trial using similar techniques it has been shown that at high relative work loads it is primarily the size of the glycogen stores that limits the capacity for strenuous work to be prolonged.[20]

Dietary manipulation as an aid to preparation for competition

In other investigations in which the glycogen stores in healthy subjects had been exhausted by heavy exercise it was shown that the glycogen content of muscles could be varied in individual subjects by varying the subsequent diet. Thus, by giving a fat plus protein diet—consisting of bacon, eggs, meat, butter and vegetable oils together with small amounts of tomato and lettuce—the glycogen content remained low at about 6 g/kg of muscle. But, by feeding a high carbohydrate diet consisting of bread, potatoes, spaghetti, sugar, fruit and juices the glycogen content rose to as much as 47 g/kg muscle.[21, 22]

The results obtained in the various investigations described above led Åstrand to recommend that athletes should first exhaust their stores of muscle glycogen by fairly heavy work, remain on a high protein–fat diet for a short period, and then consume a high carbohydrate diet for the last few days before a competition.[23] This appears to be an effective way of building up a high glycogen content in the muscles and one which will be effective for improving athletic performance.

A further recent trial has shown that besides a beneficial effect on the rate of running, an increase of muscle glycogen can affect endurance as well.[24] This trial was carried out with ten physical education students, some of whom were only slightly trained and others who were regular cross-country runners. The subjects twice ran a distance of 30 km, once after a normal diet and once after a high carbohydrate one. For the first three days of the week of the first race, six competitors ate a diet without carbohydrate; for the next three days a high carbohydrate diet provided a minimum of 2500 kcal (10·55 MJ) per day and no heavy exercise was permitted. The remaining four competitors had a normal diet before the first race. The dietary patterns were reversed prior to the second race, which took place three weeks later. Biopsy specimens were collected from the quadriceps muscles before and after each race. Before the race glycogen averaged 35·2 g/kg muscle in those subjects having the high carbohydrate diet, and only 17·7 g/kg in those on the normal mixed diet. These values were reduced to 19·0 g/kg and 5·2 g/kg respectively after the race. One subject only who had had the high carbohydrate diet had a low glycogen level after the race, but the stores of six of those who had had the normal diet were almost depleted. In every case the best performance of each runner occurred after he had consumed the high carbohydrate diet, so there was little doubt that ability to keep a good pace was directly connected with the higher levels of glycogen initially. In contrast, there was a marked reduction in running speed when glycogen levels were low, and it was impossible to maintain a rapid and continuous pace when values fell below 5 g/kg muscle. This study confirmed, therefore, that by first depleting glycogen stores with a low carbohydrate diet, then following this with a very high carbohydrate diet for three or four days immediately prior to an endurance race, the athlete can build up an additional reserve of glycogen in his muscles that will be beneficial to his performance. As such this is a tangible example of how nutrition can aid the athlete in his performance.

Timing of meals

Another aspect of the subject of nutrition in sport and one that is of practical importance to the athlete is the time that should be allowed after a meal before participating in sports. Putting it another way—since the time of the particular activity may already have been decided—how long should the last meal be taken before an event?

Large bulky meals should certainly be avoided shortly before exercise; this is especially true for the competitor in an endurance event or in hot climatic conditions. During the period immediately following the ingestion of food, blood is directed to the alimentary tract to aid the process of digestion and a reduced amount is therefore available for muscle activity. This may be partly responsible for the feeling of lethargy that follows the ingestion of a large meal. If exercise is attempted under these conditions cramp or intestinal stasis may well result, and if the practice is continued, nausea and abdominal pain and even vomiting and diarrhoea may follow. It is therefore recommended that a period of at least two hours should elapse after a heavy meal before participation in strenuous exercise. It is usually suggested that a sportsman's main meal should be taken in the evening after the conclusion of the day's physical activity. A substantial breakfast may be taken but luncheon should be light and easily digested. In view of the fact that most sporting activities will probably take place in the afternoon care should be exercised to see that the luncheon is taken at least one hour and preferably at least two hours before physical work is begun.

Summary and conclusions

The athlete requires a good all-round diet which should be palatable and supply all nutrients in adequate quantities as recommended for daily intake. There is little evidence that quantities in excess of those recommended for the normal subject are required by the athlete. However, the advantage of a high carbohydrate diet to build up glycogen stores will be of practical importance for the long distance or marathon runner. Meals should generally be taken at least two hours before training or participation in an athletic event.

I.M.S.

References

1. Harris, H. A. (1964) *Greek Athletes and Athletics*. London: Hutchinson.
2. Harris, H. A. (1966) Nutrition and physical performance: the diet of Greek athletes. *Proc. Nutr. Soc.*, **25,** 87.

3. Mayer, J. and Bullen, B. (1963) Nutrition and athletics. *Proceedings 6th International Congress Nutrition.*

4. Department of Health and Social Security (1969) Recommended intakes of nutrients for the United Kingdom. *Reports on Public Health and Medical Subjects*, **No. 120.** London: HMSO.

5. Kodicek, E. (1973) Recommended intakes of vitamins for normal growth and development. *Biblphy Nutr. Diet*, **No. 18,** 45.

6. Pettenkofer, M. and Voit, C. (1866) Untersuchungen über den Stofferbrauch des normalen Menschen. *Z. Biol.*, **2,** 459.

7. Sharman, I. M., Down, M. G. and Sen, R. N. (1971) The effects of vitamin E and training on physiological function and athletic performance in adolescent swimmers. *Br. J. Nutr.*, **26,** 265.

8. Percival, L. (1951) Vitamin E in athletic efficiency. A preliminary report. *Summary,* **3,** 55.

9. Prokop, L. (1960) Die Wirkung von natürlichem Vitamin E auf Sauerstoff-verbrauch und Sauerstoffschuld. *Sportärztl. Prax.*, **1,** 19.

10. Thomas, P. (1957) The effects of vitamin E on some aspects of athletic efficiency. *Ph.D. Thesis.* University of Southern California, Los Angeles.

11. Sharman, I. M., Down, M. G. and Norgan, N. G. (1976) Alleged ergogenic properties of vitamin E. *Proceedings XXth World Congress Sports Medicine, Melbourne.*

12. Shephard, R. J., Campbell, R., Pimm, P., Stuart, D. and Wright, G. R. (1974) Vitamin E, exercise, and the recovery from physical activity. *Europ. J. appl. Physiol.*, **33,** 119.

13. Lawrence, J. D., Bower, R. C., Riehl, W. P. and Smith, J. L. (1975) Effect of α-tocopherol acetate on the swimming endurance of trained swimmers. *Am. J. clin. Nutr.*, **28,** 205.

14. Brown, B. S. and Moore, G. C. (In press) The effects of chronic vitamin E intake on muscular strength, maximal aerobic capacity and blood chemistry measures. *Proceedings 1st International Symposium Athletes' Nutrition,* Leningrad 1975.

15. Gey, G. O., Cooper, K. H. and Bottenberg, R. A. (1970) Effect of ascorbic acid on endurance performance and athletic injury. *J. Am. med. Ass.*, **211,** 105.

16. Baldwin E. (1963) *Dynamic Aspects of Biochemistry.* Cambridge: Cambridge University Press.

17. Margaria, R. (1972) The sources of muscular energy. *Scient. Am.*, March, 84.

18. Christensen, E. H. and Hansen, O. (1939) Zur Methodik der Respiratorischen Quotient-Bestimmungen in Ruhe und bei Arbeit. *Skand. Arch. Physiol.*, **81,** 137.

19. Saltin, B. and Hermansen, L. (1967) Glycogen stores and prolonged severe exercise. *Symposia of the Swedish Nutrition Foundation*, **v,** 32.

20. Hermansen, L., Hultman, E. and Saltin, B. (1967) Muscle glycogen during prolonged severe exercise. *Acta Physiol. Scand.*, **71,** 129.

21. Bergstrom, J., Hermansen, L., Hultman, E. and Saltin, B. (1967) Diet, muscle glycogen and physical performance. *Acta Physiol. Scand.*, **71,** 140.

22. Hultman, E. and Bergstrom, J. (1967) Muscle glycogen synthesis in relation to diet studied in normal subjects. *Acta Med. Scand.*, **182,** 109.

23. Åstrand, P-O. (1967) Diet and athletic performance. *Fedn Proc. Fedn Am. Socs exp. Biol.*, **26,** 1772.

24. Karlsson, J. and Saltin, B. (1971) Diet, muscle glycogen and endurance performance. *J. Appl. Physiol.*, **31,** 203.

12

Doping

Drugs are substances which alter the body's natural chemical environment and actions. They are given in normal clinical practice for predetermined clinical objectives such as cure of infection, augmentation of deficiency, or correction of functional disorders. The clinician, knowing that almost all effective drugs may have potentially serious side-effects, is constantly balancing the benefits of treatment against the hazards of unwanted drug reactions.

Drugs are found in some situations to benefit human performance directly (e.g. the direct stimulant effect of amphetamines), or indirectly (e.g. the disinhibiting side-effect of alcohol in marksmen). Both situations imply risks of misapplication, most dramatically seen in amphetamine abuse. 'Doping' is the application of chemical substances with the deliberate intention or effect of altering performance.[1, 2]

However, sporting competition is a controlled trial—of man or team against rival—within a positively defined framework of rules.[3] The proliferation of rules in sport partly reflects man's tendency to strive for any possible advantage in competition against his rivals.

If one party introduces a new variable into a sports competitive situation, there may arise fair advantage to the innovator (e.g. new training methods), or unfair disadvantage to the rival. The latter could be in respect of new equipment, as when new vaulting poles were available only to some competitors, or in biochemical or physical terms where a rival might be at a biological disadvantage. This would occur if the innovator used a performance-boosting drug, or doped his rival with a performance-impairing substance.[4]

Because of differences in personal or political opinions or moral values, it may be difficult to find universal agreement on doping controls in sport. However, if the fundamental objective of sport is recalled—to match like with like on fair terms— then at least the obvious drug abuses can be curtailed. As there is no point in all sportsmen being equally doped, the aim is that they should be free of dope, and dope detection methods should identify those who cheat. This need not debar fair treatment of many medical disorders, and does not involve drugs involved in menstrual control. These, where necessary, remove the biological disadvantages of the menstrual cycle in less fortunate women, and therefore make for fairer competition between all women.

Other objections to doping include the legal aspects of drug abuse and the moral deception—and self-deception—inherent in such practice.[5] It should be remembered that there may be very powerful pressures on doctor, sportsman, and coach to resort to doping. Firmly and fairly applied regulations protect participants from the stress of these pressures. Too often the sportsman, using drugs because of the fear of competitive disadvantage, wishes to be free of the burden of guilt 'if only all the others were stopped from cheating too'.

Doping practices

There are presently three ways in which drugs are used to enhance or modify human sporting performance.

Stimulants

In the first instance stimulant drugs are used to delay the onset of fatigue and make the athlete feel more alert and physically powerful.

Psychotonics

Psychotonic substances are those which have their primary effect on the brain and central nervous system; the most important are the amphetamines. They are all taken to increase psychological 'tone', to increase motor activity, and to delay the onset of subjective feelings of fatigue. They do not improve muscular performance as such, and their use involves excessive expenditure of energy. Their effect in improving the totality of performance is variable, and their toxic effects both from the short-term and the long-term point of view make them dangerous and detrimental to health. Caffeine (which is also an analeptic) is the least dangerous of these agents but is also one of the least effective. It forms part of the normal diet of most people, being present in such beverages as tea, coffee, cocoa, and 'colas'.

Analeptics

Analeptics act on the cardiac and respiratory regulating mechanisms, and may be considered also to include drugs of the adrenaline–ephedrine series. Of chief interest are ephedrine, coramine, caffeine, and camphor, all of which have been used in attempts to improve performance and none of which does so safely or effectively, though the studies of Smith and Beecher[6] and of Karpovich[7] with amphetamines do suggest a true improvement. However, the use of drugs for this type of doping is now almost unknown since the introduction of effective methods of control using chromatography.

Sedatives

The second way in which drugs are used is to 'destimulate', particularly in events requiring calmness, precision, and control. Shooting is perhaps the best example, whether with rifle, pistol or bow and arrow! (In the Munich Olympic Games there was a scandal because some Modern Pentathletes used diazepam as a relaxant during the shooting phase of the competition.) Such drugs are used because performance in sports requiring a calm temperament can be severely impaired when the individual becomes too highly excited. Ethyl alcohol, usually given in the form of brandy or rum before a game, may improve performance by disinhibiting the subject from the psychological restraint of the particular sporting occasion. The use of drugs for this type of performance modification is again becoming almost unknown because adequate and effective methods of detection and control are available.

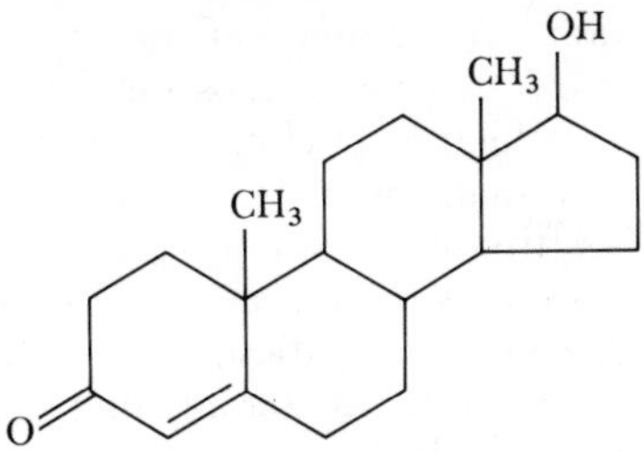

testosterone
(17β-hydroxyandrost-4-en-3-one)

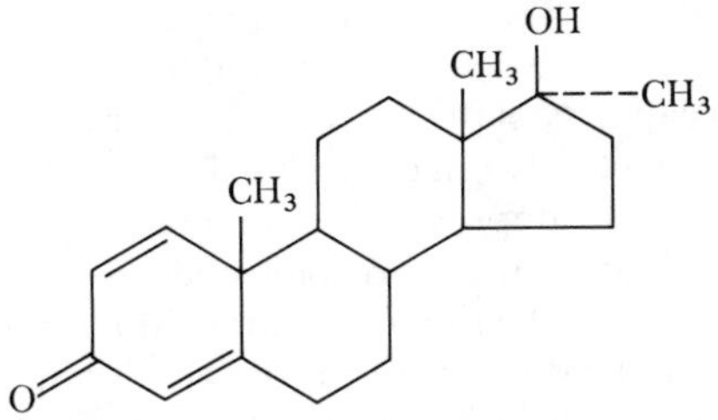

methandienone (Dianabol)
(17β-hydroxy-17α-methylandrosta-1,4-dien-3-one)

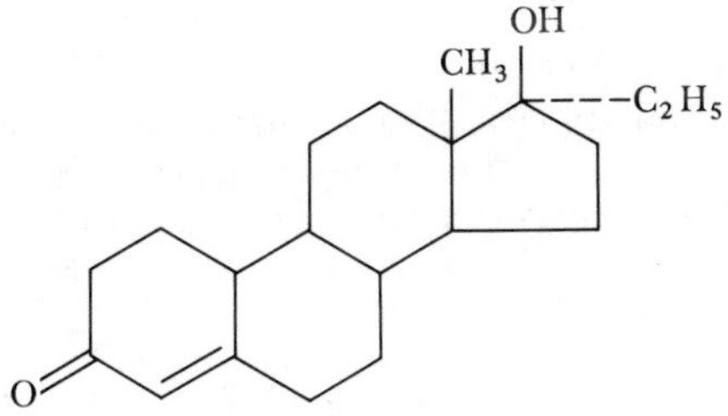

norethandrolone (Nilevar)
(17α-ethyl-17β-hydroxyoestr-4-en-3-one)

Fig. 12.1 Anabolic steroids—modified male sex hormones—as depicted by their ring formulae.

Anabolic steroids

The third and most troublesome drugs presently used in sport are the anabolic steroids (modified male sex hormones—see Fig. 12.1) for promoting muscular development in sportsmen engaged in power events, for example putting the shot or weight lifting. The evidence of the effectiveness of anabolic steroids is conflicting,[8] [12] but practical experience suggests that regardless of the exact mechanism, these drugs do cause considerable improvements in performance in these athletes.[13] Anabolic steroids are typically taken during the close season as part of heavy general body build-up programmes, rather than during the competition season. They are taken in courses of four to six weeks and only occasionally used in the middle of the competitive season for 'topping up'. The exact mechanism by which they work is not certain.[14] It is, however, possible that, in addition to any purely anabolic effect, there is also a euphoriant effect which assists in recovery after training and makes the athlete feel better (the 'ergogenic' effect). Thus, apart from any actual body building, the drug seems to have a positive effect in relation to the individual's attitude to training and therefore the quality of the training he does. Anabolic steroids present a special problem because they may be taken at a time remote from competition.

As sportsmen strive to gain further and progressively smaller advantages over their opponents in increasingly intense competition, both at national and international level, other means of utilizing drug actions will doubtless become apparent. In this context, a bizarre innovation has been attempts to improve physical performance by auto-transfusion.[15] Blood is withdrawn from an individual and stored for re-transfusion shortly before the competition, so as to produce a boost in the oxygen carrying capacity of the blood in time for the event. Grave risks attend this procedure and it is clearly unacceptable if only because of the possibility that it will *impair* rather than improve performance.

Other steroids have been considered in sport. Cortisone and its synthetic derivatives may have a euphoriant effect but the side-effects, including salt and water retention, osteoporosis, and adrenal suppression, make them dangerous. Testosterone causes testicular and pituitary suppression and its virilizing effects are undesirable in females. ACTH injections to boost natural steroid output tend to exaggerate cortisone effects, and while injections of gonadotrophins and growth hormones might boost natural anabolic effects they are impracticable in the sports context and may not be free of pituitary suppressive side-effects.

More recently, interest has centred on appetite-stimulating drugs such as the antihistaminic cyproheptadine (Periactin), but there is no evidence of beneficial effects in healthy athletes, and the side-effects of the antihistamine drugs should be borne in mind.

Techniques of detection

Most drugs taken to act during the time of competition can be detected by some form of chromatography, either thin-layer or gas–liquid[16, 17] (Figs 12.2 and 12.3). In some cases of doubt, further identification is possible using the mass spectrograph[18] (Fig. 12.4). Drugs which may act 'at a distance' such as anabolic steroids and which may be discontinued some time before competition make for greater problems, although the technique of radio-immunoassay for screening, as applied by Brooks,[19] has been proved successful. This is up to one hundred times more sensitive than chromatography and can thus detect the presence of anabolic steroids or derivatives far longer after ingestion. The principle upon which this technique presently works is the identification of 17α-ethyl and 17α-methyl side chains on the steroid nucleus (characteristic of orally taken synthetic anabolic steroids or their derivatives) by the use of antisera. (Antisera to other anabolics including those that are injected are being developed.) When steroids containing either of these side chains are present in appropriate biological samples, they will react with the prepared antibody. The test antibody/sample mixture is then titrated against a known amount of radio-labelled antigen. The amount of anabolic steroid in the test sample can be determined from the difference in take-

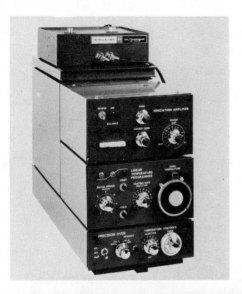

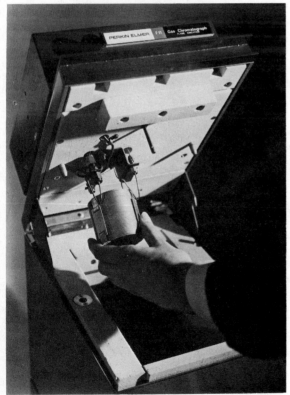

Fig. 12.2 Gas chromatography: the apparatus (photos: Perkin Elmer).

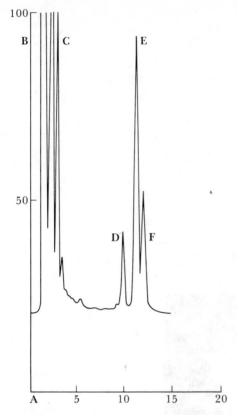

Fig. 12.3 Reproduction of chromatogram from an analysis of a racing cyclist's urine showing the presence of methylamphetamine and its metabolite amphetamine (after Beckett, Tucker and Moffat[16]). A, time; B, detector response; C, ether+urine constituents; D, *N,N*-dimethylaniline (internal marker); E, methylamphetamine; F, amphetamine.

up of labelled antigen as between the control and test samples (Fig. 12.5). This radio-immunoassay technique is only a screening test and does not identify the particular steroid taken. Clearly there may be confusion with other steroids which have 17α-methyl or 17α-ethyl side chains. Furthermore, it is not yet effective for all injected anabolic steroids. This screening test is essentially one to clear athletes of any possibility of having used oral anabolic steroids. Positives on the screening test must then be submitted to further investigation when specific identification of the steroids concerned is carried out by mass spectrography, a technique too complicated to use for screening purposes (Fig. 12.6). The anabolic screening test is only retrospective to a limited degree and to be effective must be repeated at regular intervals.

Drug control
Effective control of the use of drugs in sport demands accurate and efficient detection. As this is now available, it is possible to keep sport effectively dope-free.

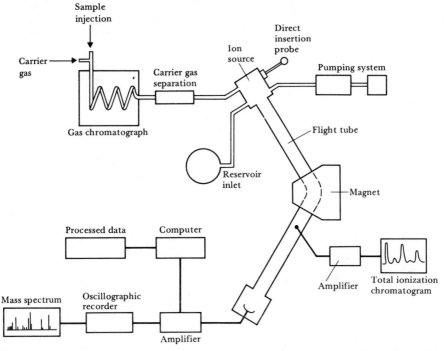

Fig. 12.4 Mass spectrography: diagrammatic layout of the system (after Ward, Shackleton and Lawson[18]).

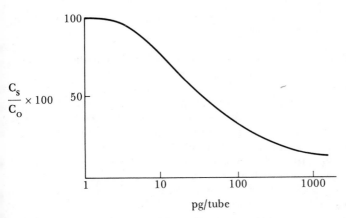

Fig. 12.5 Estimation of anabolic steroid level—concentration read from standard (after Brooks[19]). C_s, counts per minute sample or standard tube; C_0, counts per minute in zero tube.

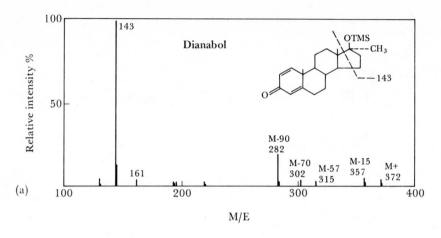

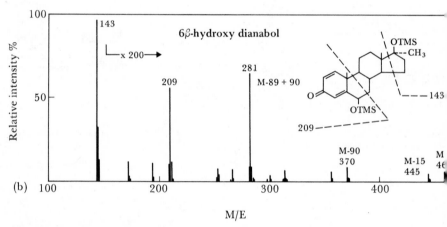

Fig. 12.6 Mass spectrograph tracings identifying (a) Dianabol, and (b) 6β-hydroxy-Dianabol (after Ward, Shackleton and Lawson[18]).

The stages by which control is carried out may be referred to as the 'Four D's', definition, detection, disqualification and deterrence.

Exact definition of doping has been a major problem for many years. Currently, that drawn up by the Council of Europe's working party on Doping of Athletes[20] is the basis of the variations used by governing bodies of sport. Unhappily, no universally agreed definition is presently available, although attempts at standardization are being made if only to facilitate the work of dope control teams required to look after different sports in different countries. The essence of any definition, however phrased, must be that it is open, because any inclusive list of forbidden drugs implies that any drug not on the forbidden list is permitted (Table 12.1). An open definition is workable if coupled with a rule that *any* form of drug taken for any reason must be cleared in advance with the dope control authorities. It is then possible to give guidelines as to what drugs will *never* be acceptable *under any circumstances*.

Table 12.1 Substances classified as Dope by the Medical Commission of the International Olympic Committee for 1972 Olympic Games.

(a) Psychomotor stimulant drugs, e.g.	(c) Miscellaneous central nervous system stimulants, e.g.
amphetamine	amiphenazole
benzphetamine	bemigride
cocaine	leptazol
diethylpropion	nikethamide
dimethylamphetamine	strychnine
ethylamphetamine	and related compounds
fencamfamin	
methylamphetamine	(d) Narcotic analgesics, e.g.
methylphenidate	heroine
norpseudoephedrine	morphine
phendimetrazine	methadone
phenmetrazine	dextromoramide
prolintane	dipipanone
and related compounds	pethidine
	and related compounds
(b) Sympathomimetic amines, e.g.	
ephedrine	
methylephedrine	
methoxyphenamine	
and related compounds	

This list is not complete. Other substances may still be added.

Following definition, the process of detection is automatic. The handling of biological samples for dope control demands a strict protocol which is clearly established by forensic experience, and should present no practical problems to sport. Once the use of a banned drug has been detected, disqualification must follow automatically. The whole concept of dope control falls into disrepute when disqualification does not occur.

A clear definition of what is and is not permissible (yet to be universally achieved), an accurate and effective means of determining what is or is not used, and a strongly enforced policy of disqualification for breach of the regulations must lead to effective deterrence. Such deterrence guarantees that dope and drug taking cannot interfere with the strictly controlled trial which is the essence of sports competition.

J.G.P.W.

References

1. Williams, J. G. P. (1963) Doping of athletes. *Phys. Educ.*, **55**, 39.
2. Raynes, R. H. (1969) The doping of athletes. *Br. J. sports Med.*, **4**, 145.
3. Williams, J. G. P. (1975) Drugs and sport. *Med. Sci. Law*, **15**, 9.
4. De Schaepdryver, A. and Hebbelinck, M. (1964) *Doping: Proceedings of an International Seminar*. London and Oxford: Pergamon.
5. Goulding, R. (1969) Drugs—their use and abuse. *Br. J. sports Med.*, **4**, 111.
6. Smith, G. M. and Beecher, H. K. (1959) Amphetamine sulfate and athletic performance. *J. Am. med. Ass.*, **170**, 542.

7. Karpovich, P. V. (1959) Effect of amphetamine sulfate on athletic performance. *J. Am. med. Ass.*, **170,** 558.
8. Ariel, G. (1974) Residual effect of an anabolic steroid upon isotonic muscular force. *J. sports Med. phys. Fitness*, **14,** 103.
9. Fahey, T. D. and Harmon Brown, C. (1973) The effects of an anabolic steroid on the strength, body composition and endurance of college males when accompanied by a weight training programme. *Med. Sci. Sports*, **5,** 272.
10. Ward, P. (1973) The effect of an anabolic steroid on strength and lean body mass. *Med. Sci. Sports*, **5,** 277.
11. Ariel, G. and Saville, W. (1972) Anabolic steroids: the physiological effects of placebos. *Med. Sci. Sports*, **4,** 124.
12. Johnson, L. C., Fisher, G., Silvester, L. J. and Hofheim, C. C. (1972) Anabolic steroid: effects on strength, body weight, oxygen uptake and spermatogenesis upon mature males. *Med. Sci. Sports*, **4,** 43.
13. Freed, D. L. J. and Banks, A. J. (1975) A double-blind cross-over of methandienone (Dianabol, CIBA) in moderate dosage in highly trained and experienced athletes. In Symposium: Anabolic steroids in sport, ed. Sperryn, P. N. *Br. J. sports Med.*, **9,** 78.
14. Hervey, G. H., Adamson, G. T., Birkenshaw, L., Hayter, C. J., Hutchinson, I., Jones, P. R. M. and Knibbs, A. V. (1975) Are athletes wrong about anabolic steroids? In Symposium: Anabolic steroids in sport, ed. Sperryn, P. N. *Br. J. sports Med.*, **9,** 74.
15. Ekblom, B., Goldborg, A. N. and Gullbring, B. (1972) Response to exercise after blood loss and reinfusion. *J. appl. Physiol.*, **33,** 175.
16. Beckett, A. H., Tucker, G. T. and Moffat, A. C. (1967) Routine detection and identification in the urine of stimulants and other drugs some of which may be used to modify performance in sport. *J. Pharm. Pharmac.*, **19,** 273.
17. Becket, A. H., Tucker, G. T. and James, R. J. (1967) Report on the testing for artificial stimulants in urine samples from football players in the World Championships (Jules Rimet Cup) in 1966. *Bull. Br. Ass. sports Med.*, **2,** 113.
18. Ward, R., Shackleton, C. H. L. and Lawson, A. M. (1965) Gas-chromatographic–mass-spectrometric methods for identification of anabolic steroid drugs and the metabolites. In Symposium: Anabolic steroids in sport, ed. Sperryn, P. N. *Br. J. sports Med.*, **9,** 93.
19. Brooks, R. V. (1975) Detection of anabolic steroids by radio-immunoassay. In Symposium: Anabolic steroids in sport, ed. Sperryn, P. N. *Br. J. sports Med.*, **9,** 89.
20. Council of Europe (1963) Report of Working Party on Doping of Athletes. CCC/EES (63) revised 91.

13

Injury in sport

Introduction

While in terms of morbid anatomy the majority of injuries in sport vary little from those met in domestic and industrial practice, there are none the less certain subtle but significant differences which stem from the nature of 'fit' tissues. There are also a number of specific injuries which seem to be peculiar to certain sports and to be rarely met elsewhere.[1]

In the past it has been customary to refer to all injuries received in sport collectively as 'sports injuries' but such a practice leads to confusion. For example, a sprain of the anterolateral ligament of the ankle joint or a fracture of the shaft of the tibia, are common injuries, both in sport and elsewhere, although the patients may present particular problems in respect of their occupations, whether sporting or otherwise. Such injuries *should* be dealt with effectively by readily available traumatology services and should not of themselves require the deployment of any special facilities except perhaps in the rehabilitation phase; a number of orthopaedic surgeons have tended to describe[2, 3] such injuries as 'sports injuries' rather than as 'injuries occurring in sport', thereby unconsciously contributing to false ideas of adequacy with regard to treatment facilities for those true sport-specific injuries or 'technopathies' which may actually seldom come before them. The majority of these technopathies are of the overuse type, but also included are a few others deriving from very peculiar movements carried out in sport: for example, the throwers' fracture of the humerus is hardly seen except in a sporting context. Such injuries, because of their specific aetiology and peculiar pathology, do require special attention if they are effectively to be managed.

Classification

Classification of injuries has in the past been somewhat haphazard. Corrigan[4] has indicated a form of classification which tends to be over-simple and does not relate directly to the causative factor. La Cava's concepts[5] are much closer to actual practice but do not tabulate easily. The nomenclature suggested by the American Medical Association[6] while fairly comprehensive, is not a true classification and remains in effect a descriptive list. Recently, a classification of injuries based on aetiology[7] has been found useful both in terms of identifying the mode of production and of indicating the most effective approach to management. This classification is readily understood and easily applied, as shown in Table 13.1.

In this classification, most true sports injuries are found in the 'intrinsic' or self-inflicted category of the major primary consequential group. Unlike the extrinsic injuries which involve outside agents and therefore greater damaging

Table 13.1 Classification of injury in sport by aetiology. (Published by permission of the Editor, *Br. J. sports Med.*)

Consequential injury
(1) PRIMARY
(A) *Extrinsic*
  (i) Human
    (front row rugby forward's 'black eye')
  (ii) Implemental
    (a) Incidental
      (cricket ball into silly mid-off's midriff)
    (b) Overuse
      (oarsman's hand blisters)
  (iii) Vehicular
    (Steeplechase Jockey's fractured collarbone)
  (iv) Environmental
    (Highboard diver's sprung back)
(B) *Intrinsic*
  (i) Incidental
    (track sprinter's pulled hamstring)
  (ii) Overuse
    (a) Acute
      (canoeist's tenosynovitis of wrist extensors)
    (b) chronic
      (middle distance runner's chronic Achilles' peritendonitis)

(2) SECONDARY
(A) *Short-term*
  (weak quadriceps syndrome)
(B) *Long-term*
  (degenerative joint disease)

Non-consequential injury
(discus thrower's sprained ankle falling down stairs at home)

---

forces, these injuries are relatively minor and so are usually chronic, although acute incidental intrinsic injuries are well represented by muscle tears.

From a logistic point of view it is the management of the true sport-specific injury that demands special facilities and expertise as compared with those other injuries that fall within the scope of orthodox traumatology.

Incidence
The relative sizes of the two injury groups is not easy to assess and will depend to some extent on selection, i.e. local patterns of sports activity. It is difficult to arrive at an accurate figure for the incidence of sporting injuries. In the United Kingdom various pilot studies have been undertaken, including those of Robson and Williams,[8] Morris,[9] and more recently, Weightman and Browne.[10] It appears that approximately 5 per cent of all cases seen in accident departments of British hospitals are due to a sporting injury. It has been estimated that the annual injury rate throughout the United Kingdom is 2 000 000 of sufficient severity to preclude the victim from participating in sport for at least one week. Of these it is further estimated that some 10 per cent involve time off work. The total size of the problem is therefore quite considerable.

Figures for other countries are remarkably similar, and those differences that exist are probably due to variation in national patterns of sports participation. In a recent British study of patients attending clinics for sports injuries,[11] it was found that approximately one-third could have been treated in an orthodox traumatology service, and one-third by recognized specialists in orthopaedics and physical medicine, leaving a final third that required management by clinicians specifically trained in sports technopathy.

General effects of injury

Physical fitness is an 'artificial' state in so far as it is specifically cultivated rather than inherent in the individual. The development of physical fitness not only produces changes in the capacity of the individual to cope with physical work but these are associated with altered metabolism at tissue level. Injury will therefore result not only in a fall in the general level of fitness (because the resultant disability interferes with training) but it may also produce a significantly different lesion because of the changes that have taken place in the tissues as a result of training. The acute muscle strain illustrates this: training has two important effects on muscle (from a micro-anatomical point of view)—it increases the bulk of the muscle fibres, and it increases the vascularity of the interstitial tissues. The result is that bleeding into the muscle and haematoma formation are likely to be more marked in trained than in untrained muscle. At the same time, the physiological mechanisms by which extravasated fluid is removed from the muscle are more efficient in trained muscle, so that absorption of a haematoma may be more rapid. Thus, the same injury in a trained as opposed to an untrained muscle can be more rapidly absorbed, and this will modify the treatment. This oversimplification illustrates the general rule that treatment of the highly trained individual must often differ from treatment of the unfit 'man in the street' by virtue of the differences in the tissue involved. It is by and large with the resultant loss of training time together with the purely local failure of function that the injured sportsman is chiefly concerned.

Prevention of injury

'Prevention is better than a cure' nowhere holds better than in the case of sporting injuries. Many of them are unnecessary and the harm that they do, not only in terms of loss of earning capacity (to say nothing of occasional loss of life) but also in terms of wasted effort and frustration is quite disproportionate to their severity. In addition, the very circumstances under which they are sustained will make the patient liable to recurrence or further injury.

An appropriate level of fitness is in itself the most valuable factor in the prevention of injury. Not for nothing is unaccustomed exercise said to be 'occasionally fatal, frequently injurious and always painful'. If the body is prepared for activity, it can cope satisfactorily with the forces which produce strains, sprains or worse. Strength, speed and endurance to say nothing of flexibility are all in their way safeguards against injury. They are of particular significance because their development and maintenance will have beneficial effect on the level of general fitness of the individual.

Skill is, however, the factor of paramount importance in safety. It involves not only the physical control to make the body do what the mind wills, but also the mental ability to 'read' the situation, to realize the risk and know how to offset it as well as be able physically to take the necessary actions. At a purely physical level the player's object is to develop effective and efficient movement patterns to the level of conditioned reflexes. Many factors, some physical such as fatigue, some mental such as 'nerves', can conspire to break down this reflex nature of a physical skill. Lack of skill not only renders the individual liable to self-injury, it renders him also more vulnerable to extrinsic injury. To take one example only, it takes considerable skill to bring off a hard, low tackle in rugby football—balance, timing and the ability to ride the hand-off are necessary if the shoulder is to be brought against the opponent's legs and the pinioning embrace completed. A perfectly executed tackle will injure neither party. But suppose the timing is at fault, suppose the hand-off is not evaded, suppose the shoulder misses the target ... Performance of a skill requires the back-up of the other components of fitness. Thus, an individual may well possess a high degree of skill (which, once acquired is virtually never lost), but not the degree of general fitness needed for its realization under conditions of stress. He may certainly perform well at a leisurely pace, and his skill may protect him from intrinsic injury, but lack of speed, strength, agility or endurance may prove the deciding factor in case of extrinsic injury. Skill alone will not protect him against conditions resulting from over-exertion if he undertakes activity beyond the limit imposed by his level of general fitness.

Prevention by control

The most important aspect of injury prevention by control is self-control. If a person loses his temper and thus his self-control, he is liable to injure not only himself but others. Self-control is the essence of self-discipline, and without self-discipline no one can aspire to any degree of physical fitness, since training is in effect self-discipline. But discipline in sport is not a purely individual matter. The practice of any sport or game is governed by rules and regulations to which every participant must subscribe on pain of disqualification. These rules are primarily intended to preserve the nature and spirit of the sport, but at the same time they are framed in such a way as to protect the participant both from his fellows and from himself. Rules may be clearly set out and defined by the governing bodies, or may simply be established informally according to precedents and 'lore'.

Regulation in sport is both remote and immediate. Remote control is exerted by the governing body of a sport through the rules it administers. In most cases adequate provision is made for prevention of injury. Some may argue that there are too many rules in every sport and that prevention of injury is a matter for the individual—that he does not have to take part in a sport if he is apprehensive of injury. Up to a point this may be true, but in the first place the majority of participants in any sport are quite unaware of the risks they may be running, and in the second, if they are aware of them they are prepared to accept them on an 'it couldn't happen to me' basis. Perhaps the risks of serious injury or even death are small, but when a large population is at risk, somebody somewhere is going to suffer. It is the responsibility of sports' administrators to legislate so as to minimize these risks.

But however well framed the rules of a sport, they can but exert a distant control. Immediate control is in the hands of the umpire or referee, and upon him rests a responsibility which he may not immediately appreciate. Generally speaking the rules of most sports, particularly those involving body contact, make provision for disciplinary action to be taken against anyone involved in a major infringement (Fig. 13.1). Such action may be in the form of disqualification, dismissal from the arena or field of play, and perhaps also suspension or kindred sanctions. Various forms of dangerous play including the application of unnecessary or unlawful violence carry such penalties, but it is remarkable how often such violence passes unpenalized. In so far as any particular action is expressly excluded by regulation, then the proper penalty should be applied.

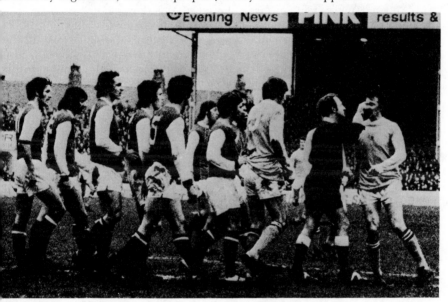

Fig. 13.1 Immediate control is in the hands of the umpire or referee.

It may be true that to adopt an inflexible and legalistic approach in the application of the rules may detract from the enjoyment of a game for both the player and the spectator, but this is only a half-truth, because what is basically the cause of the detraction is the sort of play that necessitates the strict application of the rules! If every player adhered to the rules there would be little need for an umpire or referee. It is only because, human nature being what it is, players will inevitably infringe the rules in some way that an arbiter must be present to interpret and apply them. His strictness or otherwise does not, however, fundamentally determine the course of the game—that is determined solely by the attitude of the players.

Another objection sometimes raised to the tight control of a game and the application of sanctions against dirty players is that fisticuffs and so on are usually only a matter of a brief flare-up. But such conduct is contrary to both the letter and the spirit of the rules, and if someone 'gets away with it' it encourages others to forget themselves, and so a serious injury can follow earlier and 'trivial' incidents of rough play. Certainly there is no excuse whatever for sloppy refereeing any more than there is for resentment on the part of any player penalized for dangerous play.

Protective clothing and equipment

In many sports and games the participants may or indeed must wear some form of protective clothing or use protective equipment. Such clothing or equipment may be to protect themselves or to protect others with whom they come into contact; moreover, any form of gear used for individual protection must offer no danger to anybody else.

Although there are many forms of protective clothing available it is remarkable that so few are subject to minimum standards of safety. For example, there are available on public sale male genital protectors (known colloquially as 'boxes') made of a plastic material in the form of a basket. These are provided for insertion into a special pocket in some jock-straps. They would seem to provide excellent protection except to the surgeon faced with the necessity of removing fragments of such a box from a scrotum when it has been fractured by impact from a ball. The requirements for protective clothing should be clearly defined, and any item that is not up to the task for which it is designed should be banned.

Protective clothing should:

(a) Provide complete or adequate protection to the appropriate part of the body under the conditions of use. It should withstand any foreseeable impact, and any distortion which may take place under stress should be within clearly defined limits.

(b) Be made of such a material as to allow proper cleansing and retain its properties for a reasonable period of time. Protective clothing is not acceptable if it progressively loses its capacity to protect.

(c) Be so designed and made as to allow the wearer the appropriate freedom of action, and not to interfere with his activities in such a way as to constitute a source of danger to him.

(d) Be so designed and made that its use does not in any way constitute a source of danger to anyone with whom the wearer comes into contact. In general this latter requirement should be fulfilled by any item of sportswear.

If these criteria of suitability are applied it will be found that many available items are in some way or other unsatisfactory It is common to find articles o sports equipment advertised as being designed in consultation with this or tha famous sports personality. Such advertisements mean nothing, as the articles in question may often be medically unsuitable. What is important is that sportswear and protective clothing should be designed in consultation with some medica authority.

A word about footwear: the design of footwear for various sports is often highly unsatisfactory, being dictated by fashion rather than any consideration of basic functional requirement. As examples may be quoted 'cut away' football shoes that contribute so much to the incidence of sprained ankles; track running shoe in which the emphasis is on lightness at the expense of firmness of sole and freedom of toe movement; and cricket boots that give either too little or too much adhesion

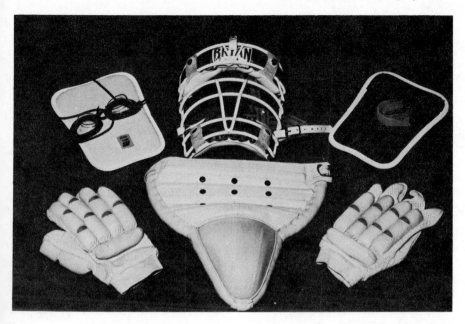

Fig. 13.2 Examples of protective clothing: face mask (hockey—goal keeper), shin pads (football), goggles (swimming), gloves (cricket—batting), genital protector (cricket—wicket-keeping) gum shield.

to the ground. There is considerable scope for improvement in the design of footwear so as to provide not only greater safety but also greater efficiency—the two are by no means mutually exclusive.

Protective equipment must be designed and manufactured to the same standards as clothing, and should in all respects perform to its design characteristics. Poor protective equipment, in addition to being dangerous in itself can engender a false sense of security. Where protective equipment requires skilled setting up, for example safety ski bindings, fail-safe mechanisms should if possible be incorporated.

Principles of prevention of injury

The following principles if conscientiously applied must inevitably result in a decrease in the incidence of sports injury. They are:

(1) Be fit for the sport or game. Remember that fitness involves both general and specific fitness. Skill, speed, strength, flexibility and endurance all exert a protective influence.
(2) Obey the rules both written and unwritten. Control yourself and accept control from referee, umpire or other official.
(3) Wear the right sort of apparel, keep it in good condition, and choose only that which permits freedom and safety of activity. See that protective clothing fulfills the four basic requirements.

To these three may be added a fourth which in a way summarizes them all—'use your common sense'.

Safety in sport, sensibily sought, contributes materially to the pleasure and satisfaction of player and spectator alike.

J. G. P. W.

References

1. Williams, J. G. P. and Sperryn, P. N. (1972) Overuse injuries in sport and work. *Br. J. sports Med.*, **6,** 50.
2. Wilson, J. S. (1972) Specific injuries of sports. *Physiotherapy*, **58,** 194.
3. Smillie, I. S. (1969) Knee injuries in athletes. *Proc. R. Soc. Med.*, **62,** 937.
4. Corrigan, A. B. (1968) Sports injuries. *Hosp. Medicine*, **2,** 1328.
5. La Cava, G. (1961) A clinical and statistical investigation of traumatic lesions due to sport. *J. sports Med. phys. Fitness*, **1,** 8.
6. American Medical Association (1968) *Standard Nomenclature of Athletic Injuries*. Chicago: American Medical Association.
7. Williams, J. G. P. (1971) Aetiological classification of injuries in sportsmen. *Br. J. sports Med.*, **5,** 228.
8. Robson, H. E. and Williams J. G. P. (1961) *Sports Injuries Survey—a Pilot Study*. Communication to British Association of Sport and Medicine.
9. Morris, M. (1963) A sports injuries survey of Greater Birmingham. *Phys. Educ.*, **55,** 41.
10. Weightman, D. and Browne, R. C. (1974) Injuries in Rugby and Association Football. *Br. J. sports Med.*, **8,** 183.
11. Sperryn, P. N. and Williams, J. G. P. (1975) Why sports injuries clinics? *Br. med. J.*, **3,** 364.

14

Bones

Structure of bone

Bone is a highly vascular, constantly changing, living connective tissue with a high mineral content. It is noted for its hardness, resilience, and power to regenerate. It grows, is subject to disease, and when fractured it heals itself.

Bone develops in two ways, either by the direct transformation of condensed mesenchyme, or the formation of a cartilaginous model which is later replaced by bone.[1]

Bones have an organic framework of fibrous tissue and cells, amongst which inorganic salts, mainly calcium phosphate, are deposited. The fibrous tissue gives the bones resilience and toughness, the salts give them hardness and rigidity, and because of the salts they are opaque to X-rays. Bone exists in two forms, compact or ivory bone which is hard and dense, cancellous or spongy bone which consists of a spongework of trabeculae arranged in patterns best adapted to resist the local strains and stresses. Alteration of the strain on a bone results in a rearrangement of the trabecular pattern. Ossification or bone formation consists of the direct mineralization of a highly vascular connective tissue laid down beforehand, and the process of ossification commences at certain constant sites known as centres of ossification. The process of laying down bone or apposition of bone is carried out by osteoblast cells. To ensure that the shape of a bone is maintained and that bone is adapted to meet the altering stresses and strains applied to it, remodelling or resorption of bone is constantly being carried out by osteoclasts.

A few bones are developed in condensed mesenchyme, e.g. the clavicle and bones of the skull, but generally the bones of the skeleton are preformed in hyaline cartilage and centres of ossification for each bone appear over a period of time, some developing about the eighth week of embryonic life, some appearing just before birth, others at intervals after birth until the age of ten or eleven. Small bones such as the carpal and tarsal bones develop from a single centre; most other bones develop from several centres, the first appearing near the centre of the future bone in the embryo and from it ossification proceeds towards either end. The ends of the bone, which are still cartilaginous, develop separate centres from about the time of birth onwards, the so-called secondary centres as opposed to the first or primary centre (Fig. 14.1).

The long bones of the skeleton are developed in this way, and at birth consist of a shaft ossified from the primary centre, and two extremities or epiphyses in which ossification is taking place from the secondary centres. The plate of carti-lage which persists between the shaft and epiphyses is called the epiphyseal carti-lage, and growth in length takes place at this growth plate. A layer of hyaline

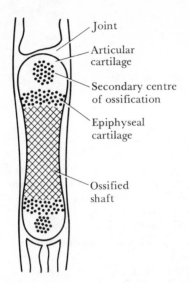

Joint

Articular
cartilage

Secondary centre
of ossification

Epiphyseal
cartilage

Ossified
shaft

Fig. 14.1 Ossification in cartilage. A cartilaginous model of the bone is ossified first in the shaft then at the epiphyses. Growth in length continues at the intervening epiphyseal cartilage.

cartilage remains over the end of the epiphysis and constitutes the articular cartilage of the joint which it will form.

Growth of bones continues until maturity when the epiphyseal cartilage ossifies, the shaft and epiphysis become continuous, and growth ceases.

All bones have an outer casing of compact bone, the interior being filled with spongy bone except where replaced by a medullary cavity. In long bones the compact bone is thickest near the middle of the shaft and becomes progressively thinner as the bone expands towards its articular extremities. These consist essentially of spongy bone covered by a thin shell of compact bone (Fig. 14.2). Spongy bone extends for a variable distance along the shaft but leaves a tubular space— the medullary cavity. The plates of spongy bone or lamellae are arranged in lines of pressure and tension; in the shafts of long bones the lamellae are arranged in concentric cylinders around small blood vessels, the so-called Haversian system, while the cylinders lie parallel to the long axis of the bone.

Bone cells lie in spaces (lacunae) between the lamellae. Capillaries, nerve fibres, and lymphatics run within the Haversian canals and communicate with each other through a wide network of minute canals. Bone marrow which is involved in the manufacture of blood cells, is found at birth in the interstices of spongy bone and medullary cavities of long bones.

Periosteum

Bone surfaces are covered with a thick layer of fibrous tissue in the deeper layer of which blood vessels run. This layer is the periosteum and the nutrition and growth of the underlying bone depends on the integrity of its blood vessels. The periosteum also has osteogenic properties and has the ability to produce new bone, e.g. in the repair of fractures. Periosteum does not cover the articulating

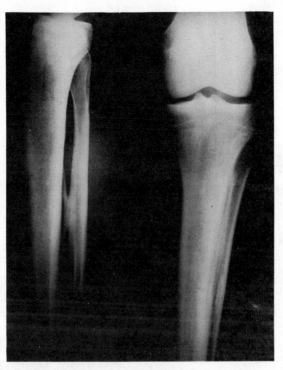

Fig. 14.2 X-rays of tibia and fibula of professional footballer. The outer casing of compact bone is very thick at mid-shaft and thins towards the knee joint. The trabecular markings of the lower end of the femur and upper end of tibia (spongy bone) are well demonstrated. There is new bone formation between tibia and fibula due to old football injury. The ossified epiphyseal lines are seen.

surfaces of the bones in synovial joints. It has a good nerve supply and is very sensitive.

Blood supply of bones

In the adult the nutrient artery of the shaft supplies mainly the bone marrow. The compact bone of the shaft and the cancellous bone of the ends are supplied by branches from the periosteum which are numerous at points where muscles and ligaments find attachment to the periosteum. The epiphyses are supplied from the circulus vasculosus, a vascular plexus which lies between the capsule and the synovial membrane adjacent to the epiphyseal line.

Bone growth and repair

Bone growth and repair are most marked during childhood and adolescence; thus fractures in childhood unite rapidly and even when there is considerable deviation from normal alignment after fracture, this can be corrected by the remodelling process which fashions the bone to meet the stresses and strains to which it is subjected (Fig. 14.3).

New bone formation may fail in certain conditions, e.g. where there is a failure

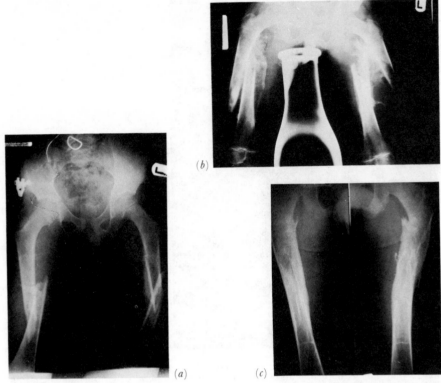

(a)   *(b)*   *(c)*

Fig. 14.3(a) A boy aged 7 was knocked down by a bus. He had severe head injuries, was decerebrate and spastic. He had fractured femora but was so ill and spastic no active treatment could be given. (b) Three months later he was still comatose and incontinent. The fractures are uniting with overlap and displacement. (c) Seven years later the fractures are well united and remodelled and the shortening has been made good.

of an adequate dietary intake and absorption of calcium, phosphorus and vitamins (particularly A, C, and D) or if there is an endocrinal upset. In rickets and osteomalacia, osteoid tissue, the precursor of bone, is laid down abundantly but there are insufficient bone salts available to complete its calcification (Fig. 14.4). In osteoporosis there is failure to lay down osteoid so that even if calcium salts are available, there is no organic structure in which they can be deposited (Fig. 14.5).

Fractures

A fracture of bone is a rupture of living connective tissue, and its repair is achieved by cellular growth as is repair in all living tissues. The repair process is described[2] in the following stages:

(a) Repair by granulation tissue. A blood clot forms between the ends of the fractured bone, and within a few days is invaded by cellular granulation tissue.

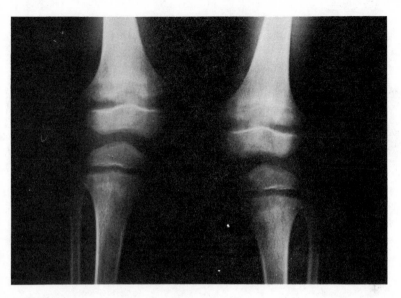

Fig. 14.4 Active rickets in a Pakistani boy: there is widening and irregularity of the growing epiphyses of femur and tibia.

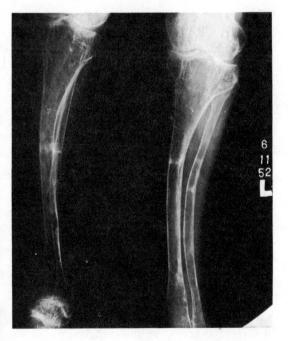

Fig. 14.5 Severe osteoporosis with stress fractures of tibia and fibula. There is practically no compact bone. Lamellar formation along lines of stress can be seen at the knee.

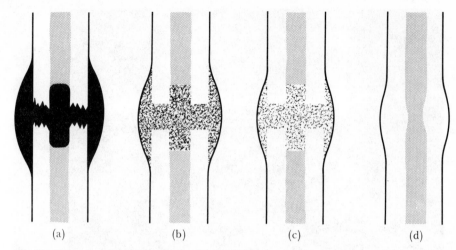

(a)   (b)   (c)   (d)

Fig. 14.6 Stages in healing of a fracture. (a) Haematoma formation between bone ends. (b) Granulation tissue. (c) Conversion of granulation tissue to Osteoid. (d) Union by bone and remodelling.

(b) Replacement by osteoid tissue. The granulation tissue is converted into fibrocartilage.
(c) Deposition of bone. Bone is now laid down in the osteoid tissue.
(d) Resorption and remodelling. There is always excess bone or callus formation at the fracture site and this is now removed by the osteoclasts to restore the shape and size of the original bone (Fig. 14.6).

The time taken for union of a fracture depends on a great number of variable factors. Whenever an athlete is admitted with a fractured bone the first question asked is 'How long will it take for the fracture to heal?' Small bones such as the metatarsals or metacarpals can be united in about four weeks as there is seldom any displacement. When it comes to fractures of the larger weight-bearing bones, such as the tibia or the femur, then it is wise never to forecast a specific time. Simple spiral fractures, where there is a large area of bone contact between the fragments, will unite rapidly and without much trouble. Where the fracture is transverse, comminuted, displaced, or complicated by damage to the overlying skin, to nerves or blood vessels, it may be impossible to give even an approximate estimate (Fig. 14.7).

Causes of fractures

Such fractures as are seen in sporting activities are usually due to the application of violence to the injured limb. The violence is described as:

(a) Direct, where the force causing the break is applied directly to the limb. In football, a direct kick on the shin may break the tibia, or when two heads meet while heading a ball, the skull may be fractured.
(b) Indirect, where the force causing the break is not applied directly to the

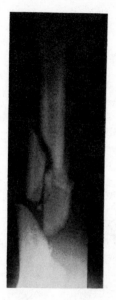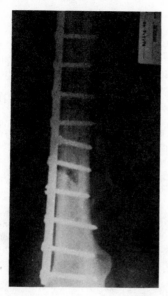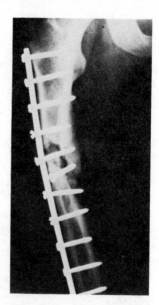

Fig. 14.7(a) Comminuted fracture shaft of femur—skiing injury. (b) Treated by long metal plate and screws. (c) Extensive stripping of periosteum to insert plate and screws has interfered with blood supply of fragments, causing collapse at fracture site with bending of plate.

injured bone but at a distance. A fall on the outstretched hand may break the forearm, the head of the radius, or the collar bone by transmitted force.

The nature of the force can determine the type of injury; fractures due to direct violence may be comminuted, displaced by the force applied, and the overlying tissues may be traumatized or even breached, exposing the fractured bones. When a fracture is exposed to the external environment by a wound of the skin and tissues overlying it, the fracture is said to be compound; such a fracture is liable to be contaminated by dirt and debris and subsequently become infected. In such cases the risk of tetanus is very real. The treatment of such a fracture must include the careful removal of all contamination, foreign bodies, and necrotic tissue, and meticulous wound toilet. When the skin overlying a fracture is intact, the fracture is said to be simple. The various descriptive terms applied to fractures, oblique, spiral, transverse, comminuted, are merely describing the appearance of the fracture on the X-ray. They are helpful to the surgeon in making a decision as to the method of treatment.[3]

Complications of fractures
Some of these have already been referred to. A fracture which is compound requires special attention. Involvement of nerves or arteries by the broken bones can occur at the time of injury or subsequently through injudicious movement of the injured limb. All fractures must be splinted before the patient is moved, in order to prevent this.

Pathological fractures

When a bone is the site of some disease process, it may break spontaneously. This occurs when a tumour is present, either a simple lesion such as an enchondroma or a malignant growth. Such problems do not arise in athletics as a rule, although children do occasionally sustain fractures through simple bone lesions while taking part in games.

Stress fractures

These fractures occur in young healthy athletes who are undergoing training in which repetitive strains are applied to a particular bone[4, 5]; young army recruits subjected to long route marches while carrying equipment may sustain stress or fatigue fractures of the metatarsals, particularly the second and third which are

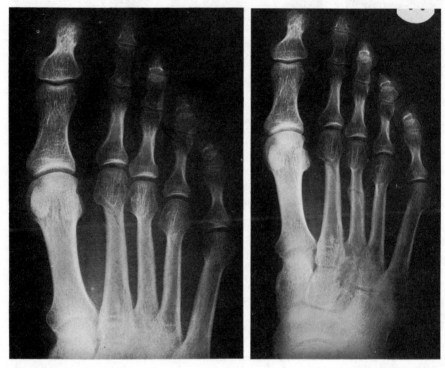

Fig. 14.8(a) Stress fractures are present in 2nd and 3rd metatarsals. (b) Two weeks later the fractures are more clearly visible.

exposed to trauma in certain feet (Fig. 14.8). Fatigue fracture of the fibula is seen in footballers and affects the lower third of the bone where torsional strain is applied when turning rapidly (Fig. 14.9). Ballet dancers and runners may also develop such fractures in the tibia. Other bones affected are the clavicle, femur and ribs but these are not so commonly seen in athletes, and are usually an indication of some underlying bone defect.

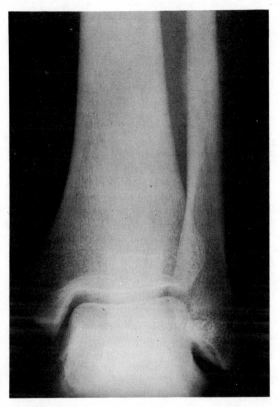

Fig. 14.9 Stress fracture of the fibula of a professional footballer. Can only be recognized by subperiosteal new bone formation.

Treatment of fractures

First Aid treatment should be applied at the scene of injury. Fractures of the clavicle (common in rugby) and fractures of the humerus and forearm bones can be treated by placing a soft pad in the axilla and between the arm, forearm and the chest, and then binding the arm to the side. Elbow injuries must be handled with care, the arm being bound in the most comfortable position without attempting to bend the elbow.

Fractures of the lower limbs are dealt with by strapping the limbs together after placing some soft material between them to prevent pressure on damaged structures. If a wound is present it must be covered with a clean and, if possible, sterile bandage. All athletes should be immunized against tetanus, especially those taking part in sport in open fields. The trainers and others responsible should encourage players to be immunized and keep records for reference in case of injury; the disease is not very common, but it still occurs. The outcome can be disastrous, while prevention by immunization is simple and lasting.

The definitive treatment of fractures is undertaken by surgeons trained in this speciality. To enable a fracture to heal, the broken bones must be immobilized, with the fragments in close apposition and retained in this position until healing occurs as described above. It has been said that non-union of fractures is due to the failure of surgeons much more than the failure of osteoblasts.

The healing process whereby the haematoma between the fractured bones is transformed into bone takes time, and any injudicious movement of the fracture or attempts to mobilize the limb too early can interfere with the process. Fractures in athletes as a rule heal rapidly and well because the athlete is young and fit, has good musculature, is experienced in performing the exercises so necessary in the rehabilitation programme, and is anxious to get back to sport.

General principles are to reduce the fracture, that is to say the broken bones are brought into contact, the alignment of the bones is restored, and any shortening of the limb due to overlap of the broken bones is overcome and full length regained; these aims can in the majority of cases be attained by the application of traction and countertraction to the limb. Exact anatomical reduction of the broken bones is not always possible, and is not necessary as the repair process can remodel fractures with displacement, especially in young people.

This conservative approach to bone injuries in the young yields excellent results. There has been a tendency in recent years to advocate operative reduction as it is felt by some surgeons that the bone fragments can be reduced accurately under direct vision, and they can then be fixed firmly by metal plates and screws.

Certain fractures where, for instance, there is interposition of muscle or tendon between the bone fragments, require open operation. It should be remembered that when a fracture is comminuted, the stripping of the fragments at operation may be sufficient to deprive them of the remaining blood supply and lead to delayed or non-union. The chance of introducing infection at operation, while not great, must be borne in mind; it has been said that there is no antibiotic to equal intact skin over a fracture.

In the treatment of fractures certain points must be borne in mind. A tight unyielding form of splint or bandage should not be applied to an injured limb likely to swell, otherwise circulatory damage may occur (Fig. 14.10). While the affected limb must be immobilized, a full regime of exercises for the rest of the

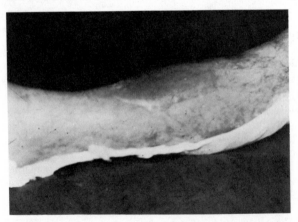

Fig. 14.10 Following a fracture of tibia and fibula on the field an unpadded cast was applied to the leg. Twenty-four hours later there was severe blistering due to swelling.

body must be prescribed. This will encourage the circulation to the affected part, reduce stasis, ventilate the lungs, and materially shorten the time of convalescence once the plaster has been removed.

When treating atheletes for injury irrespective of its nature, the physiotherapist, coach or trainer is encouraged to be present, so that instructions regarding the type and range of rehabilitation exercises and the equipment available for these is known. Whenever possible, swimming under supervision or formal hydrotherapy should be instituted at the earliest possible moment as a means of mobilizing joints and strengthening muscles without subjecting them to direct strain.

Conditions affecting epiphyses

Growth of bones takes place at the epiphyses and therefore during the growth phase these areas are centres of tremendous cellular activity. Epiphyses help to form joints at the ends of long bones, so joint capsules are found attached in these areas together with muscles and tendons controlling the joints. The young vascular growing epiphyses are, therefore, subjected to considerable stresses and strains, and in bones where these strains are great, changes can affect them. Such changes are termed osteochondritis and are characterized by fragmentation of the affected

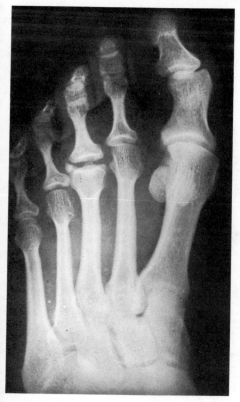

Fig. 14.11 Freiburg's osteochondritis of head of 3rd metatarsal.

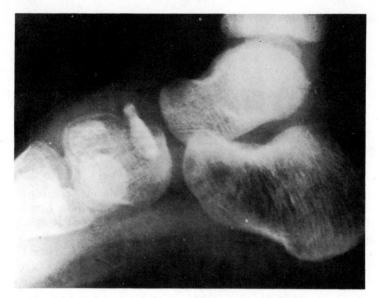

Fig. 14.12 Köhler's osteochondritis of the tarsal navicular.

bone, distortion, and collapse and, after some time, ossification of the bone in its irregular form. As each condition was first noted and described by various authors so their names were attached to the conditions, and these eponyms have remained. In the foot the metatarsal heads are affected by Freiberg's disease (Fig. 14.11), the tarsal navicular by Köhler's disease (Fig. 14.12), Sever's apophysitis

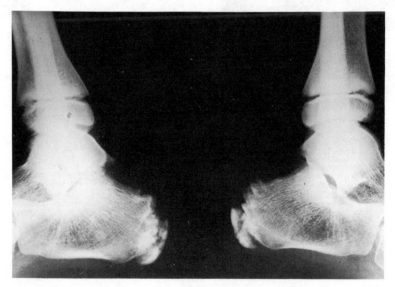

Fig. 14.13 Sever's calcaneal apophysitis.

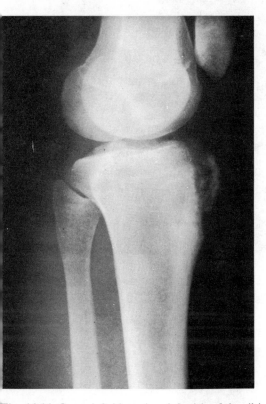

Fig. 14.14 Osgood–Schlatter's epiphysitis of the tibial tubercle.

is found in the heel (Fig. 14.13), and osteochondritis affecting the tibial tubercle to which the ligamentum patellae is attached is called Osgood–Schlatter's disease (Fig. 14.14). A similar condition affecting the femoral capital epiphysis in young children is named after Perthe, while in the spine an adolescent epiphysitis of the vertebral plates is named after Scheuermann. The one likely to be met with in athletes is mainly osteochondritis of the tibial tubercle which affects a lot of young footballers, but is also found in girls who are active in athletics. A tender swelling is present over the tubercle. It may look hot and red if the condition is very active. The complaint is of pain after activity, inability to kneel, and the presence of the swelling. It should be stressed to the individual patients concerned that this is not a disease, and clinicians should refrain from using the term. Rest from the sport and activities which are causing pain will allow the knee to settle; there is no necessity to immobilize the knee in a plaster cast; crêpe bandages and advice as to the daily regime of activities are sufficient.

Scheuermann's osteochondritis gives rise to a form of backache associated with round shoulders. Treatment to be successful requires extensive supervision in an Orthopaedic Department.

When violence is applied to an epiphysis it can be displaced in the region of the growing cartilaginous plate. Common displacements seen are at the wrist

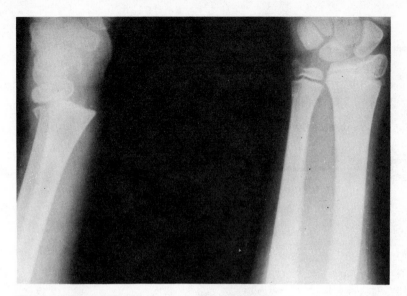

Fig. 14.15 Dorsal displacement of radial epiphysis.

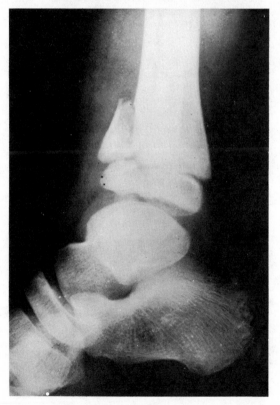

Fig. 14.16 Displaced lower tibial epiphysis in a boy aged 10. A triangular fragment has also been broken off. Sledging injury.

where the radial epiphysis is displaced by a fall (Fig. 14.15). At the ankle the lower tibial epiphysis usually takes with it a triangular fragment of the tibia (Fig. 14.16). At the knee the lower femoral epiphysis is displaced by a violent fall on the knee as from a motor cycle crash. In the hip joint the femoral capital epiphysis can be displaced by violence. For example a boy jumped from a haystack and was unable to rise because he had displaced his femoral epiphysis. The type of displacement of this epiphysis which interests orthopaedic surgeons is one which appears to take place spontaneously, and first manifests itself by pain in the knee (Fig. 14.17). Many young surgeons have overlooked an early slipping of this epiphysis because the complaint initially was directed entirely to the knee. Unexplained pain in the knee at any age calls for an examination of the hip

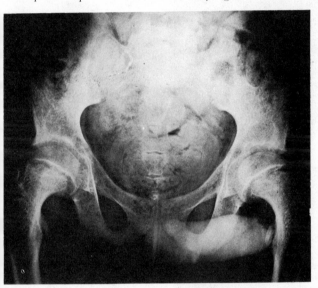

Fig. 14.17 Bilateral slipped upper femoral epiphysis.

joint as instanced by two girls treated within a period of months who were 'national' highland dancers, and who developed slipped upper femoral epiphyses; the first one had finished dancing at a competition and was on her way home when she found she was unable to walk. The second one over a period of time found that her dancing was becoming more difficult, but many months passed before she gave up and reported to hospital with pain in her knee.

Traumatic displacements of epiphyses are treated along normal lines as for fractures which indeed they are; spontaneous displacement of the femoral epiphysis can be replaced if seen early and then fixed by wires or nails. If seen later it may be impossible to replace the displaced epiphysis and more detailed surgical procedures are required.

Periostitis and ectopic bone formation
Often an athlete will be seen who has sustained an injury in the region of a joint, commonly the knee. When seen there is marked swelling around the affected

region. There may be bruising, the area is painful to touch, and movements of the joint are restricted. At first glance it would appear that there has been a fracture, but X-ray examination is negative.

The condition is periostitis, due to a severe strain at a muscle or tendon insertion. The underlying periosteum is damaged. It may be detached, so that subperiosteal haematoma formation takes place and contributes to the pain and swelling. Ossification can now occur in this haematoma and manifests itself in the form of a hard indurated swelling. X-ray examination shows the new bone forma-

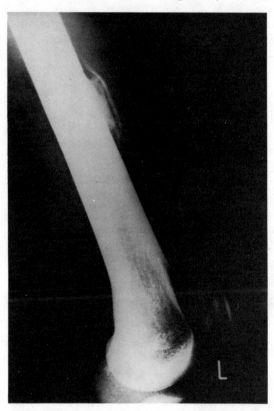

Fig. 14.18 Ectopic new bone formation in the thigh at the site of periosteal bruising— 'myositis ossificans'.

tion (Fig. 14.18). This lesion can lead to a very prolonged period of incapacity to the athlete, usually a footballer. Treatment consists of aspiration of the haematoma, if seen early enough, to be followed by firm bandaging with crêpe and cotton wool. Once the bone is formed, however, an adequate period of rest from sport must be taken so that further haemorrhage does not occur and extend the process. The player can usually return to football. It is only necessary to remove the ectopic bone on a few occasions when it is very large and interfering with function. Given adequate time the amount of bone is usually reduced by gradual absorption.

Bone infections

Osteomyelitis is not common in the athlete, other than complicating compound fractures which become infected or caused by penetrating injuries by equipment such as javelins, or arrows. Occasionally, osteomyelitis presents in schoolboys and girls where the cause is considered to be an injury at games with subsequent infection. Anyone who has suffered from osteomyelitis should not be allowed to take part in sport unless the infection has been completely eradicated. Treatment today with the antibiotics available can result in a cure, and there are many people who have been able to return to sporting activities after treatment.

Bone tumours

Benign bone tumours are rare, although osteoid osteomas, non-ossifying fibromas, chondromas, and exostoses may be encountered.

Osteoid osteoma frequently presents problems of diagnosis. The patient complains of pain—well localized and worse at night, but relieved by aspirin. Although this 'tumour' is described as a self-limiting disease, symptoms may warrant local excision or curettage. X-ray changes are not obvious at first; there may be a slight periosteal reaction, and a small radio-translucent nidus surrounded by a dense sclerotic halo may be seen, particularly on macrogram or tomogram.

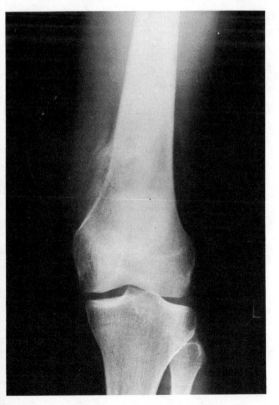

Fig. 14.19 Osteosarcoma presenting initially as a 'knee injury' after netball.

Chondromas may present as swellings or because of associated (pathological) fracture. Treatment may be expectant—excision and replacement by bone graft or chips may be indicated in selected cases. When they occur in the hands it is best to advise the patient not to play cricket or hockey or to box, as these sports are especially likely to produce hand injuries.

Solitary exostoses are not uncommon. When swelling is the only symptom it is better to leave them alone, since operative intervention may leave a painful scar or adhesions. Otherwise simple exostosectomy may be performed.

Multiple exossis (metaphysical achalasia) presents special problems. Body contact sports should be avoided. The local lesions should be dealt with as necessary.

The chief problem of other bone tumours is early diagnosis. Onset of symptoms is often insidious, and when presenting in a sportsman may easily be mistaken for minor soft tissue injuries (Fig. 14.19). The tragedy which may result if such tumours are permitted to progress undiagnosed is a further stimulus to the proper investigation of sports injuries.

A. McD.

References

1. Warwick, R. and Williams, P. L. (1973) *Gray's Anatomy*, 35th Edn. London: Longmans.
2. Wiles, P. (1960) *Atlas of Fractures, Dislocations and Sprains*. London: Churchill.
3. Adams, J. C. (1972) *Outline of Fractures*. Edinburgh: Churchill Livingstone.
4. Devas, M. B. (1958) Stress fracture of the tibia in athletes or 'shin soreness'. *J. Bone Jt Surg.*, **40B,** 227.
5. Burrows, H. J. (1956) Fatigue fracture of the tibia. *J. Bone Jt Surg.*, **38B,** 83.

15

Joints

Structure and function

Anatomically a joint is described as the union between adjacent bones whether this enjoys movement or not.[1] A joint is classified by its structure, and may be described as fibrous, where fibrous tissue unites the bone ends. Where some slight movement occurs it is called a syndesmosis (Fig. 15.1), and where no movement occurs, a suture (Fig. 15.2).

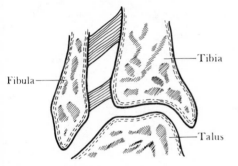

Fibula —

— Tibia

— Talus

Fig. 15.1 Fibrous joint; syndesmosis.

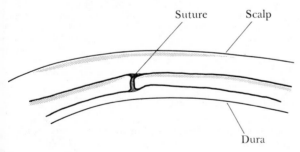

Suture   Scalp

Dura

Fig. 15.2 Fibrous joint; suture.

Where cartilage unites the bones, either temporarily (as in an epiphysis) or permanently (as in the vertebral column, the symphysis pubis, or the manubriosternal articulation) the joint is termed cartilaginous (Fig. 15.3).

Synovial joints are those surrounded by a fibrous capsule where the bones can move easily upon each other because they are plated with smooth articular cartilage, and lubricated and nourished by synovial fluid (Fig. 15.4).

The fibrous capsule of a joint may be thickened in areas of stress to form a

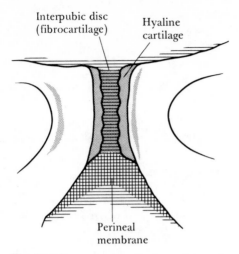

Interpubic disc
(fibrocartilage)

Hyaline
cartilage

Perineal
membrane

Fig. 15.3 Secondary cartilaginous joint; the symphysis pubis.

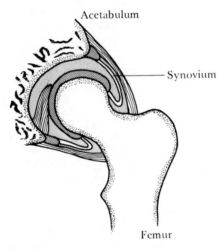

Acetabulum

Synovium

Femur

Fig. 15.4 The hip joint; an example of a cotylical joint.

ligament. Sometimes accessory ligaments are found within the joint to give added strength, for example the cruciate ligaments in the knee.

The synovial membrane lines the inner surface of the joint capsule, but does not encroach onto the articular cartilage. Protrusions of the synovial membrane may occur through the capsule to form bursae to reduce friction between the capsule, bone, and adjacent tendons. In addition, plates of fibrocartilage may extend from the margins of the capsule into the joint to prevent jarring, or to mould more accurately the bony surfaces to fit each other, as in the temporomandibular joint and the knee. Whatever the anatomical structure and shape, the stability of synovial joints is maintained essentially by the activity of the surrounding muscles.

A joint performs three functions; to transmit stress, to fix part of the limb whilst other joints are moving, and finally, itself to permit movement. Joints transmit stress while stabilized by muscular activity, and the least muscular activity is required when the stress is transmitted through the centre of the joint. If repeated or excessive stress is placed on a joint away from the position of minimal effort, muscles fatigue or are strained, and ligaments stretch or tear. Stabilization of joints is essential so that muscles can obtain maximal leverage for movement. Every joint has its own range of movements, which may be gliding, angular, or rotational.

The synovial lining of a joint is a mesothelium, secreting synovial fluid, having the capacity of regeneration if damaged and having also some phagocytic power. It can assimilate red blood cells and some intra-articular foreign materials. Synovial fluid is lubricant, nutritive, anticoagulant and bacteriostatic.

Joint injuries

A joint may be injured in a number of ways, including a direct blow leading to contusion of the capsule or injury to cartilage or bone.[2] An unexpected or excessive force to which the protective mechanism of the joint does not have time to react, or cannot develop the tension to withstand, may cause damage, as may overuse of an unconditioned joint, or faulty or abnormal techniques leading to low grade repetitive stresses on the joint. External penetration of the joint may occur as well as damage to supporting structures.

Diagnosis of joint injuries should be possible in most cases from careful eliciting of the history, symptoms, and signs. Ancillary methods of diagnosis such as X-ray, blood tests, arthroscopy and biopsy should be used for confirmation as appropriate.

The history is all important. It is necessary to determine from the patient how and when the injury occurred; what stresses were on the joint at the time of injury; where the pain was first felt; whether the injury was sufficient immediately to incapacitate him; the progress of symptoms after the initial onset of pain; the history of any previous similar injury, and if positive what treatment had been given. The physical examination of the joint should be meticulous, particular attention being paid to local tenderness, swelling, deformity, instability, and altered range of movement. If after the joint has been thoroughly examined gently and without stress, the diagnosis is still uncertain the joint should be subjected to a functional test. This is particularly important and should reproduce the pain in cases of doubt. It also allows technical faults to be noted, and a suitable rehabilitation programme to be instigated where injury is already recovering or is minor.

X-ray findings
X-rays are essential and should be repeated after 14 days if satisfactory progress is not being made. Only exceptionally should manipulations be carried out without preliminary X-rays

Types of injuries

Fracture

Such fractures are intra-articular and commonly involve the articular surface, damaging the articular cartilage.[3] Accurate reduction is essential to minimize the risk of later osteoarthrosis. Where a displaced fragment is present it may be left provided it does not impinge on the joint surface, otherwise removal is indicated. Tilting of the joint surface must be realigned and any irregularity of load bearing surface must be actively corrected, if necessary surgically. Avulsion injuries of insertions of tendons and ligaments to bone require careful assessment of joint stability, so as to decide whether or not surgical repair is required.

Fracture dislocation

Difficulty in handling these injuries arises for two reasons, firstly because the fracture, being intra-articular, is often unstable even though impacted. In attempting to reduce the dislocation, disimpaction occurs and the intra-articular fragment may rotate into a bad position, so that operative reduction is then re-

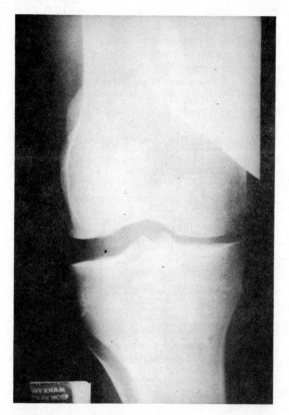

Fig. 15.5 Capsular damage revealed by stress X-ray after spontaneously reduced subluxation of the knee joint.

quired. The second reason is that since the fracture line is at the joint level, instability of the fracture still remains after reduction of the dislocation, and operative repair to the bone may have to be carried out to stabilize the fracture. Further, callus formation is poor if the fracture line is exposed to anticoagulant synovial fluid.

Dislocation

These injuries may be complete or partial (subluxation). In the latter case the bones may spontaneously reduce and the condition go unrecognized unless X-rays are taken while stress is applied to the capsule and ligaments (Fig. 15.5).

Dislocations of both types inevitably mean damage to capsular ligaments, synovial membrane and often articular cartilage. Instability in the joint may be present after reduction. This must be treated by adequate immobilization (in the upper limb three weeks, in the lower limb six weeks), or by surgical repair of the ligaments. Less positive treatment gives a risk of recurring dislocation in the joint, requiring subsequent operative repair which at this stage rarely gets the joint back to pre-injury mobility, strength, and stability. This is particularly so in shoulder and ankle injuries.

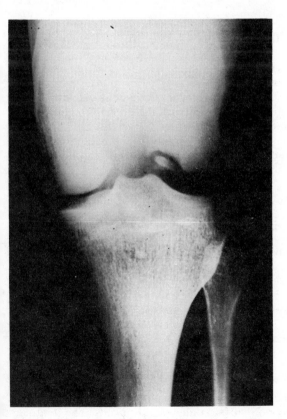

Fig. 15.6 Osteochondritis dissecans; a common site on the femoral condyle.

Separated epiphysis

This condition occurs in children, and displacement may occur some time after the initial trauma.[4, 5] Accurate replacement of the epiphysis must be achieved by manipulation or open operation and pinning. The injury is then treated as if the bone had been fractured.

Osteochondritis dissecans

Many theories have been put forward as to the cause of this condition.[6, 7] That trauma is a major one seems logical in that the lesions are almost always in the bone at the point where contact is made in jarring injuries. Damage occurs to the articular cartilage and subchondral bone. The bone and cartilage are devitalized by avascular necrosis, and flakes of cartilage and/or of bone can be extruded into the joint as loose bodies which may require operative removal. In some cases revascularization can take place before extrusion occurs. The joints commonly affected are the knee, ankle, and elbow (Fig. 15.6).

Injuries affecting the cartilage

Chondromalacia

This is a condition of the articular cartilage where fibrillary flaking occurs.[8] It is commonest in the knee on the patella (see Chapter 25).

Damage to the fibrocartilage

By far the most common lesions are to the menisci of the knee.[9] The only satisfactory treatment for these lesions is surgical removal of the meniscus, although in the older athlete a compromise of physiotherapy with the emphasis on quadriceps re-education may avoid operation.

Damage to fibrocartilaginous discs in the temporomandibular joint, lower radio-ulnar joints, and sterno-clavicular joints, although rare, can be crippling to sportsmen, and should be treated surgically if troublesome.

Capsular injuries

A sudden unexpected force, either in the normal plane of movement or acting in an abnormal plane, can result in capsular tears. At the same time damage to the synovial membrane can occur. Tearing of the fibres of the capsule leads to haemorrhage and tenderness locally, whereas damage to the synovium leads to an effusion in the joint and sometimes haemarthrosis. Provided the stability of the joint is retained these lesions respond very well to measures indicated in the general outlines of treatment—ice, pressure, muscle re-education and, after initial rest, a graduated exercise programme. After 48 hours, movement must be encouraged and contrast baths and heat in the form of short wave diathermy can be used.

Contusions

Direct blows lead to bruising of the periarticular tissues as well as to sprains if the force pushes the joint beyond its normal range of movements. The treatment is the same as for sprains.

Pinching of the intracapsular soft tissues

Not uncommonly a sudden movement, often with a rotational factor, causes soft tissue to be crushed between the bones of the joint. This is particularly common in the knee joint where the infrapatellar pad of fat is very vulnerable. An effusion which is often haemorrhagic then occurs. It is treated as for a sprain, but resumption of movement is more guarded as the fat is slow to heal and is often replaced by inelastic fibrous scar tissue which is easily irritated. In severe cases the infrapatellar pad is sheared off the upper end of the tibia. Surgical intervention is sometimes necessary. A long-term effect of this condition is that portions of the pad may become pedunculated and adherent by bands to the femur. Torsion and gangrene can occur, leading to haemarthrosis or locking. Calcification of the tag may also occur. Surgery offers a swift cure.

Traumatic bursitis

Irritation of the numerous periarticular bursae lined by synovium, which may or may not directly communicate with a joint, either by direct trauma[10] or overuse of tendinous structures near them, can lead to chronic effusion (Fig. 15.7). Healing is possible if the treatment used is ice, pressure, aspiration, and cessation of the irritating movement but should thickening of the bursa occur, surgical removal offers the only relief. In the more superficial bursae absorption of the effusion may be stimulated by short wave diathermy.

Ligament sprains

Clinically it is of major importance to determine to what extent the ligament is torn.[11] If only a few fibres are torn the only treatment necessary is to apply ice to minimize the swelling, support the joint to prevent further stretching, and allow full activity. Stability of the joint is fully maintained. Where there is a

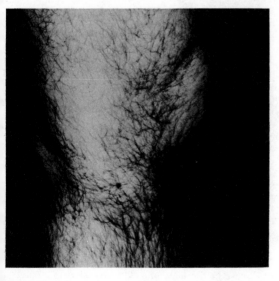

Fig. 15.7 Popliteal cyst (semi-membranosus bursa) causing swelling behind the knee.

substantial number of fibres torn but the tear is incomplete and stability is still retained, the same first aid treatment and subsequent support is carried out, but activity is initially restricted to gentle movements in the normal plane of the joint, starting first with non-weight-bearing exercises and swimming, and progressing to weight-bearing straight-ahead exercises. Finally rotational twisting movements are introduced after 2–3 weeks. Many authorities use infiltration with hydrocortisone in these lesions believing that healing is speeded up. It is this type of lesion also that some practitioners are inclined to infiltrate with local anaesthetics so as to allow the competitor to continue to play. This is disastrous as the risk of completing the tear is extremely high. *The only use for a local anaesthetic is where doubt occurs whether a full tear or a partial tear exists.* As a diagnostic test, infiltration allows the surgeon more accurately to determine whether instability exists. If a complete tear is present surgery or a plaster immobilization for at least six weeks is necessary.

Rheumatic and degenerative conditions

The first important fact is that sportsmen are not immune to these conditions. It is therefore necessary to guard against diagnosing every joint condition as trau-

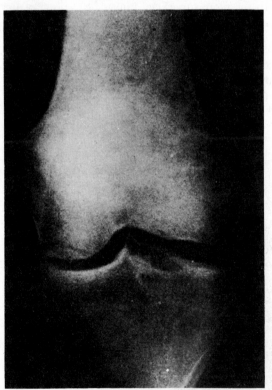

Fig. 15.8 Severe degenerative joint disease in the knee of a 32-year-old tennis player. There was a history of recurrent injury and two meniscectomies.

matic because it occurs in a sportsman. There is no doubt that injury can precipitate an acute episode in a joint where a degenerative or infective lesion is present. This is particularly so in osteoarthrosis.

Gout

Sport is quite compatible with this disease provided the disease has been adequately controlled medically. Should injury occur to a joint, immediate prophylactic increase in medication should be undertaken over the first seven days. It should in this context be noted that a high serum uric acid may be a normal phenomenon in athletes.

Osteoarthrosis

This is a disease of attrition affecting primarily the articular cartilage and later the bone around the edges of the articular cartilage. It most commonly involves the weight bearing joints, and is markedly precipitated by irregularity of the articular surface, damage of the articular cartilage due to trauma or infection, or where deformity of the bones leads to excessive stress being exerted on a part of the joint—genu varum leads to osteoarthrosis of the lateral compartment of the knee. Do sportsmen develop arthritis in joints more quickly than the sedentary population? It is certain that joints which have been subject to repeated trauma, recurrent sprains or fractures, or are the subject of surgical interference have a higher incidence than joints spared injury (Fig. 15.8). However whether a normal joint subjected to normal or even heavy exercise wears out more rapidly is not easy to prove. Should an athlete then cease activity because of developing osteoarthrosis? Frequently osteoarthrosis (Fig. 15.9) is symptomless and is not aggravated clinically by exercise, so that it may be better to balance the risk of later osteoarthrosis against the cardiovascular dangers of a less active way of life.

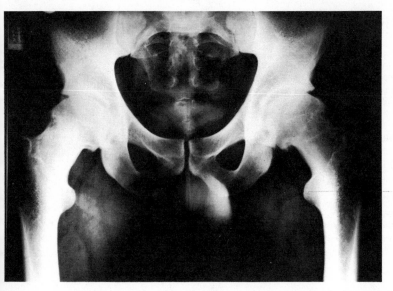

Fig. 15.9 Bilateral osteoarthrosis of the hip joints in an active professional rugby player.

Periarthritis
This group of diseases is ill-defined. Usually they are associated with an active disease process elsewhere, and may collectively be referred to as rheumatic. The tissues around the joint are infiltrated, there is a slight increase in temperature of the joint, and generalized pain and tenderness are present. Small effusions are not uncommon and movement is painful. Rest is indicated and heat, in the form of hot packs, appears to relieve the condition. Formal investigation to establish the cause will lead on to appropriate management.

Loose bodies
Occasionally loose bodies form in a joint as a result either of trauma, degeneration, or inflammation. They may be bony, cartilaginous or synovial, single or multiple (as in chondromatosis), and free or attached (Fig. 15.6). They are harmless unless they interfere with movement (locking), in which case they should be removed surgically.

Infection

Infection may be primary from a penetrating wound (accidental or surgical) or secondary, being blood-borne and infecting a pre-existing haemarthrosis or haematoma about the joint. Specific infections such as tuberculosis may also occur in sportsmen. Absolute rest and energetic treatment of the infection take precedence over joint activity. Resumption of activity must be carefully planned and graduated.

Aims of treatment of joint injuries

Correct deformity
Any deformity must be corrected so that normal configuration of the joint is obtained, irregularity of bony surface minimized, and mechanical obstruction to movement of the joint removed. Stability of the joint must be restored either by proprioceptive neuro-muscular re-education, or where necessary, by surgical repair of torn structures.

Minimize swelling
Early treatment with ice, pressure, elevation of the joint and rest will greatly lessen the risk of excessive swelling. Heat is contraindicated as is massage. Aspiration is indicated for diagnostic purposes and for the relief of tension—it does, however, introduce the risk of infection and its consequences. Aspiration should therefore always be carried out with full aseptic precautions.

Minimize muscle wasting
Inhibition or wasting of muscle groups quickly follows joint injury, classically of the quadriceps group in knee injuries (Fig. 15.10). Preventive exercise is essential.

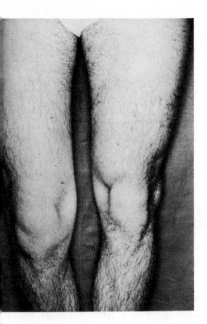

Fig. 15.10 Muscle wasting after joint injury; loss of quadriceps bulk after injury to the right knee joint.

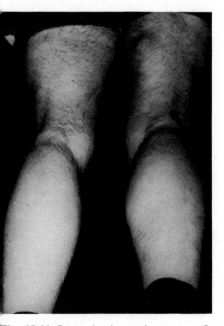

Fig. 15.11 Protective hamstring spasm after injury to the right knee joint.

Reabsorb swelling

This is achieved by joint and muscle activity together with local pressure. The aim is to prevent development of capsular laxity due to chronic effusion.

Periarticular swelling must be absorbed to allow full joint movement and normal tendon activity. Contrast baths (after 48 hours) and exercise are the best methods.

Overcome muscle spasm

Protective muscle spasm frequently interferes with rehabilitation, particularly hamstring spasm after knee injuries (Fig. 15.11). In such cases the spastic muscle must be treated with local ice and spasmolytics.

Instigate normal movements

All remedial exercises must be designed to restore movements in the normal plane. Support to the joint must be such that movement in this plane is not restricted. Limps or trick movements must be eliminated before extra strains are placed on other joints, tendons, and ligaments.

Regain normal strength

As the joint regains a normal painless range of movements, exercise should be introduced to redevelop muscle strength. Return to full activity before this is achieved can only lead to recurrence of injury.

Re-educate to full technical function

Once movement and strength has been regained, technique training must be resumed. Breakdown will occur if the muscles and joint are not re-educated into the rhythm of the movement.

Minimize the risk of infection

This is particularly important in the penetrating wound. Thorough surgical cleansing of wounds must be undertaken—reliance on antibiotic cover is not adequate.

During these stages of rehabilitation, attention must be paid to the general conditioning of the patient. Whilst it is essential to modify and restrict movements in the affected joint, every opportunity should be taken to continue normal training of the rest of the body.

Finale

Whilst this chapter has been written about joint injuries, it is timely to point out that many joint injuries are preventable by accurate basic training to condition the joint, understanding the role of the joint in the sport to be performed, developing adequate muscle strength for the task, and meticulous attention to technique training. It is better *to prevent* than cure.

H.C.T.

References

1. Warwick, R. and Williams, P. L. (1973) *Gray's Anatomy*, 35th Edn. London: Longmans.
2. Polacco, A. (1971) In *Encyclopedia of Sport Science and Medicine*, ed. Larson, L. A., London: Collier-Macmillan.
3. Harmon, P. H. (1945) Intra-articular osteochondrial fractures as a cause for internal derangement of the knee in adolescents. *J. Bone Jt Surg.*, **27A,** 703.
4. Sideman, S. (1943) Traumatic separation of the lower femoral epiphysis. *J. Bone Jt Surg.*, **29,** 913.
5. Larson, R. L. and McMahan, R. O. (1966) The epiphysis and the childhood athlete. *J. Am. Med. Ass.*, **196,** 607.
6. Green, W. T. and Banks, H. H. (1953) Osteochondritis dissecans in children. *J. Bone Jt Surg.*, **35A,** 26.
7. Green, G. P. (1966) Osteochondritis dissecans of the knee. *J. Bone Jt Surg.*, **48B,** 82.
8. Wiles, P., Andrews, P. S. and Devas, M. B. (1956) Chondromalacia of the patella. *J. Bone Jt Surg.*, **38B,** 95.
9. Helfet, A. J. (1959) Mechanism of derangements of the medial semilunar cartilage and their management. *J. Bone Jt Surg.*, **41B,** 319.
0. Larson, R. L. and Osternig, L. R. (1974) Traumatic bursitis and artificial turf. *J. sports Med.*, **2,** 183.
1. Allman, F. L., Jr. (1967) Classification of sprains and strains. In *Proceedings of the Eighth National Conference on the Medical Aspects of Sport*. Chicago: American Medical Association.

16

Tendons

Anatomy and physiology

Tendons are composed of compact bundles of longitudinally disposed collagenous fibres. In the resting state the fibres have a slightly wavy appearance suggesting that they are capable of a certain amount of stretch. The fibroblast nuclei are spindle-shaped and are arranged along the collagenous bundles with their long axes parallel to those of the collagenous fibres. The tendon is invested in a tubular sheath, the paratenon, which is a smooth membrane lined with mesothelial cells and there is a small amount of interstitial tissue, the endotenon which carries the nutrient vessels to the tendon fibres.

In some areas the paratenon forms the visceral layer of a true tendon sheath for example around the flexor tendons of the fingers, but in other sites such as the Achilles tendon there is no synovial sheath. A tendon gains attachment to bone by the paratenon becoming continuous with the periosteum and the tendon fibres entering the cortical bone. A junctional zone exists between the cortical bone and tendon, in which chondrocytes are seen and this area of fibrocartilage is separated from the tendon by a line of demarcation with basophilic staining properties, the 'blue line'. At its other extremity, the tendon fibres blend with the striated muscle fibres. This is the weakest point of a muscle tendon unit.

The blood supply to a tendon is tenuous. Nutrient arteries which are small in calibre enter the paratenon at the musculo-tendinous junction and from the periosteum. Branches extend into the endotenon to supply blood to the deepest fibres. It will be seen that the midpoint of the tendon which is at the end of the supply lines is most likely to suffer the effects of any interference with blood flow. Increase in tension in the tendon has been shown to decrease and finally stop the blood flow in veins and capillaries.[1] The capillary bed decreases with age and inactivity.[3]

The metabolic activity of tendons is low[4], of the order of $0\cdot1\,\mu l/mg/h$ and the mature collagen fibres and fibrocytes are thought to be able to withstand anoxic conditions for some hours. The possible relationships between blood supply, blood flow, ageing, tension, and excessive use on the one hand, and degeneration and rupture on the other, have never been adequately explored.

Great intrinsic strength is required if a tendon is to perform its function of transmitting the power of a muscle contraction to the joint over which it operates. This strength may be of the order of $5-10\,kg/mm^2$ as in the case of the Achilles tendon.[5] This great intrinsic strength is usually sufficient to tolerate the stresses of muscle contraction, but the tendon may be most vulnerable when a sudden and unexpected stretching force is applied, as when missing a step or the edge of a kerb. In general, however, the tendon is protected by the presence within its substance of stretch receptors (the Golgi tendon receptors) which when stimulated by excessive stretch have an inhibitory effect on muscle contraction. This counterbalances the other main muscle stretch receptor system (the muscle spindles) which responds to stretch by exciting muscle contraction.

Continuous remodelling of the collagenous fibres and secretion of new collagen takes place. Thus, provided that the tendon is not deprived of its blood supply, exposed to over-use, or weakened by a generalized disorder of connective tissue, e.g. rheumatoid disease, rupture or degeneration would appear to be an unlikely event. Nevertheless, partial and complete rupture of tendon is not uncommon.

Pathology of tendon degeneration and rupture

There is increasing evidence that spontaneous rupture of tendon occurs only when the tendon has undergone degeneration.[6-8] Spontaneous rupture is an uncommon event in youth and early adult life, but becomes increasingly common in the older sportsman and may occur with comparatively trivial stress. Experimentally it was found possible to produce ruptures by persistent exercising on a treadmill, but unfit rats were apparently unable to generate sufficient muscle power to enable rupture to take place. Ljungqvist[9] has provided evidence that rupture may be partial, a condition analogous to ligamentous strains. More recently central degeneration of the Achilles tendon has been described.[10] In all these conditions histological examination reveals areas of degenerate collagen with pyknotic fibroblast nuclei and, in the case of central degeneration of the tendon, there are areas of granulation tissue with a few mononuclear cells and collections of thin-walled blood vessels (Fig. 16.1). Repair in the form of proliferation of young fibroblasts is strikingly sparse.

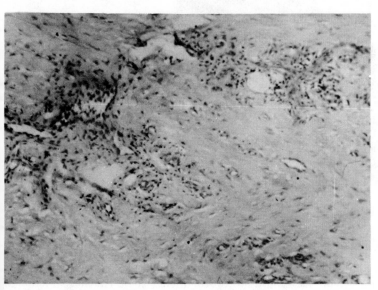

Fig. 16.1 Histological appearances of degenerate tendon showing necrotic collagen fibres, pyknotic fibroblast nuclei and thin-walled blood vessels.

Ossification of tendon

Not uncommonly cracks occur in the cortical bone at points of tendinous insertion, and the adjacent fibrocartilagenous region and the tendon itself may be invaded by osseous tissue including bone marrow elements. Compact bone may then be found to extend for up to 2 or 3 cm along the tendon. These lesions do not cause pain or interference with function *per se* but are apt to fracture, in which case pain persists until the ossicle is excised.

Calcific tendinitis

Deposits of calcium in the form of calcium apatite are commonly observed in the tendons of the rotator cuff of the glenohumeral joint but may also be observed in other sites, for example the common extensor origin at the elbow (Fig. 16.2).

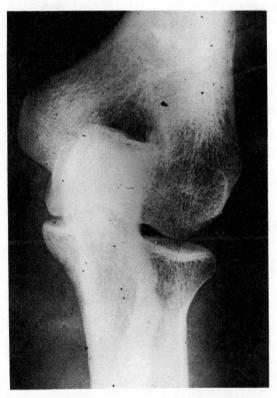

Fig. 16.2 Tennis, elbow; ectopic calcification of the common extensor origin.

The abrupt deposition of these salts is accompanied by an acute inflammatory reaction in the capsule and synovial membrane of the joint, and causes intense pain, muscle spasm and limitation of joint movement. Deposits may also slowly accumulate over a period of years, presumably in areas of degenerate tendon, and cause little or no discomfort. Not uncommonly acute calcific tendonitis is spontaneously relieved by the deposit of calcareous material rupturing into the joint cavity or subacromial bursa.

Tenosynovitis and tenovaginitis

Where a true synovial sheath is present, certain conditions such as over-use and compression may induce a tenosynovitis. Usually this is an acute condition which settles with rest, but it may become chronic and the pathological features then are not dissimilar to those seen in rheumatoid arthritis, that is reduplication of the lining cells with increased numbers of blood vessels, oedema, and infiltration of mononuclear cells. Where there is no parietal synovial layer, the paratenon apparently becomes thickened with fibrinoid degeneration and formation of dense fibrous adhesions to the tendon fibres.[11] In some areas the presence of inflammation in the tendon sheath leads to stenosis: a typical example of this occurs at the point in the wrist where the tendons of abductor pollicis longus and extensor

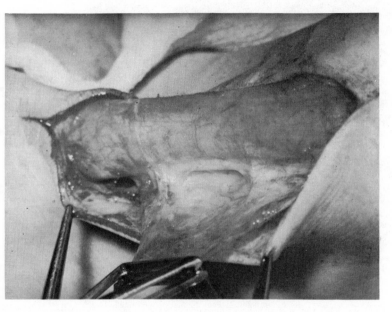

Fig. 16.3 Peritendonitis; inflammatory reaction between paratenon (of Achilles tendon) and surrounding tissues.

pollicis brevis cross. In this site, chronic inflammation leads to thickening and stenosis of the sheath with pain on movement of the wrist or thumb, a condition known as De Quervain's disease. In other situations where there is a single layer of paratenon (such as the Achilles tendon) the inflammatory reaction appears to be between the paratenon and the surrounding tissues, a peritendonitis (Fig. 16.3).

Where tendons pass around bony prominences and are required to alter direction, they are usually secured in place by a retinaculum. Apparently baffling cases of intermittent pain may be found to be due to rupture of the retinaculum allowing a tendon to slip out of its normal alignment as may occur with the peroneal tendons at the ankle.

Enthesopathies

In a number of situations the tendinous insertion of a muscle into bone may be the site of persistent pain. This condition, known as an enthesopathy, is particularly common where the common extensor tendon arises from the lateral epicondyle ('tennis elbow'), and at the origin of adductor longus from the pubis. The aetiology is not fully understood but enthesopathies appear to arise from causes such as chronic over-use, a sudden and unexpected strain on the muscle attachment, and perhaps contusions. Histologically, they consist of areas of necrotic collagen, granulomatous changes with thin-walled blood vessels, and

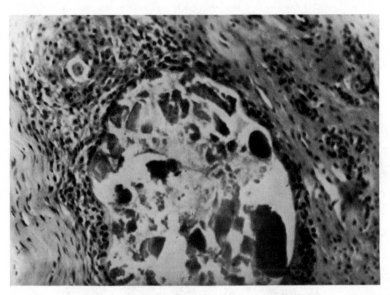

Fig. 16.4 Histological changes in tennis elbow—an enthesopathy; note chronic inflammatory cells, fibroblast proliferation, and necrotic collagen.

chronic inflammatory cells, small areas of active fibroblastic proliferation, and sometimes calcification (Fig. 16.4).

Goldie,[12] and Conrad and Hooper[13] have carried out detailed analyses of lateral epicondylitis, and their papers justify careful consideration. Goldie draws attention to the numerous conditions, apart from epicondylitis, which are lumped together under the title 'tennis elbow'. These include osteoarthrosis of the radiohumeral joint, entrapment of the posterior interosseous nerve, and nipping of synovium between the bone ends.

Clinical features of tendons and their sheaths

The Achilles tendon provides an excellent example of the ways in which disorders of tendons and their sheaths may present, and its pathological manifestations will be described in some detail (see also Chapter 25).

Tendon rupture

Rupture of the Achilles tendon is a relatively common disaster, the majority of cases occurring in the older athlete, particularly those over the age of forty. Rupture usually occurs during strenuous activity, almost always without any premonitory pain or tenderness. Occasionally, rupture may occur due to direct violence, for example a kick on the heel while the triceps muscle is actively contracting. Sometimes ill-advised intratendinous hydrocortisone injections may be an aetiological factor. As previously stated, the theoretical strength of the Achilles tendon in a healthy state is far in excess of any load which can be applied to it by physiological circumstances, and the conclusion that rupture is the result of degeneration of the tendon is in some cases supported by histological evidence. Rupture usually occurs approximately 3 cm above the insertion of the tendon into the os calcis. There is a sharp pain and a feeling of a thud which often prompts the victim to feel that somebody has shot him in the heel or kicked him. Subsequently, pain is not a prominent symptom but there is a weakness of the ankle with a typical flat-footed gait.

There are two schools of thought regarding the correct treatment of this condition. It has always been assumed in complete tendon rupture that the best results are obtained by approximation of the torn tendon ends with sutures after debridement. It has been customary to repair the Achilles tendon, and then to immobilize the lower leg and foot in a plaster of Paris walking splint with the foot in full equinus, for eight to twelve weeks after which a slowly increasing amount of activity is allowed. However, training cannot usually be resumed for many months. Complications of this procedure include failure of the skin incision to heal, rerupture of the tendon, wound sepsis, and calcification or ossification of the scar in the tendon. Adherence of skin to the tendon may also be a problem leading to persistent pain. In some series these complications have been very frequent.[6] The protagonists of conservative management point to these various complications, and claim that at follow-up, patients who have been treated merely by immobilization of the foot and lower leg in the equinus position in plaster of Paris for eight to twelve weeks, have a final result as good as or better than those treated surgically although return to sport is delayed by six months or more.[14] Most doctors who have the responsibility for athletes would feel, however, that accurate surgical repair leads to quicker return to activity, smaller chance of recurrent rupture, and less risk of persistent weakness of triceps surae. Prognosis is usually very good with full training possible within three to four months and very little chance of recurrence.

Partial rupture

It has recently been pointed out by Ljungqvist[9] that partial rupture of the Achilles tendon is not uncommon Fig. 16.5). This condition is heralded by sudden onset of pain during activity which persists whenever any stress is applied to the tendon.

Commonly the symptoms are at their worst when the patient first arises in the morning, tending to improve with walking, but any attempt to walk rapidly or run usually results in increasingly severe pain which precludes such activity. A tender swelling can be palpated at the site. Ljungqvist (1968) has reported typical EMG and X-ray findings which may be of some value in diagnosis. As in complete rupture, localized degeneration of the tendon, possibly due to an

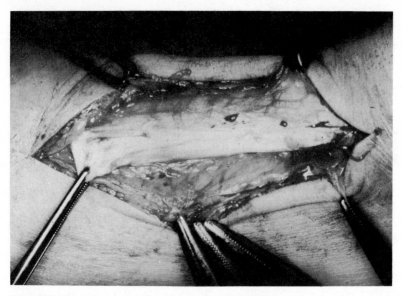

Fig. 16.5 Partial rupture of tendon (tendo Achilles).

inordinately severe training schedule, contusion and intra-tendinous hydrocortisone injection may be factors (see also Chapter 25).

Central degeneration

One of the more obscure causes of pain in the heel has been revealed as a degeneration of the central fibres of the Achilles tendon (Fig. 16.6). This condition, in which granulomatous changes appear but repair fails, is seen at the midpoint between musculo-tendinous junction and insertion of the tendon. Usually the most centrally placed fibres of the tendon are involved. It is probably no

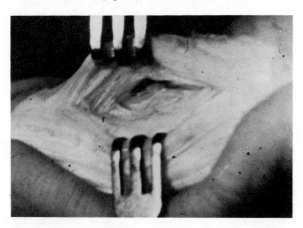

Fig. 16.6 Central degeneration of the Achilles tendon with failure of repair and cyst formation.

coincidence that this point has been shown to have the lowest blood supply of any portion of the Achilles tendon, and ischaemia is likely to be the pathogenetic mechanism.[15] The condition is usually seen in athletes undertaking very strenuous training programmes. The use of low heeled boots and running shoes has been cited as a cause of this problem, but probably more important is a change to training on hard surfaces such as road or board, a sudden marked increase in the severity of a training programme, and a change from the heel-strike type of foot placement of middle and long distance running to the toe-strike style employed in sprints and shorter middle distance events.

At first pain is felt only in the morning but tends to wear off after a few minutes walking. When training is attempted there is usually pain in the warm-up period, but in the early stages this may pass off and full training and even competition in endurance events may be possible. However, with the passage of time, pain becomes more prominent and persistent, particularly during sprinting, and usually ultimately forces withdrawal from competition. A period of rest from training may induce temporary relief of symptoms, only to be followed by a depressing relapse as soon as the level of activity is increased. Thus the clinical course is usually one of comparative freedom of symptoms after periods of rest, followed by relapses. The only sign is a small nodule in the tendon which is exquisitely tender to compression.

If the diagnosis is made very early, a complete rest for two weeks, with physiotherapy consisting of ultrasonic therapy and massage, may be helpful. On the whole, however, conservative management is disappointing and repair only takes place after a lengthy period of rest, with or without plaster of Paris, splinting or surgical intervention. For best results in these chronic cases the tendon should be opened and the necrotic fibres and granulations identified and excised (see Chapter 25). Some residual tenderness and thickening of the tendon can be expected in the first months after return to training.

Peritendonitis

Sudden increases in training may lead to a peritendonitis, that is, inflammation of the areolar tissue surrounding the tendon. This is characterized clinically by pain and swelling, the pain tending to disappear with activity. Examination reveals diffuse swelling around the tendon, sometimes with palpable crepitus on movement (Fig. 16.7). There is diffuse tenderness throughout the region. The condition almost always resolves with rest and physiotherapy, but occasionally requires infiltration of the peritendinous tissue with corticosteroid. Stubborn recurrent cases require operative treatment (see Chapter 25).

Rupture at the musculo-tendinous junction

Sudden acute pain of an intense stabbing nature, followed by swelling and severe pain when attempting to contract the affected muscle, is likely to indicate rupture of part of the muscle. In the calf, this condition has tended to be misdiagnosed as rupture of the plantaris tendon, but it is exceedingly unlikely that such a condition could be associated with so severe a pain and frequently vast haematoma formation, if indeed it exists at all. In some cases there may be a fairly substantial amount of muscle torn, and as the haematoma disperses a gap may become apparent in the muscle. This is of no great importance and surgical intervention

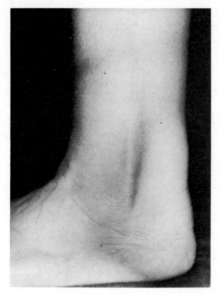

Fig. 16.7 Peritendonitis; pain and swelling around affected tendon as typified in this case of Achilles peritendonitis.

and attempted repair is certainly not indicated. Treatment is as described for muscle injuries (Chapter 17).

Other tendons

The conditions described above in relation to the Achilles tendon may be found in other tendons elsewhere in the body, e.g. the patellar tendon. They tend to present with very similar clinical features.

H.C.B.

References

1. Schatzker, M. D. and Branemark, P. I. (1969) Intravital observation on the microvascular anatomy and microcirculation of the tendon. *Acta orthop. scand.*, Suppl. 126.
2. Rothman, R. H. and Parke, W. W. (1965) The vascular anatomy of the rotator cuff. *Clin. Orthop.*, **14,** 176.
3. Rothman, R. H. and Slogoff, S. (1967) The effect of immobilisation on the vascular bed of the tendon. *Surg. Gynec. Obstet.*, **122,** 1064.
4. Peacock, E. E., Jr. (1959) A study of the circulation in normal tendons and healing grafts. *Ann. Surg.*, **149,** 415.
5. Elliott, D. H. (1965) Structure and function of mammalian tendon. *Biol. Rev.*, **40,** 392.
6. Arner, O. and Lindholm, A. (1959) Subcutaneous rupture of the Achilles tendon— a study of 92 cases. *Acta chir. scand.*, Suppl. 239.
7. Konn, G. and Everth, H. J. (1967) Morphologie der Spontanen Sehnengerreissungen. *Hafte Unfalheilk*, **91,** 255.

8. Judet, R., Judet, J., Letournel, E. and Rigault, P. (1963) A Propos de la rupture du tendon d'Achille' *Mém. Acad. Chir.*, **89**, 298.
9. Ljungqvist, R. (1968) Subcutaneous partial rupture of the Achilles tendon. *Acta orthop. scand.*, Suppl. 113.
10. Burry, H. C. and Pool, C. J. (1973) Central degeneration of the Achilles tendon. *Rheum. Rehabil.*, **12**, 177.
11. Snook, G. A. (1972) Tenosynovitis in long distance runners. *Med. Sci. Sports*, **4**, 166.
12. Goldie, I. (1964) Epicondylitis lateralis humeri. *Acta chir. scand.*, Suppl. 339.
13. Conrad, R. W. and Hooper, W. R. (1973) Tennis Elbow: its course natural history, conservative and surgical management. *J. Bone Jt Surg.*, **55A**, 1177.
14. Lea, R. B. and Smith, L. (1972) Non surgical treatment of tendo-achilles rupture. *J. Bone Jt Surg.*, **54A**, 1398.
15. Lagergren, C. and Lindholm, A. (1959) Vascular distribution in the Achilles tendon. *Acta chir. scand.*, Suppl. 116.

17

Muscles

Structure and function

The individual contractile elements of skeletal (voluntary) muscle are bound together into fasciculi or bundles by the connective tissue sheath called the perimysium, and these bundles are further bound together by the denser epimysium to form the muscle itself. Between the fasciculi lie the ramifying vessels and nerves, and a varying amount of fat.

Contractile elements

The muscle fibre consists of a firm tubular sarcolemma within which is contained the contractile substance[1] which presents a striated appearance. Each fibre is up to 40 mm in length and from 0·01 to 0·1 mm in diameter. The fibres do not branch; their spindle-shaped ends interlock with other fibres or the tissues of the muscle origin or insertion.

In voluntary muscle the striations consist essentially of alternate bands of actin and myosin arranged in pallisades. During contraction the actin strands slide between the myosin rods like the graphite rods in a nuclear reactor. Interaction is greatest at about 50 per cent overlap and least at extremes, which accounts in part for the muscles' maximum tension development in the middle range.

Two main types of fibre have been described, the red fibres—rich in myohaemoglobin and poorly striated—and the markedly striated pale fibres. The former have a more prolonged contraction after an extended latent period, are found in the more deep-seated muscles, and are thought to be primarily concerned with the maintenance of posture, whereas the pale fibres with their more rapid action, initiate movement. Fast and slow twitch fibres show specific responses to different training methods.

Non-contractile elements

The vascular capillary bed of skeletal muscle is most extensive, forming a network between the fibres. The degree to which these vessels are patent, and hence the vascularity of the muscle, depends on the type of training to which it has been submitted.[2] Lymph vessels have not been demonstrated in voluntary muscle. The amount of interstitial fat varies with the degree of training and is most marked in atrophied muscle.

Mechanics

Force is developed when a muscle contracts in the long axis of its fibres, or in the line of the long resultant (parallelogram of forces) in the case of multipennate muscles.

In order that movement may occur, the muscle requires two points of attachment (origin and insertion) separated by a mobile joint. Such points of attachment may be tendinous, aponeurotic, or fleshy (in which the perimysium, not the fibres, is fused with the periosteum or perichondrium). When muscle contracts to produce a movement the tension in the muscle during the movement remains generally more or less constant, and the contraction is called isotonic. Isometric contraction takes place in the absence of movement when tension increases without shortening of the fibres.

The power of a muscle is approximately proportional to the number of constituent fibres and to its cross-sectional area, and is of the order of 120 to 140 lb/in² (828–966 kPa).[3] During contraction the fibres may shorten to 60 per cent of their length when fully stretched.[4]

When muscle functions at almost full shortening it is said to be working in the inner range; when at about half-length, in the middle range; and when almost fully stretched it functions in the outer range. Because of the obvious mechanical factors as well as the greatest actin/myosin strand interaction, maximum tension is developed only in the middle range. Muscle is less powerful and efficient in the inner and outer ranges.

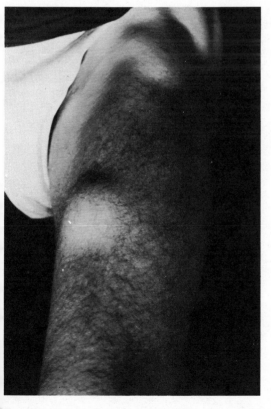

Fig. 17.1 Complete rupture of the rectus femoris. Note two retracted muscle ends in the middle and upper part of picture.

Muscle injury

Damage to a muscle, whether intrinsic or extrinsic in origin, will result in tearing and disruption of the muscle fibres, connective tissue, and vessels, and may occur in the belly of the muscle, or at the origin or insertion of the fibres into tendon, aponeurosis or periosteum. (Not to be confused with periosteal detachment from bone at the site of a muscle tendon or ligament attachment—see Chapter 16.)

Complete rupture with solution of anatomical continuity and the production of a demonstrable gap in the muscle is uncommon (Fig. 17.1). This may be confused with muscle hernia in which there is a split in the muscle sheath which allows the belly of the muscle to bulge up through it during contraction (Fig. 17.2). Rarely, a peculiar ladder or ripple pattern may be observed as an incidental finding. It is not associated with injury and causes no disability. Edwards[5] has shown this to occur on passive stretching with the muscle silent on electromyography. It is probably due to banding of the overlying fascia (Fig. 17.3).

Most commonly injury is restricted to only a few muscle fibres and their supporting connective tissues, in which case it may be called a 'pull', 'tear', or 'strain'.

When a tear or strain occurs, both contractile and non-contractile elements

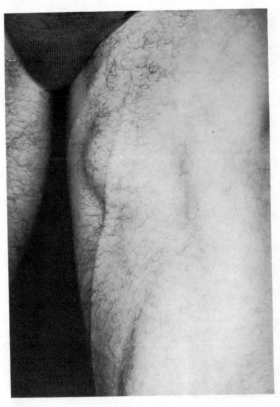

Fig. 17.2 Muscle hernia. Hernia of adductor in left thigh bulging up under the saphenous vein. The quadriceps is also contracted in this view.

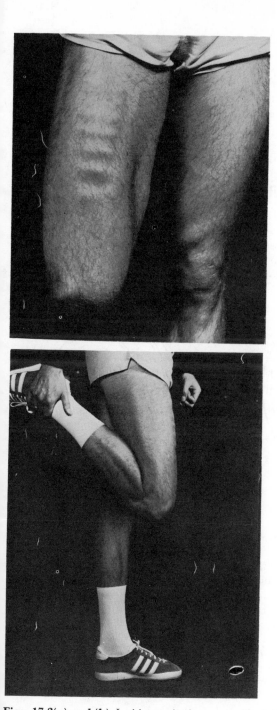

Figs. 17.3(a) and (b) Ladder or ripple muscle. Fascial bands stand out with the muscle passively extended. (Photo: R. H. T. Edwards.)

are damaged, but such is the comparative strength of the muscle fibres that the major damage is probably incurred by the connective tissues, particularly the blood vessels. As a result of this injury, blood (and to a lesser extent tissue fluid) escapes into the extracellular and interstitial spaces of the muscle already somewhat engorged as a result of the hyperaemia of exercise, thus producing the haematoma. In the more severe cases where the muscle sheath has also been damaged, this haematoma may expand into the potential space between the muscles. The degree of haemorrhage and haematoma formation is directly proportional to the vascularity of the muscle, and inversely proportional to the degree of general muscle tone.

When extrinsic violence is applied to a muscle the subcutaneous and deep connective tissues are damaged as well, and also become the site of haematoma formation. Thus, intramuscular haematomas are more commonly produced by intrinsic tears, interstitial haematomas by external bruising (Fig. 17.4). Bruising is also most commonly the cause of muscle hernia. In open wounds involving muscle, the haematoma tends to be more localized since haemorrhage to the surface occurs in preference to 'tracking' in the deep tissues.

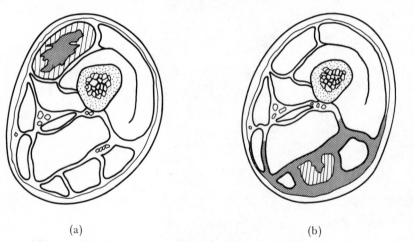

(a)　　　　　　　　　　　　　　　　　　(b)

Fig. 17.4 Muscle haematomas; A, intramuscular; B, interstitial.

Haemorrhage from the site of injury will cease as intramuscular tension builds up, thus compressing the bleeding points. In normal subjects clotting is complete within a few hours although, while the clot is still friable (two or three days), further haemorrhage is likely in response to additional trauma, for example massage! Resolution of the haematoma takes place by a process of absorption and fibrosis, leaving some degree of scarring and, in the tissue planes, adhesion. Because of their length, only part of the muscle fibres in an area of tear or bruising may be damaged. In such cases regeneration can take place with restoration of muscle fibre structure. The process takes about three weeks.[6]

Aetiology of muscle tears

At present the exact cause of muscle tears remains unknown. Various explanations have been put forward to account for the occurrence of these essentially intrinsic injuries.

Tucker[7] regards muscle tears as being due to a postural fault—he suggests that movements are carried out by the activators and synergists against a background of general postural alertness in the prime fixers. He goes on to point out that analysis of this type of injury shows that the activators are 'thrown into action hurriedly before the prime fixers are alerted and a sudden strain is imposed on the prime fixers'. This theory might explain the incidence of muscle tears in football, but not of those occurring in track runners.

Abrahams[8] postulated some sort of circulating toxin as the cause of muscle strains, but brought forward no evidence in support of this theory.

Lloyd[9] does not regard defective skill as the full answer to intrinsic muscle injury. He considers that 'speed of muscular contraction is a greater factor than actual work done during contraction' in the production of muscle injury, and suggests that tearing is most likely when rapid maximum contraction is demanded of a fully stretched muscle which has to overcome increased frictional resistance resulting from the changing shape of the muscle.

Archer[10] quotes certain American coaches as considering that tearing takes place during the relaxation phase, when the pull of the strongly contracting antagonist is applied too vigorously, thus increasing the frictional resistance against the passively stretching muscle to such a point that it 'sticks', and tearing takes place.

Travers[11] blames technical inadequacy for the production of muscle tears, and suggests that the incidence of muscle injuries will diminish as technical faults are corrected. In the case of hamstring tears he considers 'overstriding' to be the chief cause and states that these injuries may be eliminated by training the

Table 17.1 Distribution of muscle strains in the legs of 45 athletes sustaining intrinsic injuries.

	Sprinters	Middle distance	Cross country	Hurdlers & Jumpers	
Adductors	1	3			4
Tensor fasciae latae				2	2
Rectus femoris	5	2		2	9
Vasti					0
Biceps femoris:					
Deep					0
Superficial	4	2		1	7
Semi membranosus/tendinosus	7	2		2	11
Sartorius				1	1
Gastrocnemius	1	6	1	1	9
Soleus					0
Anterior tibials			2		2
Totals	18	15	3	9	45

athlete to ground the leading foot no further forward than directly beneath the leading shoulder.

Some differentiation must be made between those injuries associated with external violence such as the 'blocking' of an active movement, e.g. the effect on the quadriceps of trying to kick a wet and heavy ball, and those purely intrinsic tears such as the sprinter's hamstring pull. A pointer to the mechanism lies in the actual muscles affected.

There can be no doubt that muscle tears occur most commonly in the lower limb. It is interesting to note the distribution of leg injuries, including muscle tears, in different types of track athlete (Table 17.1).

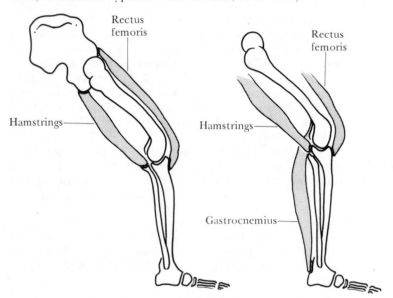

Fig. 17.5 Diagrammatic representation of the layout of the 'two span' muscles of the lower limbs.

When such figures are studied, it is noted that there is one anatomical property shared by those muscles which received intrinsic injury which is missing from those which escaped—they all span two joints. It follows, therefore, that they are all capable of producing movement at more than one joint (Fig. 17.5).

It will also be noted that those muscles most commonly torn, namely rectus femoris, gastrocnemius, and the hamstrings, when contracting during the action of running are 'paradoxical' in their actions. That is to say, of the two joint movements each produces when contracting, one is required in the activity (knee extension by rectus femoris, plantar flexion of the foot by gastrocnemius, extension of the hip by hamstrings), while the other (hip flexion by rectus femoris, knee flexion by gastrocnemius and hamstrings) is inimical to the desired activity (Lombard's paradox). For example, were rectus femoris and the hamstrings to contract in isolation without the backing of their associated single-span muscles (vasti and glutei) no movement would take place at either hip or knee joint, the muscles remaining in tension like the springs of an Anglepoise lamp to produce a sort of dynamic equilibrium. This state of equilibrium should be compared with the positive supporting reaction. However, visual analysis of muscle action during running (which is most easily done by means of the analysing projector and film loops) suggests that these two span groups *are* used to produce joint movement in addition to maintaining a background of postural equilibrium. This is seen in the case of the hamstrings which contract vigorously during the running cycle, firstly in flexing the knee during the pick up as the leg is brought through, and again in extending the hip as the foot is grounded at the beginning of the stride. It is obvious that the neuromuscular activity during a compound action such as running is extremely complex. Detailed analysis awaits development of more sophisticated techniques of electromyography.

Even so, it is possible to argue that most of this activity is carried out at reflex level; indeed the whole object of technical training is the development of the movement cycle, in whatever form it may take, as a conditioned reflex. Now the running action closely resembles a series of crossed extensor reflexes, an essential feature of which is reflex antagonist inhibition. When this reflex inhibition is blocked, it will follow that the prime mover and its antagonist will be contracting together instead of the one 'giving way' to the other to permit movement. Such a situation is more likely to exist in the case of two-span muscles, whose actions are governed by the demands of movements at more than one joint, than in the case of the single-span prime movers or activators. In tetanus, rabies, and strychnine poisoning there is a failure of reflex inhibition, and so muscles contract violently and antagonistically with resultant tears in many cases. It seems that muscle tears are caused by a breakdown in co-ordination of reflex inhibition leading to synchronous contraction of antagonist muscle groups. Such a breakdown may follow the bombardment of the spinal centres with impulses arising in the higher centres, which occurs when the athlete is mentally as well as physically 'flat out'; in other words straining for the last ounce of effort. This straining manifests itself clinically by loss of form (of which overstriding is a symptom), as the reflex nature of the athlete's actions gives way under intense pressure and he concentrates on moving one leg after the other as fast as possible rather than simply on running fast. Fatigue, lack of fitness, and weakness of basic technique all contribute to this breakdown which is particularly liable to involve the most delicately co-ordinated muscle groups, namely the two-span muscles (Fig. 17.6).

In injuries or tears involving *external* violence the mechanism is apparent—in such cases single-span muscles or activators (prime movers) are frequently affected.

Symptoms and signs of muscle injury

As a rule muscle damage occurs suddenly and the patient is able accurately to pinpoint in time the provocative incident, which may be a blow or an unexpected strain. Initially a sudden searing pain is felt which quickly fades away to a dull ache (exactly similar to that felt after an intramuscular injection). Movement of the affected part is painful, particularly under conditions of load. It is unusual for there to be any actual weakness.

On examination the affected muscle is tense and tender to the touch and there may be considerable local spasm. Sometimes swelling is marked, and in cases

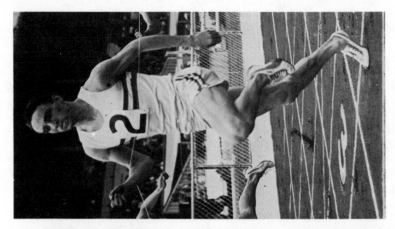

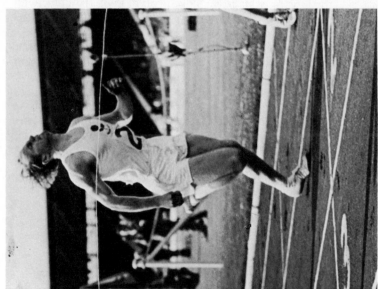

Figs. 17.6(a) and (b) Two sprinters at the finish of a race; one shows a picture of strain, the other relaxation. (Photos: Sport and General.)

of complete rupture a gap may be felt between the muscle ends. In muscle hernia a bulge appears in the long axis of the muscle (generally one of the thigh muscles) on vigorous contraction. Pain may be produced by passive stretching (depending on the degree of haematoma), and is invariably provoked by active contraction of the muscle against resistance. Skin discoloration is a late sign which may be quite remarkably extensive and appear at a site some distance from the original lesion.

The signs and symptoms of muscle bruising are similar, but there is a history of direct trauma, and localization of the injury is less definite as more than one muscle may be damaged.

Muscle stiffness

The foregoing injuries should not be confused with muscle stiffness although the mechanism by which pain is produced is similar, namely raised intramuscular pressure. Stiffness is due to accumulations of extracellular fluid in the muscle as a result of raised capillary filtration pressure in unaccustomed exercise. In such cases the vascular bed in the muscle is unable to cope adequately with the return of blood to the veins, and in the absence of lymphatics, dispersal of this increased extracellular fluid is delayed. Stiffness is a disease of the unfit, but may also occur in the trained sportsman under abnormal conditions, for example in the forearm muscles of a sculler racing into a cross-head wind. In the latter case resolution is rapid after cessation of exercise and the discomfort is only transitory.

Under certain circumstances the condition may be more disabling—the classic example is the Anterior Tibial syndrome. Here intramuscular tension is exaggerated by the unyielding surrounding tissues (see Chapter 25) to such an extent that local infarction may take place—in rare instances leading to massive local necrosis or a form of Volkmann's contracture. Alternatively raised tension within muscle fibres may so modify the internal frictional resistance of the muscle that fast movements become impossible and local tears occur if 'seizing up' of the whole muscle does not supervene.

The patient with muscle stiffness complains of gradually increasing pain, swelling, and in extreme cases difficulty in moving the affected muscle group. There is no evidence available to support the theory that these symptoms are due to local accumulation of lactic acid—indeed, all the evidence opposes it.

Hypertrophic states

Occasionally the muscle hypertrophy resulting from prolonged heavy training may produce local symptoms due to a 'space-occupying lesion effect'. For example hypertrophy of the lowest fibres of tibialis anterior may cause blocking of the upper extensor retinaculum of the ankle, while hypertrophy of the long thumb extensors may embarass excursion of the wrist extensors beneath. Treatment is by appropriate decompression.

The treatment of muscle injuries

In all cases the predominant symptom is pain which may be out of all proportion to the actual extent of the damage. Loss of function is usually a secondary phenomenon as complete ruptures are rare and even they may produce remarkably little functional disability.

Pain is due to the presence of a 'space-occupying' haematoma within the muscle, which produces stretching of the fibres and connective tissues in all directions. The only sensory nerve endings in muscles are stretch receptors, though it is suggested that the actual presence of irritating extravasated blood may also be a factor in symptom production.

The purpose of treatment is first to prevent haematoma formation, and second to promote rapid resolution of any haematoma which does form, with the two-fold object of getting rid of the pain (which is the chief initial disability) and preventing the formation of excess scar tissue and adhesions (which are the chief delayed disabilities). In addition, in cases of intrinsic muscle injury, treatment is not complete until the underlying cause of the injury has been elicited and any preventive measures indicated brought into action.

First aid

Immediately, or as soon as possible after injury occurs, pressure is applied to the site by means of a soft sponge rubber or Gamgee pad held in place by an elastic bandage. If available, ice cold water should be used to soak the dressing or alternatively an ice bag may be applied.[12] Proprietary cold (or hot) bags are on the market which contain chemicals that react endothermically (or exothermically) on mixing—these are useful in the First Aid kit, as are cold storage packs, e.g. Cryogel, although the latter need to be precooled. The effect of this cooling is to diminish blood flow and hence bleeding in the injured area by an 'axon reflex', not by the direct action of cold. (The subcutaneous fat acts as an insulator against direct cooling.)

When the lower limb is involved the dressing should be applied with the leg elevated, and ideally bandaging should start from the base of the toes working proximally. This will prevent venous engorgement distal to the pressure dressing. For injuries below the knee Elastoplast strapping is generally preferred to a crêpe bandage.

In dealing with the treatment of muscle injury Woodard[13] stresses the importance of restoring what he calls balance, and advises that following a muscle tear the patient should continue his exercise by gentle jogging round until the pain fades away. This routine may be successful in minor tears such as those in the calf muscles, but is inadvisable when swelling 'blows up' immediately. It should never be undertaken without strict medical supervision, and it must be remembered that as this is a painful procedure strong and persistent motivation is required!

Definitive treatment

The pressure pad is retained for 48 to 72 hours, being reapplied as necessary when it works loose, and the patient is encouraged to persist in gentle, active, unresisted exercise (for example, with a hamstring tear lying prone and gently flexing and extending the knee). An enzyme preparation of the Varidase or Chymoral type may be given, but treatment with these drugs is unlikely to be successful unless started within 24 hours of injury.[14] Topical preparations such as heparinoid and adrenaline creams have been used, but any enzyme absorbed can clearly only reach the tissues by carriage through the blood and not by direct diffusion.

If the injury is severe and bruising is extensive, bed rest for the first few days may be necessary.

On the second or third day after injury physiotherapy may be started. First heat is given, preferably as short wave diathermy but failing this as infrared, with the double object of promoting local vasodilatation (either directly or by axon reflex) and hence speeding up absorption of the haematoma, and of producing reduction of spasm and relaxation as a subjective response to the feeling of warmth.[15]

Massage, initially as gentle surface effleurage but progressing to more vigorous pétrissage as local tenderness diminishes, further encourages dispersal and re-absorption of the haematoma.[16] After massage, progressive resistance exercises are carried out, the load and number of repetitions being adjusted to produce maximum effort at minimum discomfort. These exercises are carried out in such a way as to ensure that the joints spanned by the injured muscle or group are put through their full range of active movement. Finally, the treatment session is concluded with full-range passive joint movements and muscle stretching.[17]

At this stage of treatment ultrasound is of considerable value, although much controversy persists as to dose level and whether or not the stimulus should be pulsed. Practical experience suggests that a daily session of 10 minutes unpulsed at $2 \cdot 5$–$3 \cdot 0$ Watts/cm^2 is both safe and effective.

Extravagant claims have been made for pulsed short wave diathermy but it has been impossible to reproduce the results claimed. The technique is time-consuming, expensive, and erratic in outcome.

As improvement continues and the patient regains confidence heat and massage become less important and are gradually discarded, while the exercises are increased in vigour and variety until they merge almost imperceptibly with the normal training routine.

In cases of complete tear, repair of the torn muscle may be attempted surgically as an emergency procedure, but results tend to be disappointing and convalescence is prolonged. Surgical repair of the muscle sheath in muscle hernia is sometimes successful and should be seriously considered when the fascia lata is split.

Rehabilitation

During the phase of definitive treatment general supporting activities are carried out by the patient which enable him to maintain his general level of fitness while throwing no strain on the injured muscle group. The type of activity required will depend on the site and severity of the injury. When normal training is resumed the patient's technique should be studied closely to discover if there is any gross fault which may be predisposing towards injury or persistence of post-traumatic residual disability. Minor faults in technique are of little significance and, in the better class athlete, any attempts to correct them will do more harm than good. What is important is to see that the technique is sufficiently well developed to ensure that the patient keeps his form under all conditions, particularly severe competitive stress.

Before the patient is finally discharged from treatment he must be put through and pass a strenuous fitness test. The value of this test is not only that it enables the clinician to assess the effects of his treatment, but also that its successful outcome will enormously restore the patient's confidence. Rehabilitation is not complete until the athlete is fit, and knows he is fit, to resume his full competitive schedule.

The basic requirements of the fitness test are that it should prove the patient's general level of fitness, and impose on the injured region loads comparable to those born in competition. The actual type of test will vary with the individual

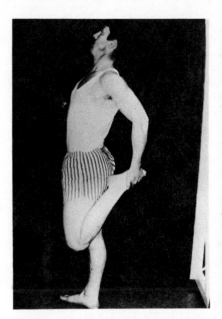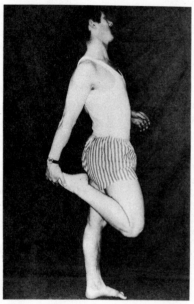

Figs. 17.7(a) and (b) Loss of extensibility after muscle tear. Contrast the extended hip and flexed knee of the left leg with the flexed hip and less extended knee on the injured side.

but must include full-range joint movements, passive stretching, maximal static contractions, and a full work-out of the appropriate sporting activity (sprinting, jumping, kicking, etc.) all of which must be encompassed without the slightest discomfort. Above all, recovery of full muscle extensibility must be demonstrated before resumption of serious training or competition can be permitted (Fig. 17.7).

Late cases

Cases of muscle injury presenting for treatment some time after injury are treated by a programme of progressive mobilization after the exclusion of the presence of complications. In chronic cases with marked fibrosis and a well-localized tender spot, injections of hydrocortisone (50 mg) in local anaesthetic with Hyalase (1500 units) are of value. Rehabilitation of such cases is liable to be more protracted.

Complications

Complications are rare if the injury is correctly treated from the outset, since they are due to excessive haematoma formation which the proper treatment is specifically designed to prevent.

Infection

Occasionally a haemotoma becomes infected with subsequent suppuration. This may occur in subjects with a mild bacteraemia (for example patients with focal skin sepsis) when the haematoma is sited in a relatively avascular area. It is therefore uncommon in muscle unless the haematoma is enormous, and is most frequently seen in subcutaneous lesions. Infection may result from an open wound, or following intramuscular injection or aspiration. Infected haematomas are treated by rest and systemic antibiotics before localization is complete. Once pus has formed surgical drainage is required, and this is to be preferred to aspiration as it allows further collections to escape. When drainage is free exercises may be started. Normal training is resumed when healing is complete, and it is frequently remarkable how little scarring remains.

Cyst formation

When a haematoma forms in lax tissues, or where the amount of bleeding is excessive, absorption may not take place. Clot retraction leaves a serum-filled cavity lined with organizing fibrin deposits. This fluctuant swelling persists and absorption is seldom completed. Drainage by aspiration is usually insufficient as the cavity contains clots which will not pass through even a wide bore needle, so that incision in the line of the muscle fibres is required. Strict asepsis is observed during this procedure, and antibiotic 'umbrella' is justifiable if the haematoma is large. When the cavity has been evacuated a firm pressure dressing is applied and exercises started. It is generally unnecessary to leave any form of drain *in situ*, if a sufficiently wide incision is made.

Myositis ossificans

Probably the most unpleasant complication of intramuscular haematoma is myositis ossificans in which calcareous deposits are laid down in the haematoma, later to be converted into a species of cancellous bone. The quadriceps group is most commonly affected, and this type of lesion is also found around the elbow joint after dislocations. The patient presents some time after injury (usually a bruise but occasionally a tear) with a hard tender swelling at the site of injury. X-ray confirms the diagnosis which can seldom be made with assurance on clinical grounds alone (Fig. 17.8). In early cases complete rest is required as exercise provokes extension of the calcareous deposits. Normal exercise can only be resumed after repeated clinical and X-ray examinations show the lesion to have 'burnt out'.

Treatment is by short wave diathermy together with gentle mobility exercises but the eventual outcome is never certain. Some disability almost invariably remains which is seldom amenable to excision of the bony deposits or any form of myoplasty.

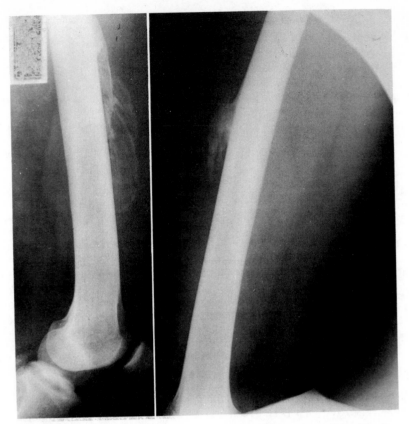

Fig. 17.8(a) The early radiological appearances of myositis ossificans in the quadriceps group.

Fig. 17.8(b) X-ray photograph of the thigh showing appearance of 'burnt out' myositis ossificans. The new bone has now developed a definite structure (compare with Fig. 17.8(a)).

On the basis that prevention is better than cure this condition must be anticipated when muscle bruising is due to direct violence, and progress of treatment should be cautious particularly if the haematoma becomes firmer to palpation as it localizes.

Aneurysm and arteriovenous fistulae

If major vessels are involved in direct trauma and subsequent haematoma formation, aneurysmal dilatation or fistulous connections may result. Such lesions are extremely rare, the popliteal vessels being most usually involved. These vessel injuries should be distinguished from traumatic aneurysm (pulsating haematoma), which is not a true aneurysm but is a haematoma fed by a ruptured arteriole, and is quite often seen. Pulsating haematomas may be treated by exploration and ligature. Aneurysms and fistulae require specialist treatment from a vascular surgeon.

Phlebitis and phlebothrombosis

Superficial venous thrombophlebitis is a relatively common sequel of bruising, particularly on the inner side of leg and thigh. The lesion is generally well localized and embolic phenomena are excessively rare. As the lesion is well limited rest and local heat are all that is required for treatment. Anticoagulants are quite unnecessary unless the thrombotic process is actively spreading. A crêpe bandage should be worn until the symptoms have subsided when normal training may be resumed. Anti-inflammatory drugs such as phenylbutazone (100 mg after meals thrice daily) may be given if the reaction is severe.

Other forms of treatment

Electrical stimulation

Faradism may be useful to reactivate and re-educate inhibited muscle.[18] The range through which it is applied should be carefully chosen and it should not be used if myositis ossificans is present or suspected.

Injection

Acupuncture is generally useless, though in skilled and experienced hands it can help to overcome spasm.

The use of local anaesthetics such as xylocaine which temporarily diminish pain is dangerous and should be avoided in muscle injury. The routine treatment of pulled muscles by injection, however immediately effective in diminishing pain, is contrary to the basic principles of management of these injuries in that the size of the 'space occupying lesion' is increased. There is, in addition, the risk of provoking further more severe damage on exercise. Such injections may be permissible in extreme cases, for example to permit an athlete to take part in an Olympic event, but even then only under certain conditions, namely (a) that the patient is made fully cognizant of the risks (of further irreparable damage) and accepts them, and (b) that the patient is taking part in an individual event and not competing as a member of a team.

In such cases 5 to 10 ml of 2 per cent xylocaine in 1/10 000 adrenaline to which has been added 1500 units of Hyalase, is injected directly into the tender area which may be gently massaged for a few minutes afterwards.

The use of hydrocortisone has already been indicated.

Aspiration

'Aspiration' of the acute haematoma is probably a waste of time and no more effective than the first aid measures outlined above. Even the largest and most fluctuant haematomas will resolve, at least in part, on conservative measures. Later drainage of a localized encysted pocket may be necessary but is best accomplished with the knife as described.

Rest

The role of rest is strictly circumscribed. After the first 48 to 72 hours it has no place in the definitive treatment of muscle injuries, except in the rare cases of myositis ossificans and following complete rupture. Not only will it produce muscle atrophy with consequent delay in rehabilitation, but scarring and adhesion formation are more likely to occur, with consequently a high recurrence rate. Too many athletes are told by their medical advisers to rest a muscle tear or 'pull'—it is perhaps not surprising, therefore, that many of them have little confidence in doctors!

Prevention of injury

It will never be possible completely to eliminate extrinsic muscle injury which is one of the accepted hazards of sport, particularly the body contact sports, although some degree of protection may be gained from the maintenance of a reasonable level of physical fitness and the care of personal accoutrements, especially footwear. Many of these injuries are exaggerated because the patient is not wearing the right type of shoe or boot for the ground and weather conditions, which result in him slipping from lack of adhesion, or straining himself because he is stuck.

Intrinsic muscle tears are largely if not entirely preventable, since they are essentially due to technical failure. From the moment an athlete or sportsman of any kind starts training he or she must constantly bear in mind that strength and guts are never enough—that if the body cannot work efficiently the sportsman will not 'tear up' the opposition but instead tear himself. Lloyd[9] in his analysis of injuries at the 1958 Empire and Commonwealth Games suggests that muscle tears are not commonly seen in cyclists and oarsmen because the rate of muscular contraction in these groups is slower. But cyclists and oarsmen do tear muscles. The reason why such injuries were uncommon at Cardiff is that the sports in question demand such a highly technical skill (as compared with running) that in the international class cyclist or oarsman breakdown is unlikely.

Side by side with the development of technique must go the development of the ability to retain it under pressure of competition. Such pressure may be nervous (psychological) or physical. Many are the instances of an athlete or sportsman 'falling to bits' on the big occasion, losing form and so on. The reasons underlying form loss are many and complicated, but the inevitable consequence is a breakdown in technique and co-ordination from which muscle tears are likely to result. This breakdown is not necessarily dramatic—indeed, many sportsmen are able to compete successfully and win their events in spite of it, and many more manage to avoid injury—but it is there, a kind of lowest common denominator in all cases of muscle injury.

Many athletes and coaches consider that adequate 'warm-up' will prevent muscle tears and other injuries, but like so many saying, this is only half true. Probably the most important effect of 'warm-up' is the relaxation it can induce and it is this relaxation which prevents injury. 'Warm-up' itself will not produce a relaxed performance, nor is it a necessary pre-requisite, as experience shows. The most important preventive measure is the development of the ability to relax while competing so that the body can be allowed to carry out the required activity at reflex level. This quality of relaxation characterizes the performances of all the truly great athletes and sportsmen, and is most difficult to achieve, perhaps because it is seldom if ever deliberately cultivated. Weight-training, circuit training, controlled interval activities and so on will produce a fit, strong, and durable athlete, but these very qualities, if not complemented by an adequate technique and the ability to maintain it, will tend to provoke injury and aggravate its severity.

J.G.P.W.

References

1. Bourne, G. H. (1972) *The Structure and Function of Muscle*. London: Academic Press.
2. Vanderhoof, E. R., Imig, C. J. and Hines, H. M. (1961) Effect of muscle strength and endurance development on blood flow. *J. appl. Physiol.*, **16,** 873.
3. McDonald, A. (1957) Some reflections on the 'physical' in physical education. *Phys. Educ.*, **49,** 33.
4. Haines, R. W. (1934) On muscles of full and short actions. *J. Anat.*, **69,** 20.
5. Edwards, R. H. T. Personal communication.
6. Van Linge, B. (1962) The response of muscle to strenuous exercise. *J. Bone Jt Surg.*, **44B,** 71.
7. Tucker, W. E. (1954) Injuries in sport. *Jl R. Inst. publ. Hlth Hyg.*, **17,** 245.
8. Abrahams, A. (1961) *Disabilities and Injuries of Sport*. London: Elek.
9. Lloyd, K. (1959) Some hazards of athletic exercise. *Proc. R. Soc. Med.*, **52,** 151.
10. Archer, J. Personal communication quoted various American sources.
11. Travers, P. R. in *Training, Style and Injury for Runners*, unpublished.
12. Ryan, A. J. (1969) Quadriceps strain, rupture and Charlie horse. *Med. Sci. Sports*, **1,** 106.
13. Woodard, C. R. (1954) *Sports Injuries: Prevention and Active Treatment*. London: Parrish.
14. Morrison, M. C. T. and Williams, J. G. P. (1961) The value of buccal streptokinase/ streptodornase (Varidase) in the treatment of minor injuries. *Postgrad. Med. J.*, **37,** 96.
15. Corrigan, A. B. (1965) The immediate treatment of muscle injuries in sportsmen. *Med. J. Aust.*, **1,** 926.
16. Andrivet, R. (1968) Les Accidents Musculaires Sportifs. *Ann. Med. Phys.*, **11,** 285.
17. Millar, A. P. and Salmon, J. (1967) Muscle tears. *Aust. J. sports Med.*, **2,** 435.
18. Williams, J. G. P. and Street, M. (1976) Sequential faradism in vastus medialis re-education. *Physiotherapy*, in press.

18

Head injuries

Introduction

Participation in many sports carries some risk of injury to the head, and this is more pronounced in body contact and fast vehicular sports. The injury may be of a chance or accidental nature or may be directly attributable to the nature of the competition.

An indication of the relative frequency of head injuries can be gathered from the extensive statistical investigation of lesions due to trauma in sport over four years throughout Italy by La Cava.[1] In classifying his large series by site affected he found that 11·7 per cent involved the head and neck making it one of the principal parts of the body injured, following knee (20 per cent) and ankle (15 per cent).

Boxing deserves special mention because by the nature of the contest there is an indirect head injury in which the point of impact is the chin with con- is an indirect head injury in which the point of impact is to the chin with concussive effects probably transmitted to the brain stem from the skull base. Punches to the side of the head may cause shearing damage due to the abrupt lateral or rotational movements with tearing of bridging vessels. Secondary injury may occur when the head strikes the floor of the ring as the boxer falls.

In any of the codes of football, trauma can result from hard contact between players, by striking the ground, and sometimes from an opponent's fist or boot. In hockey and other games when a bat or 'stick' is used the weapon of the assault is obvious. Even in cricket and golf and other non-contact sports, the ball or other implement may cause a missile type of injury to the head (Fig. 18.1). In motor and motor-cycle racing, the vehicle or ground causes the damage. In swimming, diving with the head extended or striking the bottom of the bath or river or sea-bed, particularly where there are rocks, may cause the injury.

Pathological effects

It is not generally realized how much of a semi-solid substance the brain is, nor how much movement of it occurs when sudden violence is applied to the skull. This was first clearly shown in 1944 by Sheldon and his colleagues who fitted a transparent lucite calvarium in monkeys and took high-speed cinematograph films of the brain during the application of violent blows and penetrating injuries to the head.[2] With blunt injuries the brain seemed to slither about like a rather loosely fitting jelly in a box, and during penetrating wounds there was a terrific

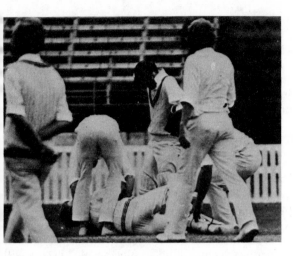

Fig. 18.1 'The ball may cause a missile type injury to the head.' Chatfield the New Zealand batsman felled by a 'bumper' in a cricket Test Match. (Photo: Associated Press.)

commotion, the brain appearing to boil and bubble during the passage of the missile. It is likely that much the same changes in the brain occur when the human skull is subjected to violence.

The commonest injury probably results from movement of the brain within the skull, and from the sudden change in momentum which occurs when the skull receives a blow. Thus a blow on the forehead will knock the skull backward; the skull begins to move before the brain, and the front of the lagging brain will, as it were, be smacked by the rapidly travelling skull. Similarly, when the back of the head strikes the ground, the skull becomes arrested suddenly just before the brain, and the back of the brain bumps into it.

Concussion

The simplest effect of injury is what is known as concussion, which is easier to define in clinical than pathological terms. Its essential feature is sudden loss of consciousness at the moment of injury with full physiological recovery within a few minutes. The loss of consciousness is so transient that there may not be time for accurate observations, but there is often pallor, slowness and feebleness of the heart beat, shallow breathing, and abolition of reflex function. In some ways it resembles syncope and surgical shock but it differs from the former in that abolition of consciousness may last longer in concussion, and from shock in the invariable loss of consciousness and the fact that the effects are of shorter duration.

The changes which occur in concussion are thus reversible, and there are no visible structural abnormalities. Electroencephalograms in a group of amateur boxers taken immediately after boxing showed that changes, chiefly increases in the interval alpha rhythm, did not persist after 4 minutes.[3]

Contusion and laceration

In more severe injuries the brain may be contused or lacerated, particularly if the skull is fractured and bone fragments are driven in, and in penetrating wounds. This damage may also occur in closed injuries without a skull fracture or with linear fractures with no displacement of the fragments. The brain is bruised or torn by violent impact against the skull, especially against the sharp edges of the sphenoidal ridge, the bony prominence of the anterior fossa and the free edge of the tentorium.

In simple contusion, the meninges are torn with the blood vessels traversing them, subarachnoid haemorrhage is profuse and clots are found in the sulci and brain. If death does not occur the bleeding stops, the clots becoming organized or liquified with accompanying oedema.

Recovery of consciousness may not take place for hours or days, and this may be followed by a period of drowsiness and confusion before the patient is fully orientated and rational. Severe headache is common in the acute stage, particularly where there has been subarachnoid haemorrhage. Giddiness is also common, characterized by a momentary feeling of unsteadiness which occurs with sudden change of posture. Focal neurological abnormalities such as hemiplegia, aphasia and hemianopia are uncommon in closed injuries. In many cases, severe neurological defects which are apparent when the patient regains consciousness clear up almost completely in a matter of days or weeks. In some cases the patient is left with some degree of intellectual defect varying from slight impairment of memory and concentration to profound dementia.

Clinical features

Although recovery may occur within a short time, complications may arise from extradural or subdural haemorrhage, and life may be endangered. Hence close observation is essential during the first few days after injury.

In the majority of cases, recovery is rapid and uncomplicated. Those with severe head injuries should be admitted to hospital immediately, preferably to a special unit.

A sportsman with a short period of unconsciousness should be put to bed for a day or two and be kept under observation. As soon as he has recovered consciousness, he should have a neurological examination. The signs to look for are weakness, sensory loss, alteration in the reflexes, defects in the visual fields (by confrontation tests), disturbance of speech, and abnormalities in the pupils and ocular movements. Even in drowsy and unco-operative patients gross abnormalities can be detected (Fig. 18.2).

Treatment

In mild concussion such as after the chin knock-out or on the football field, it may be difficult to persuade the injured athlete to go to bed. The majority of boxers who have been knocked out by a single blow usually stir at about the count of seven and try instinctively to rise. They can usually get up with or without assistance at the end of the count and are able to walk to their corners where they recover rapidly. In the dressing-room they are disappointed

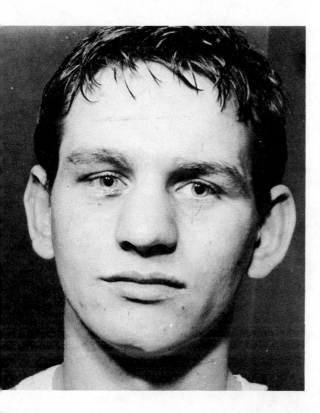

Fig. 18.2 Recovery from severe concussion. Note recent laceration under right eye, enlarged left pupil and left facial weakness, and old fractured nasal bones. This type of patient, if allowed to resume sport too soon, becomes a candidate for traumatic encephalopathy. (Photo: James-Baker Studio.)

but alert, have no retrograde amnesia and do not complain of headache or vomiting. Neurological examination is usually negative. They must always be accompanied home and advised to stay in bed and see their doctor the next day.

Where there has been a longer period of unconsciousness or retrograde or post-traumatic amnesia, the boxer is carried from the ring, or the player from the field (Fig. 18.3), and removed to hospital immediately. This type of head injury occurs after what may be called the cerebral knock-out. The boxer receives numerous blows on the head; he gets weaker and weaker; he loses his muscular control and finally goes unconscious even from a slight blow or without receiving a blow. This is caused by diffuse neuronal changes in the cerebrum which are, however, reversible but which give rise to headache, amnesia, and vomiting on recovery. It is regrettable that footballers, cricketers and hockey players are allowed to continue to play in matches after they have partially recovered from concussion of this type. Schneider and Kriss[4] have laid down useful practical guidelines for American gridiron footballers. They emphasize that with any

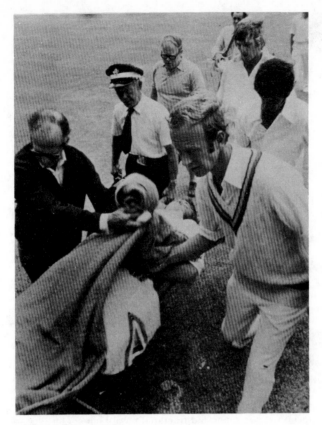

Fig. 18.3 The injured player removed from the field. (Photo: Associated Press.)

progression hospitalization and an emergency neurosurgical consultation is deemed essential.

Cerebral compression

The most urgent complication is cerebral compression from extradural haemorrhage, mostly from tearing of the middle meningeal artery. There may be dazing or unconsciousness of a few moments or minutes with full recovery of consciousness known as the 'lucid interval', lasting perhaps for some hours. There may be evidence of a local injury to the temporal region and an X-ray may show a fracture crossing a line of the meningeal vessels.

Within an hour or so the patient complains of headache which gets steadily worse. He becomes drowsy, comatose and may die. There is rapidly progressive paralysis of the opposite side of the body with dilatation of the pupil on the side of the lesion. The patient should be transferred to hospital immediately for surgical treatment.

Other complications

Other possible complications are meningitis from fractures involving one of the accessory air sinuses, permanent loss of smell resulting from torn filaments of the olfactory nerve, facial palsy due to contusion and compression of the facial nerve, diplopia from damage to the sixth nerve, nerve deafness from damage to the eighth nerve, middle ear deafness, and tinnitus.

Hemiplegia, sensory loss, aphasia,[5] and hemianopia are commonest in compound fractures and penetrating wounds.

Epileptic attacks may occur early and anticonvulsive drugs should be given which should be continued for two or three years. Traumatic epilepsy may follow in 6 per cent of severe closed injuries.

Sometimes haemorrhage may accumulate between the dura and the arachnoid. The quantity of extravasated blood may be considerable and forms an encapsulated clot termed a chronic subdural haematoma, the usual site being the frontoparietal region.

Symptoms may follow immediately or even weeks or months after a head injury. They consist of headache, intermittent drowsiness, lack of concentration, mild confusion. Hemiparetic signs and papilloedema may be present. Investigation by scanning, cerebral angiography and/or air studies of the brain would be indicated. If positive, surgical evacuation of the contents of the haematoma is carried out.

Subarachnoid and intracerebral haemorrhage may also occur after head injuries. This can be confirmed by lumbar puncture.

The electroencephalogram

The EEG is not pathognomonic.[3] Boxers who have received a large number of blows during a contest show a greater number of changes, mostly in the slowing of the alpha interval, than those who have been knocked-out. These changes usually disappear in four minutes. However, the EEG may be valuable in locating focal change and if this is persistent the boxer should be permanently banned. Incipient epilepsy may be discovered by the typical spike and wave tracing.

Abrasions and lacerations and other injuries to the head

Abrasions

These are common on the face and skull. Bleeding should be stopped by pressure; fibrin foam applied with pressure on a pad of gauze or cotton wool is usually successful in obstinate cases. Bathing of the wound with warm saline is followed by the application of cetrimide (1 per cent) and light dusting with sulphatiazole powder. Antibiotics should not be applied locally as they may cause sensitivity reactions.

Lacerations

When the wound is dry and has been cleaned as indicated above, it should be sutured to ensure sounder and more rapid healing as well as less disfigurement. Alternatively, superficial lacerations may be closed with adherent tape such as Steristrip or Ethistrip. When the laceration involves the underlying tissues, it should be formally closed in layers to prevent scar adhesion to bone.[6, 7] Fine interrupted catgut sutures are used with the knots reversed, that is, tied underneath. The skin is then closed in the normal way using silk thread. This can be obtained already threaded on fine curved needles in pre-sterilized packs. Sutures should be removed not later than five days after insertion. Small dry wounds can be held together and sealed with a plastic material such as Nobecutane or collodion—dumb-bell plaster strips applied at right-angles to the wound are also useful. Boxers should be prohibited from further competition for at least four weeks— in other sports the period off need not be so long (Fig. 18.4).

Haematomas

The common 'black eye' hardly ever needs treatment, but cold applications limit the extravasation of blood. Enzyme preparations of the Varidase type are claimed to be useful in promoting early reabsorption.[8] Haematoma of the auricle ('cauliflower ear'), if seen early, requires aspiration and the injection of 1500 units of

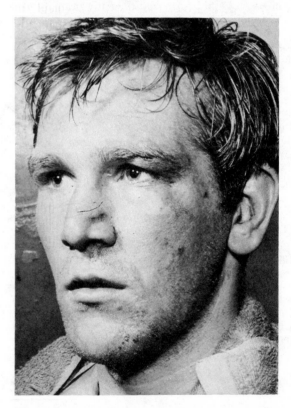

Fig. 18.4 Two typical cases of 'cut eye' resulting from boxing. (Photos: James-Baker Studio.)

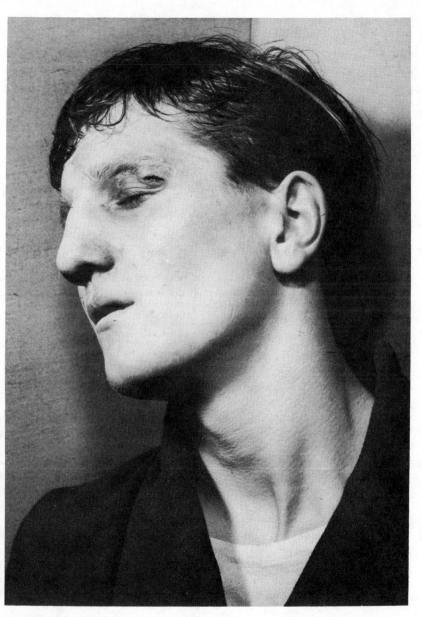

Fig. 18.4 Continued.

Hyalase; in later cases the clot must be evacuated, the wound plugged, and healing allowed to occur by granulation from the bottom (Fig. 18.5).[6]

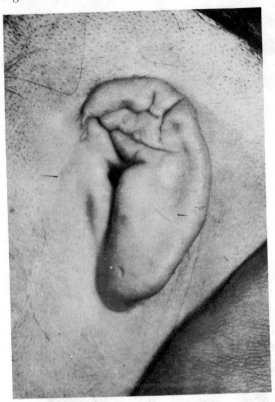

Fig. 18.5 Haematoma of the auricle; 'cauliflower ear'.

Nasal injury

A wide variety of nasal injuries occur in sport. Simple epistaxis is common and is best treated by direct pressure maintained for a few minutes. If severe, packing may be required. When bony injury is suspected, the patient must be moved to hospital as soon as possible. Subsequent management will depend on the severity of the injury and the patient's sporting interests.[9] In general, cosmetic surgery should if possible be delayed until the sporting career is over (Fig. 18.6).

Punch drunkenness

Traumatic encephalopathy or 'punch drunkenness' in boxers is supposed to have become extremely rare since the end of World War I, because contests are much shorter and the medical welfare of boxing has advanced considerably in the past 50 years. Whilst the risks have doubtless been reduced, the reports of neurologists indicate that they have not been eliminated. Critchley in 1957 described trau-

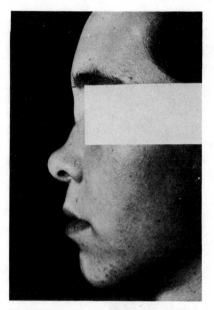

Fig. 18.6 The typical appearance of a 'broken nose'. There is bruising and depression of the bridge of the nose, and deviation to one side or the other when viewed from in front.

matic progressive encephalopathy in 69 professional boxers who had been registered between 1929 and 1955, and estimated a prevalence rate of traumatic encephalopathy which was higher.[10] He suggested too that the evidently transitory incapacity usually sustained in bouts might result in permanent, slight, but cumulative damage to delicate neuronal structures.

The term 'punch-drunk' is derived from the fact that the victim exhibits the signs of a person who has had a little too much to drink. He is unsteady on his feet, fatuous, euphoric, voluble, speech-slurred, sometimes quarrelsome, and even aggressive. Memory and intellect are impaired and moral sense is lost. Rarely frank progressive dementia develops. In advanced cases there is a coarse tremor, rigidity and ataxia. A clinical syndrome has emerged which is often predominantly either cerebellar or extra-pyramidal.

The neurological features have been ascribed to petechial haemorrhages in or near the brain stem. In addition, it is now suggested that diffuse neuronal destruction can result from the cumulative effects of minor repeated trauma.[11]

Strict supervision and administration of boxing should prevent the occurrence of this condition. These days amateur bouts only last three rounds while professional ones are not more than fifteen rounds. Referees are much more injury conscious and bouts are stopped when a boxer is obviously outclassed, dazed, cannot defend himself, or cannot possibly win. Sparring partners and the slugger type of boxer who is prepared to accept many punches so long as he can land a telling blow, are the types who most likely become 'punch-drunk'. The first signs are a slowing-up of the boxer and his reactions, and a dragging of one foot or leg. His speech may become slightly slurred and his euphoria abnormal. That

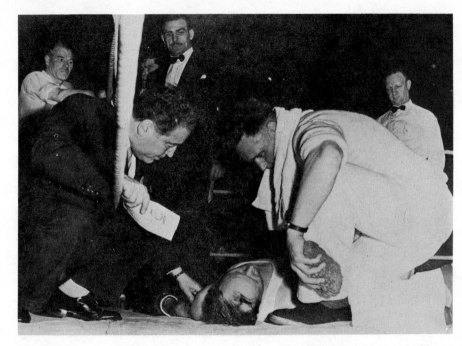

Fig. 18.7 Knock-out. The full count must be taken after the end of the round (Photo: H. W. Neale).

is the time for a complete neurological examination. An EEG may show some focal damage and the boxer must be permanently banned. It is recommended that amateur boxers should retire at 25.

The compulsory minimum period off boxing following concussion or amnesia, the compulsory eight count when the boxer is knocked down, and the continuation of the count at the end of a round when the boxer is down (adopted by the International Amateur Boxing Association-A.I.B.A.), will help considerably to eliminate permanent brain damage (Fig. 18.7).

Prevention of head injuries

It is not possible to eliminate head injuries altogether from sporting activities as even in non-contact and recreational sports accidents may occur. However, the hazards are obviously more in the combat and speed sports, and prevention depends on wearing protective headgear and adherence to the laws of the game concerned with safety in the sport. The number and severity of head injuries in motor cyclists has been considerably reduced by the wearing of crash helmets. In motor racing, drivers wear helmets which are required to comply with strict standards and these have effectively lessened the risk of serious sequels. Lighter hard skull caps are often used in sports such as horse racing, skiing and cycling (Fig. 18.8).

In boxing, the frequency and severity of head injuries has been greatly reduced by the introduction of the sorbo-rubber or felt cover, $\frac{5}{8}$ in (15 mm) thick, for

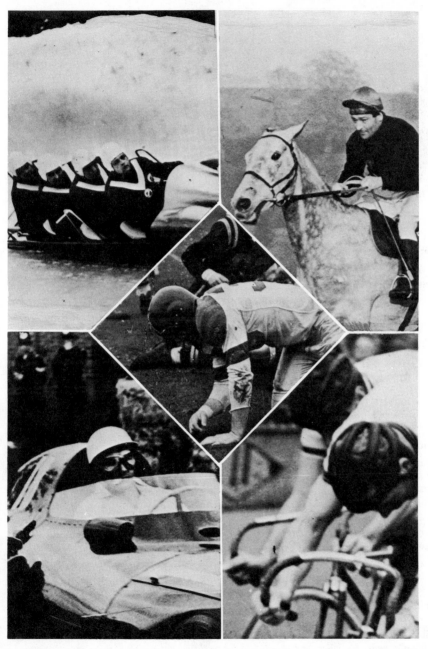

Fig. 18.8 Protective headgear for sport. Various types of protective helmet for different sports are shown in use.

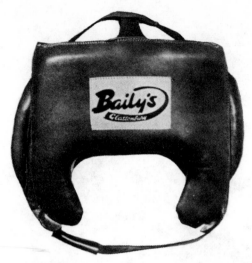

Fig. 18.9 Boxer's head guard to prevent head injuries and 'cut eye'.

the ring floor. This is covered by a tightly-stretched canvas. Many of the serious head injuries were caused by the occiput striking the floor of the ring when the boxer fell backwards. Gum shields are worn not to protect the teeth but to soften blows to the jaw which are transmitted to the skull. Head injury may also be reduced[12] with the appropriate headgear (Fig. 18.9).

Periods off sport

For mild concussion where consciousness has been regained in a few minutes with no anterograde or post-traumatic amnesia and no focal neurological signs, three or four weeks away from the particular sport is recommended. Light training should not be resumed until the last week. During the period of rest, no alcohol should be taken and plenty of sleep encouraged.

If there has been amnesia for over an hour, particularly of the post-traumatic type, or where headache, giddiness, lack of concentration, irritability, impairment of memory, and insomnia persist, then two months off games is essential. Where there has been an extradural, subdural or subarchnoid haemorrhage all forms of strenuous games, particularly skiing, boxing, football, and wrestling, and other body contact sports should be given up completely. Walking, golf, and bowls should be considered as alternatives.

A player who sustains a minor head injury such as bruising, a haematoma, an abrasion, or a superficial laceration may continue if the wound is cleaned and dressed with an adhesive dressing, providing he is not dazed, giddy, disorientated, or vomiting. If there has been any period of unconsciousness, however short, or anterograde or post-traumatic amnesia, he should not be allowed to continue.

A dazed or staggering athlete is obvious. Dilated pupils indicate a moderately severe injury. If one pupil is larger the athlete must stop immediately and be treated as a severe head injury, that is, carried off.

Another method of assessing the player's condition is to ask the score of the game, the round in boxing, and which way his side is kicking in football. Recovery from dazing is usually rapid and the player can continue.

In conclusion, it must be stressed that no head injury should be taken lightly. This is as true today as when Hippocrates first enunciated the principle: 'No head injury is so severe it need be despaired of, nor so trivial it may be neglected.'

G.K.V.

References

1. La Cava, G. (1960) *Indagine Clinico Stastica Sulle Lesioni Traumatische Da Sport.* Turin: Edizioni Minerva Medica.
2. Sheldon, C. H., Prudenz, R. H., Restavski, J. S. and Craig, W. M. (1944) Lucite calvarium—method for direct observation of brain; surgical and lucite processing techniques. *Neurosurgery*, **1,** 67.
3. Blonstein, J. L. (1960) Electroencephalography in boxers. *J. sports Med. phys. Fitness*, **1,** 30.
4. Schneider, R. C. and Kriss, F. C. (1969) Decisions concerning cerebral concussion in football players. *Med. Sci. Sports*, **1,** 112.
5. Palazzo, F. A. (1951) Aphasia resulting from cork ball injury of head. *J. Mo. St. med. Ass.*, **48,** 391.
6. Bailey, B. N. (1965) in *Medical Aspects of Boxing*. London and Oxford: Pergamon Press.
7. McCowan, I. A. (1959) Boxing injuries. *Am. J. Surg.*, **98,** 78.
8. Blonstein, J. L. (1960) The use of 'Buccal Varidase' in boxing injuries. *Practitioner*, **185,** 78.
9. Ellis, M. (1965) in *Medical Aspects of Boxing*. London and Oxford: Pergamon.
10. Critchley, M. (1957) Medical aspects of boxing, particularly from a neurological standpoint. *Br. med. J.*, **i,** 357.
11. Roberts, A. H. (1969) *Brain Damage in Boxers*. London: Pitman.
12. Schmid, L., Hajek, E., Votipka, F., Teprik, O. and Blonstein, J. L. (1968) Experience with headgear in boxing. *J. sports Med. phys. Fitness*, **8,** 171.

19

Eye injuries

Introduction

Eye injuries are usually dramatic, giving rise to immediate loss of effective vision and pain.[1]

Body contact team games, for example rugby and water polo, frequently involve direct or glancing blows to the eyes and orbits. These direct blows may be from the ball itself or from collision of heads, elbows, hands, or feet. Individual sports can equally well cause serious eye injuries from rackets and balls (especially in the game of squash rackets).[2]

It is important to understand how serious these injuries can be. The smaller the ball and the faster it travels, the greater the risk of serious eye injury. For example, the squash ball travels at considerable speed and its size is such that it can 'fit' inside the orbit, and hence cause total disruption of the eye.[3] The larger balls, such as footballs, usually cause less severe ocular damage because the bony margins of the orbit protect the eye when the ball strikes the upper part of the face.[4]

Foreign bodies may blow or be thrown into the eyes in most sports whether team or individual. Mud and grit can be thrown up into the eyes in, for example, riding, Rugby and Association football, or from the surface of tennis courts and golf course bunkers.

Prevention of eye injuries

Measures which can be taken are as follows:

(1) All sportsmen and sportswomen should ensure their vision is good enough for their particular sport, and that the correct spectacles and contact lenses are worn if required. Uncorrected poor vision can lead to serious injuries to the sportsman concerned, and also to those engaged in the sport with him.
(2) Spectacle wearers should remove their spectacles where body or ball contact is likely (boxing, Rugby and Association football).
(3) If the vision of the spectacle wearer is poor without spectacles then contact lenses should be worn.[5] Soft contact lenses are especially suitable for sports.
(4) When spectacles are worn for sports such as athletics, tennis, and cricket they should be especially well fitted with a strong frame and unsplinterable lenses (special sport spectacle frames are available).
(5) The inexperienced sportsman should be regarded with caution, especially in racket games, as wild swings at the ball can cause it to fly off at dangerous angles and velocities to strike an opponent or partner.
(6) Myopic (short-sighted) sportsmen should be discouraged from boxing for two

reasons. Firstly, uncorrected vision is not good enough to allow the boxer adequately to protect himself. Secondly, retinal detachments occur more commonly in myopic people, and blows to the head can precipitate a retinal detachment.

(7) Skiers should always wear filtering spectacles or goggles as protection against ultraviolet irradiation in sunny conditions at high altitudes. Reflection of the sun's rays from the bright snow produces a great deal of ultraviolet light scatter which can cause 'snow blindness' (multiple tiny corneal epithelial erosions). Yachting in bright sun where a great deal of sunlight is reflected from the water may also cause excess ultraviolet light scatter, and protective spectacles are usually necessary.

Recommended first aid equipment for eye injuries

The following simple pieces of equipment and medication are recommended for all first-aid boxes (Fig. 19.1):

Torch	Single-dose eye drops of:
Sellotape	fluorescein sodium
Eye pads	tetracaine (Amethocaine)
Bandage	chloramphenicol (Chloromycetin) or
Glass rod	neomycin
Cotton buds	Antibiotic eye ointment:
	chloramphenicol (Chloromycetin) or
	neomycin

Good illumination is necessary for the examination of eye injuries or for looking for foreign bodies, and a hand torch is an essential piece of equipment.

Sharp instruments should be avoided when removing superficial foreign bodies: cotton wool buds are recommended for removing corneal and conjunctival foreign bodies.

Single-dose eye drop ampoules tetracaine (Amethocaine), fluorescein, and

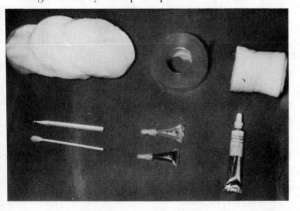

Fig. 19.1 First aid equipment for eye injuries; eye pads, Sellotape, bandage, cotton bud, glass rod, single-dose eye drops, and antibiotic eye ointment. (Reproduced by permission of the Audio-Visual Communications Department, St Mary's Hospital Medical School).

chloramphenicol (Chloromycetin) are desirable as they are always sterile and the remains can be discarded immediately after use. This means that larger drop bottles with their disadvantage of easy contamination and bulky storage are not required.

Antibiotic eye ointment should be instilled after removing a foreign body or treating a corneal abrasion. Sellotape keeps the eye pad in place before a firm bandage is applied over it.

Orbital injuries

Severe concussional blows to the orbital region usually cause bruising and oedema of the eyelids. This swelling may be so severe that the eyelid cannot be opened either by the patient or the examiner. Such patients should be seen by a specialist as soon as possible to exclude the presence of an associated injury to the eye.

Bleeding into the orbit (retrobulbar haemorrhage) causes proptosis of the eye which in turn hinders opening the eyelids; this makes an examination of the globe of the eye difficult.

Patients with severe eyelid and orbit haematomas require X-rays of the orbit to exclude fractures of the orbital walls and floor (orbital floor fractures are called 'blow out' fractures).

'Blow out' fractures are caused by concussion injuries to the orbit giving rise to fracturing of the orbital floor.[6] This gives rise to (a) enophthalmos (the soft tissues of the orbit herniate through the fracture causing the eye to sink back in the orbit), (b) diplopia on looking upwards (the inferior rectus muscle is bruised or possibly tethered to the fractured floor), (c) anaesthesia or hypoaesthesia of the skin of the cheek (due to damage of the inferior orbital nerve). No emergency treatment is usually required but as with all severe concussion injuries of the orbit, the patient should be examined by a specialist, preferably within a few hours of the injury, in order that damage to the globe can be excluded.

Eyelid injuries

Lacerations of the eyelids should be covered by a clean pad if suturing on the spot is not possible. The pad reduces bleeding and oedema a little. The suturing is best achieved before the skin and connective tissue oedema becomes too pronounced, and where skin only is involved 6/0 silk should be used. Lacerations of the medial quarter of the eyelids are especially important because of the danger of severance of the canaliculi.

Eye injuries

Subconjunctival haemorrhage

Foreign bodies or trivial injuries to the conjunctiva may cause a subconjunctival haemorrhage. Such injuries may be caused by lightly touching the eye with a finger or even a score card. The bright red and localized appearance of this subconjunctival haemorrhage is characteristic (Fig. 19.2). No treatment is required but other associated ocular injury should be sought. The subconjunctival haemorrhage usually disappears gradually over a period of 10–14 days.

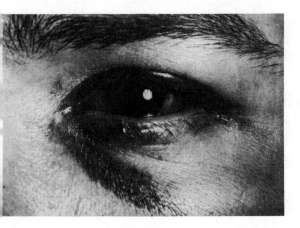

Fig. 19.2 Fist injury to left eye and orbit, with bruising of the eyelids and subconjunctival haemorrhage.

Corneal and conjunctival foreign bodies

These may be blown into the eye especially in windy conditions on dusty pitches and courts. There is an immediate sensation of pricking in the eye with watering and redness.

In a good light (daylight or using a good torch) the foreign body can usually be seen resting on the cornea or conjunctiva. Corneal foreign bodies invariably cause an associated corneal abrasion and this abrasion will show up as a bright green mark when a small fluorescein drop is instilled.

Eversion of the upper eyelid (Figs 19.3a and b) should always be performed as foreign bodies commonly lodge in the groove of the tarsal conjunctiva lining the upper eyelid.

Corneal abrasions

Corneal abrasions occur frequently in sports such as water polo, wrestling and boxing which involve a close physical contact. They are due to fingers catching the eye (in water polo especially), and the sportsman experiences a sudden sharp pain in the eye. After a few minutes the eye becomes very red, photophobic and waters a great deal.

Diagnosis is easily made by instilling a drop of fluorescein into the eye and this stains the area of the abrasion a bright green colour (the fluorescein stains only the part of the cornea where the epithelium is absent). First aid treatment is to instil chloramphenicol (Chloromycetin) eye ointment (or other antibiotic eye ointment) and place a firm pad and bandage over the eye ensuring the eyelids are closed behind the pad. The pad is renewed in 24 hours and most small abrasions are healed in about 48 hours (Fig. 19.4).

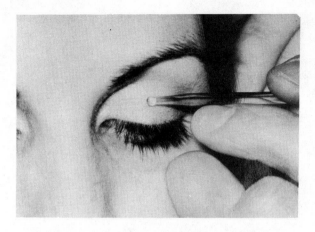

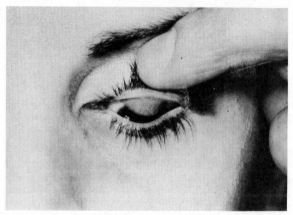

Fig. 19.3 Eversion of the upper eyelid. (a) Glass rod/or matchstick) placed gently along upper eyelid. Patient must be *looking down*. (b) Eyelid margin and lashes held and everted over glass rod (or matchstick), supporting the everted eyelid by the lashes with the index finger. (Reproduced by permission of the Audio-Visual Communications Department, St Mary's Hospital Medical School).

Hyphaema (haemorrhage into the anterior chamber)

Concussion injuries to the eyes such as with a football or tennis ball can cause haemorrhage into the anterior chamber of the eye (between the cornea and iris). The haemorrhage comes from damage to small vessels on the iris and should always be regarded as potentially serious.[7]

The patient immediately experiences severe blurring of vision and an aching pain in the eye. Within minutes the eye becomes red and photophobic. A corneal abrasion is often present. Examination reveals fresh blood in the anterior chamber preventing a clear view of the pupil and iris. The haemorrhage settles quickly to form a 'fluid level' of blood if the patient keeps still (Fig. 19.5).

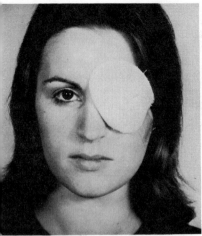

Fig. 19.4 Eye pad held in place with Sellotape. (Reproduced by permission of the Audio-Visual Communications Department, St Mary's Hospital Medical School).

An eye pad should be applied to the eye and the patient sent directly to a hospital ophthalmic department. Secondary haemorrhage into the anterior chamber may occur during the first few days after the injury, and admission to hospital is usually necessary for bed rest to help avoid this complication. The secondary haemorrhage can be more severe than the primary hyphaema and give rise to secondary glaucoma.

Most hyphaemas absorb within a week of the injury providing a secondary haemorrhage has not occurred. After absorption of the hyphaema the pupil is dilated by the specialist to inspect the retina for associated damage.

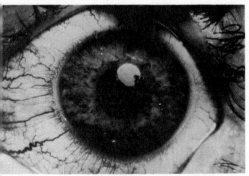

Fig. 19.5 Hyphaema (blood in the anterior chamber). Note the intense dilatation of the vessels round the cornea and the 'fluid level'). (Reproduced by permission of the Audio-Visual Communications Department, St Mary's Hospital Medical School).

Penetrating injuries

Any moderately sharp object or high velocity small ball may cause penetration of the globe. A broken racket, a fall in skiing, or a hard hit squash ball can cause rupture of the globe and urgent hospital admission is required for the patient (Fig. 19.6).

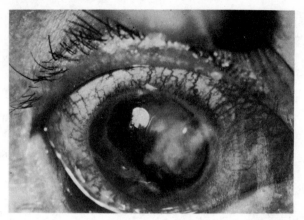

Fig. 19.6 Severe penetrating injury to the right eye. Note the corneal wound, distortion of the pupil, and cataract.

There is immediate loss of vision in the eye, pain, and redness. There is usually prolapse of iris through the wound and hyphaema.

Emergency treatment is to cover the eye with a clean pad and arrange for the patient to be admitted to hospital urgently. Antibiotic eye drops may be instilled to prevent secondary infection but ointment should be avoided as it may enter the eye in solid form through the wound.

Retinal detachment and retinal injuries

A concussion injury to the eye gives rise to retinal haemorrhages, ruptures in the choroid, retinal breaks (tears and disinsertions), and, rarely, avulsion of the optic nerve.[8] All give rise to sudden failure of vision.

Retinal haemorrhages and retinal breaks (usually in the form of a retinal disinsertion or dialysis) should be suspected in any severe concussion injury to the eye. Balls, fists, rackets, sticks, and boots are all especially liable to give rise to concussion injuries.[9]

Retinal haemorrhages

Retinal haemorrhages are fairly easy to recognize if a clear view of the retina is possible with the ophthalmoscope (a hyphaema may prevent a clear view for several days). The retinal haemorrhages and retinal oedema occur most commonly in the macular area or sometimes in the part of the retina adjacent to the blow. The temporal part of the retina is the most vulnerable therefore. Retinal oedema and retinal haemorrhages following injury ·are known as commotio retinae or concussion oedema, and usually resolve in a few weeks without treatment with complete recovery of vision in many cases.

Choroidal ruptures

These frequently occur in association with traumatic retinal haemorrhages, and their appearance with the ophthalmoscope is of whitish circumscribed areas close to the disc. This is a contrecoup effect of the injury. Their whitish appearance

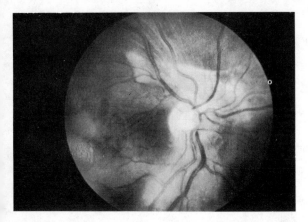

Fig. 19.7 Fundus appearance following concussion injury showing retinal haemorrhage (above and left of optic disc), choroidal ruptures (pale area below disc), and choroidal haemorrhage (upper right quarter of photograph).

is because the choroidal rupture allows the underlying sclera to be seen from its inside surface. Choroidal ruptures and retinal haemorrhages can only be treated by the patient resting at home or in hospital and avoiding strenuous physical activity for two or three weeks (Fig. 19.7).

Retinal detachments

Retinal detachments are always associated with a break in the retina, and following a concussion injury to the eye the retinal break takes the form of a retinal dialysis or disinsertion. The disinsertion of the retina probably occurs at the time of the injury but *the retinal detachment which follows this may not occur for weeks or months after the injury.*

The retinal dialysis appears as a red area, well demarcated, in the extreme periphery of the retina, almost invariably temporally because of the vulnerability of this area to injury. When there is an associated detachment the detached retina looks greyish in colour and the vessels almost black when seen with the ophthalmoscope.

If the retinal dialysis can be diagnosed before the retinal detachment occurs, then the prognosis for vision is greatly improved. A retinal dialysis can be 'sealed off' using the technique of photocoagulation (light coagulation) or cryotherapy to the retina in hospital. Once a retinal detachment has occurred then a surgical operation is required to replace the retina.

Where severe penetrating injuries to the eye occur the retina is frequently torn in several places with immediate retinal detachment occurring. The prognosis for vision in such cases is very poor and treatment is initially directed at repairing the penetrating wound.

Conclusion

All eye injuries in sport should be regarded as potentially severe and managed accordingly. Loss of sight is a grave handicap and must never be permitted to occur unnecessarily.

J.L.K.B.

References

1. Duke-Elder, S. (1972) *System of Ophthalmology. Vol. XIV: 1.* London: Henry Kimpton.
2. Ingram, D. V. and Lewkonia, I. (1973) Ocular hazards of playing squash rackets. *Br. J. Ophthal.*, **57,** 434.
3. North, I. M. (1973) Ocular hazards of squash. *Med. J. Aust.*, **1,** 165.
4. Anonymous (1973) A ball in the eye. *Br. med. J.*, **ii,** 195.
5. Fishkoff, D. (1965) The role of contact lenses in sport. *J. sports Med. phys. Fitness*, **5,** 163.
6. Converse, J. M. and Smith, B. (1960) Blow-out fracture of the floor of the orbit. *Trans. Am. Acad. Ophthal. Oto-lar.*, **64,** 676.
7. Chandran, S. (1973) Hyphaema and badminton eye injuries. *Med. J. Malaya*, **26,** 207.
8. Park, J. H., Frenkel, M., Dobbie, J. G. and Choromokos, E. (1971) Avulsion of optic nerve. *Am. J. Ophthal.*, **72,** 969.
9. Burnstein, F. (1963) Ocular injuries in sports. *J. sports Med. phys. Fitness*, **3,** 25.

20

Dental injuries

Introduction

The upper front teeth in particular are essential to a pleasing appearance, and an unsightly front tooth causes embarrassment to its owner. A simple mouth guard will prevent a high proportion of injuries, and medical advisers and sports coaches are urged to motivate those taking part in contact sports towards using this simple measure. Comparatively minor forces can lead to fracture and dislocation of the upper front teeth, and the sequelae of discoloration and loss of teeth require tedious treatments. These complicated restorative procedures are expensive, and the cost of a mouth guard is only one-thirtieth of the cost of

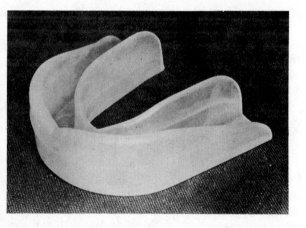

Fig. 20.1 A simple 'self-moulding' mouthguard not as satisfactory as a correctly made dental appliance which fits closely.

restoration of each damaged or lost tooth. The mouth guard should fit accurately and be made by a general dental practitioner (Fig. 20.1).

Protruding upper incisor teeth are particularly prone to injury, and about 45 per cent of the population are at risk for this reason.[1] Twenty-seven per cent of all athletic injuries at school are dental injuries[2] and the proportion of teenagers leaving school with damaged front teeth is 5 per cent.[3] Almost one-tenth (9·1 per cent) of all facial fractures are sustained as a result of sport, and 83 per cent of these occurred during football and cricket matches. Of a series of 267 fractured malars, 21 per cent occurred as a result of sports.[4]

Morphological considerations

The nomenclature of the bones of the face is applied clinically in a way which leads to confusion, and there is much to be said for adopting the simple terms 'upper jaw' and 'cheekbone'. The correct anatomical terms refer to the paired maxillae and zygomatic bones above, and the mandible below. However, clinical usage has adopted the terms 'fractured maxilla' to refer to unilateral and bilateral fractures of the maxillae, and 'fractured malar' to refer to fractures of the zygomatic bone. The 'middle third' of the facial skeleton is bounded above by the lower limit of the frontal bone, and below by the plane of occlusion of the maxillary teeth. A 'middle third facial fracture' therefore causes discontinuity of the upper dental arch as a whole from the cranium, and is often associated with a fractured malar. The alveolar process of either jaw is the part which encloses the roots of the teeth, and an alveolar fracture causes discontinuity between a group of teeth and the body of the jaw.

The strength of a tooth lies in the core of dentine containing its nutrient tissue, the pulp. The crown is covered by enamel, which is hard but brittle. The root is covered by cementum, a modified form of bone, which provides attachment for the periodontal ligament, rupture of the latter permitting dislocation of the tooth from its socket.

The stress-bearing struts of the facial bones are functionally adequate for mastication, but respiration and phonation in the middle third of the face have been facilitated by pneumatization, the consequent thinness of the bones being unable to withstand excessive external forces. However, the blood supply is good and the prospects for union excellent; so excellent, in fact, that malunion of a displaced fractured maxilla can occur within two weeks. It follows that failure to diagnose such fractures, which is not uncommon, can leave the patient with an unacceptable malocclusion of his teeth.

Patterns of injury

The displacement of the fractured bones in the middle third of the face is due to the direction of the blow, modified by gravity when the fragment is large (Fig. 20.2). Muscle spasm is less important as a displacing factor (unlike fractures of the mandible, where muscle spasm can cause considerable displacement, particularly of a posterior fragment which bears no tooth). In the context of sports injuries, the interesting entity of the 'blow-out' fracture of the floor of the orbit should not be forgotten (Fig. 20.3). This presentation can complicate fractures of the zygomatic bone, with palpable deformity at the orbital rim, but when in pure form without displacement of the orbital rim, it is easily overlooked. It arises when a blunt object strikes the optic globe with such force that hydrostatic pressure is transmitted through the fluid contents of the orbit to the weakest point, the eggshell thin orbital floor, which gives way, allowing fat to prolapse into the antrum. The typical instruments producing this fracture are a fist or a ball.[5] Its sequelae are diplopia, due to tethering of the inferior ocular muscles at the fracture line, and enophthalmos, due to loss and necrosis of orbital fat trapped in the maxillary antrum.

The mandible is a stronger bone than the maxilla, but areas of weakness are

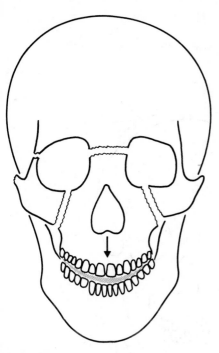

Fig. 20.2 A typical middle third facial fracture. The arrow indicates downward (and backward) displacement of the main fragment. Note step defects of orbital margins, and open bite (shaded).

present at the canine and third molar regions, and at the condylar neck. Contact sports produce fairly characteristic patterns of injury to the mandible: a blow at the angle of the jaw often produces a fracture through an unerupted third molar tooth socket; trauma at the side of the chin may produce a fracture at the site of the blow and at the opposite condylar neck (Fig. 20.4(a)); and a blow

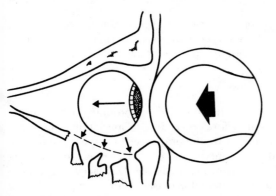

Fig. 20.3 'Blow-out' fracture of the orbit. Hydrostatic force is transmitted through the optic globe and orbital contents to the thin bony floor, which gives way. This can occur without fracture of the orbital margins.

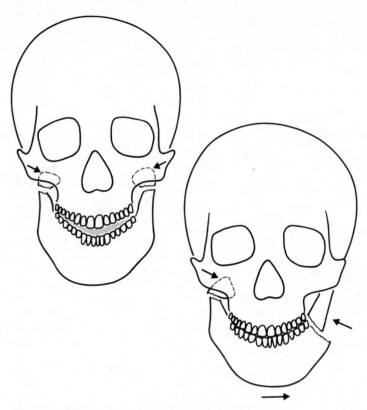

Fig. 20.4 (a) Bilateral condylar neck fracture of the mandible. Note displacement of condyles due to spasm of lateral pterygoid muscle, and open bite (shaded). (b) Fracture of the angle of the jaw due to direct violence (on the patient's left), and the condyle of the opposite side due to transmission of the blow. Note the deviation of the chin.

to the point of the chin may fracture both condylar necks if the mouth is open at the time (Fig. 20.4(b)).

In general, teeth are fractured or dislocated by direct violence to the teeth themselves, although sometimes a blow on the mandible may cause tooth fracture by the reaction to the force from the opposing dental arch.

Diagnosis

A diagnosis can usually be made on the basis of direct questioning, observation, and gentle palpation and percussion, before proceeding to special investigations. Definitive radiographs will be required by the oral surgeon responsible for the treatment; they are not essential for diagnosis, and are better reserved until specialized radiographic staff and equipment are available. Displaced fractures of either jaw produce derangement of the dental occlusion. For example, gagging at the molar teeth with separation of the incisors is usual in fractures of the maxilla, and of the mandibular condyles. Displaced fractures of the body of the mandible produce obvious occlusal derangement at the fracture site. However, where displacement is minimal, only the patient may be aware of an alteration in his bite and he should be specifically questioned on this point.

Subconjunctival haemorrhage is indicative of fracture of the zygomatic bone, when the posterior limit of the effusion cannot be defined. The patient may complain of diplopia, particularly when looking upwards, and this sign is suggestive of a fracture of the orbital floor. An epistaxis which is unilateral and transitory may arise from haemorrhage at the fracture site, the blood passing into the nose via the ostium. Periorbital ecchymosis, and bruising in the oral vestibular sulcus are usually associated with fractures in these regions. Anaesthesia of the cheek or lip may arise from trauma to the infra-orbital and mental nerves. Limitation of mandibular movement occurs due to muscle spasm, or to mechanical interference between a depressed fragment of the zygomatic arch, and the ramus of the mandible.

Palpation of the accessible bone edges, that is to say the orbital rim, the nose, the lower border of the mandible and the sulci of the mouth will elicit tenderness and step deformity. Crepitus may be found when the ends of the fragments pass over one another, but it is unnecessary and painful to elicit it as a physical sign; crepitus at the condylar neck of the mandible may be heard by the patient, or by the observer on auscultation in front of the ear. In the absence of obvious tenderness in the mandible, traction at the chin will demonstrate tenderness at the condylar neck.

To examine for a middle third facial fracture, place one hand on the vertex of the skull, and a forefinger in the vault of the palate; pressure between the hands of the observer will elicit pain or mobility at the site of discontinuity between upper jaw and skull.

Treatment

The definitive treatment of these injuries is outside the scope of this review, but initial care and referral are important.

There is very little a lay person can do to help the patient with a fractured tooth. Administration of pain relieving drugs should be followed by urgent referral to a dental surgeon. The patient's usual dental practitioner should be sought in the first instance, as it is he who will carry out the definitive treatment. When he is not available, first aid measures can be obtained in the oral surgery department of a District General Hospital. It is usual to refer the patient to the accident and emergency department, which will request the specialist opinion. The initial treatment will aim at preservation of the pulp, if feasible, by the insertion of a sedative dressing combined with splinting of the tooth if it is mobile. A dislocated tooth which is interfering with jaw movement can sometimes be manipulated gently into its correct position by the doctor on the spot. Occasionally a tooth which has been completely avulsed from its socket can be splinted, and subsequently remain firm in its socket for a number of years. The prognosis depends on the viability of the cells of the periodontal ligament, and the best course of action in the field is to wash dirt from the tooth with normal saline if available, or tap water if not, and replace the tooth in its socket until a dental surgeon can splint it. Gentle pressure from the opposing teeth may be reinforced

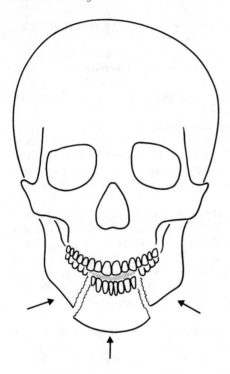

Fig. 20.5 Bilateral fractures of the body of the mandible in the premolar regions. Muscle spasm will pull the posterior fragments inwards, and may cause the anterior fragment to fall back, the latter reinforced by gravity embarrassing the airway.

by the application of a bandage to support the jaw. Antibiotic and antitetanus therapy should be commenced immediately.

Fractures of the facial bones need little first aid treatment. Pain is not usually severe, although difficulty in swallowing may distress the patient. Bleeding is not often a problem either, but can be moderated by the application of a gauze pack. A firm barrel bandage of crêpe applied over cotton wool padding will make the patient more comfortable, although consequent displacement of a large anterior mandibular fragment may embarrass the airway (Fig. 20.5). Where haemorrhage is excessive, or displacement of the fragments allows the tongue to fall back and obstruct the pharynx, the airway should be secured by transporting the patient in a face down or 'tonsil' position, without bandaging.

At the District General Hospital, the oral surgeon will treat the fracture by wiring or splinting the teeth in occlusion, a position which is maintained for about five weeks. A soft or fluid diet is taken for this period, and the patient is not fit for sport for about eight weeks. Clinical union usually occurs in about five weeks, but contact sports such as boxing should be avoided for three months.

Dislocation of the jaw is rarely seen as a result of trauma. The usual cause is an unco-ordinated contracture of the lateral pterygoid muscle during maximum excursion of the jaw in laughing or yawning for example. The condyle of one or both sides slips over the eminentia articularis, and is kept there by muscle spasm. Its reduction may be achieved by sustained downward pressure with the thumbs over the lower molar teeth, the chin being grasped with the remaining fingers of the operator's hands. The jaw will suddenly jump back into its anatomical position, and the thumbs of the operator should be padded to avoid damage.

Dental and facial pain

Dental disease is widespread, and is at its height in the first three decades of life, so that it is worthwhile to consider some conditions which may present in young athletes and affect their performance.

Pain in the teeth on taking sweet foods is usually due to decay, and may be relieved by the insertion of a filling. Pain on thermal changes in the mouth indicates inflammation of the pulp (pulpitis), which is usually reversible by treatment, but may require removal of the pulp for relief of the pain. A tooth which is tender on biting may be so because pressure is transmitted to the pulp through dentine weakened by decay, or, in an apparently intact tooth, because of inflammation of the periodontal ligament. These changes are often reversible without extraction of the tooth, although urgent treatment is required as such tenderness is an early sign of abscess formation. None of the foregoing symptoms is moderated by the administration of drugs, apart from pain relief by anodynes.

An apical abscess results from death of the pulp and suppuration in the bone surrounding the root, producing a swelling of the gum overlying the root, and if neglected, a swelling of the face. Extraction of the tooth is often indicated, although drainage of the abscess through the tooth, and subsequent root treatment may be successful, particularly in anterior teeth, and time may be bought by antibiotic therapy. Tenderness of the gum behind the last standing molar tooth in the lower jaw indicates inflammation of the pericoronal tissues (pericoronitis) of a buried or partially erupted wisdom tooth. Pericoronitis tends to recur two or three times a year until the underlying tooth is removed, and it may progress to a pericoronal abscess with facial swelling and inability to open the mouth. The application of local heat by means of hot saline mouth baths is effective in reducing inflammation; again antibiotic therapy is indicated to abort the infection and to buy time until a specialist opinion is sought.

Temporomandibular joint dysfunction, characterized by clicking, locking and pain in the affected joint is most commonly observed in females around the age of twenty years. It is a myofunctional disorder, and responds well to reassurance and simple exercises prescribed by an oral surgeon. It is associated with stress, and therefore can be expected to appear at times of maximum endeavour.

In conclusion the importance of prevention of dental pain is once again stressed. The most important instrument in preventive dentistry is a toothbrush, its correct use minimizing gingivitis and decay. Correct oral hygiene can only be taught by practical instruction by a dental surgeon or dental hygienist. It should be remembered that the hour of onset of dental pain is usually inopportune, and incapacities can be avoided if regular dental treatment is obtained. Athletes should be examined every six months, as dental fitness is essential for their peak performance. Trauma sufficient to damage the teeth and jaws can never be foreseen, and the use of a mouth guard will do much to protect those who take part in contact sports.   J.R.

References

1. Walther, D. F. (1960) Some of the causes and effects of malocclusion. *Trans. Br. Soc. Study Orthod.*, **1,** 16.
2. Kramer, L. R. (1941) Accidents occurring in High School athletes with special reference to dental injuries. *J. Am. dent. Ass.*, **28,** 1351.
3. Hargreaves, J. A. and Craig, J. W. (1970) *The Management of traumatised Anterior Teeth in Children.* Edinburgh: E. & S. Livingstone.
4. Rowe, N. L. and Killey, H. C. (1968) *Fractures of the Facial Skeleton.* Edinburgh: E. & S. Livingstone.
5. Converse, J. M. and Smith, B. (1960) Blow-out fracture of the floor of the orbit. *Trans. Am. Acad. Ophthal. Oto-lar.*, **64,** 676.

21

Ear and nose problems

Introduction

Participants in surface and underwater swimming are particularly prone to ear and nose disorders, but other sports do have these disorders to a lesser extent. Outer ear infection is more common in surface swimmers who also suffer middle ear infection, but underwater swimmers, especially scuba divers, commonly suffer outer, middle and inner ear disorders due to pressure changes in descent and ascent causing aural barotrauma. In addition to the primary ear disorders, there are a group of conditions which have their primary disorder in surrounding structures, that is the jaw muscles and the teeth, giving referred symptoms that implicate the ears, the nose and the sinuses.

The outer ear

The problems to consider in this section are otitis externa aggravated by wax collections and exostoses, and outer ear barotrauma or 'reverse ear'. The two main types of external otitis are the localized boil, and the widespread or diffuse external otitis caused by bacteria, fungi, or allergy.

Diffuse otitis externa

The predisposing causes of otitis externa are prolonged immersion in the water with the removal of the normal ear wax, probing of the ear with matchsticks or hairpins, and rubbing in or around the ear with a finger. It is known to be more common in tropical climates because the warmer water washes out the wax coating quicker, the humidity is greater, and airborne infections are more common. Wax in the ear is a normal protective secretion but where present in lumps, prevents water from draining out freely, leading to maceration of the skin making it susceptible to otitis externa. Infection from water born organisms is an uncommon cause of otitis externa; it is certainly not so in the case of chlorinated pools and it is highly unlikely in the open sea due to the dilution factor. Waterborne infection may be a factor in untreated or overloaded pools, or where sea pollution is high.

Symptoms and signs

The main symptom is the itch but there also may be an ache or discharge from the ear. This latter may be thin and run out easily, or it may be thick and look like wet blotting paper. The skin itself is reddened and sometimes swollen and tender.

Treatment

This consists of thorough aural toilet (Fig. 21.1) even to the extent of preliminary syringing, and then the use of the antibiotic/steroid eardrops, 3 per cent glacial

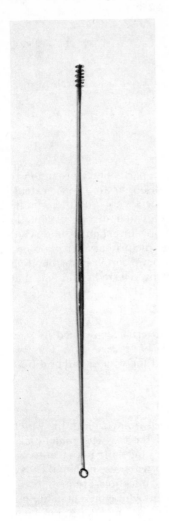

Fig. 21.1 Jobson–Horn probe useful for aural toilet. Dry cotton wool twisted onto the serated end is used for mopping whilst the ring currette is used for clearing solid material.

acetic acid in Vosol (benzethonium chloride)/Hydrocortisone, or antifungal preparations such as 'Jadit' solution or Mycostatin dusting powder. Water aids infection so that dry mopping or suction cleaning of the outer ear canal, especially after syringing, are the best methods of cleaning.

Prevention of otitis externa
(1) Do not pick at, poke or rub in or around the ear, a common practice in those who have itchy ears, a blocked ear feeling, or odd ideas about personal hygiene. Eurax antipruritic lotion should be supplied to those whose ears itch or irritate.

(2) In susceptible people it may be necessary to continue with prophylaxis for up to three months. Five per cent glacial acetic acid in spirit (SVR) used daily or weekly can prevent a recurrence, and swimming is allowed provided these drops are used after swimming.[1]

Exostoses

Another factor predisposing to otitis externa is the presence of exostoses (Fig. 21.2), which grow in susceptible people, in response to the irritation of cold water on the skin of the outer ear canal.[2] Exostoses are not related to otitis externa and are not caused by infection, but since they prevent water from draining out, make the skin susceptible to infection. The bony swellings continue to grow while

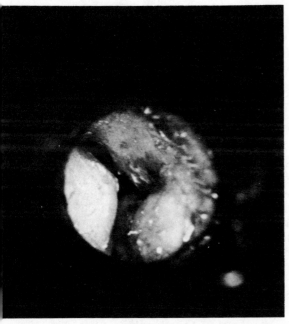

Fig. 21.2 Exostoses are localized bony swellings of the inner third of the outer ear canal, and may eventually close the canal completely (seen here through an aural speculum).

there is a continued exposure to cold water; the temperature that qualifies as cold is that found in sea water and outdoor unheated swimming pools in temperate climates. When medical examination reveals an early developing or an established exostosis, it is important that measures are taken to prevent its continued growth. If swimming in non-tropical waters, a hood should always be worn, or for surface swimmers some form of ear plug should be used.

Outer ear barotrauma

This outer ear squeeze or 'reverse ear' is not a serious condition, but can make a person unfit for scuba diving, so it has a considerable nuisance value. With

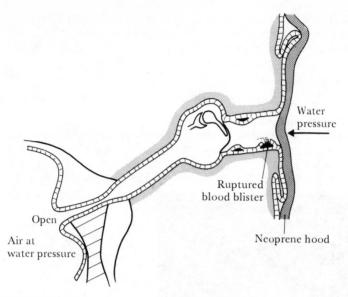

Fig. 21.3 'Reverse ear' in which barotrauma occurs to the skin of the outer ear.

the outer opening of the ear canal obstructed by the hood or ear plugs, on descent a negative pressure develops, maintained by the elasticity of the neoprene hood which prevents water from entering the outer ear canal (Fig. 21.3).

To get sufficient pressure differential to cause trouble, the diver needs to be at a depth of 30–50 ft (9–15 m) as compared to 6–10 ft (1·8–3 m) for middle ear trouble.[3] The eardrum will bulge outwards though seldom sufficiently to cause pain or rupture, and the skin capillaries rupture, forming blood blisters in the skin of the ear canal. These blisters can break spontaneously giving a tattered look to the ear canal and eardrum.

Treatment
Maintain the ear dry and use antiseptic ear drops or powder to clear or prevent infection, and, as it heals, 5 per cent glacial acetic acid in SVR. The damage seen should not be confused with a ruptured eardrum.

Prevention
If it has occurred then earplugs should not be used but a small hole can be cut in the hood over the ear, to let in water.

Otitis media

In a person without a perforation of the eardrum, infection is carried to the middle ear from the nose by way of the Eustachian tube. The symptoms are of earache and mild to severe deafness, and the treatment is by antibiotics and nasal decongestants.

Its predominance in the social swimmer[4] is due to faulty technique, resulting

n nasal congestion and infection which leads to Eustachian tube congestion and
nfection, all brought about by the physical irritation of the nasal mucosa by
the water.

Prevention of otitis media

It is recommended, and it is taught by most coaches, that the surface swimmer
should breathe out whenever the nose enters the water and that the scuba diver
should keep his face mask clear of water. With swimmers, exhalation should be
both through the nose and the mouth, and explosive expiration should not be
taught because while the buoyancy advantage is negligible, there is a decreased
blood return to the heart due to raised intrathoracic pressure. Also the level at
which the breath is held is in the throat, so there is an increased likelihood of
nasal irritation by water, leading to Eustachian tube congestion and otitis media.
Any nasal infection or congestion is a bar to scuba diving, but with the correct
technique minimal nasal infections are not a bar to surface swimming. It must
be remembered that the toxic effect of any illness, especially respiratory, has a
general effect on the body, and subjects with moderate to severe respiratory infection should not overexert themselves in any sports activity.

Otitic barotrauma or the 'squeeze'

As a result of descent, as in an aeroplane or in underwater swimming, there is
a change in the external pressure on the ear from low to high, and, if the Eustachian tube does not allow air into the middle ear, then the outside raised pressure
will push the eardrums inwards (Fig. 21.4) as the gas in the middle ear is compressed or squeezed. Pain in the ear commonly occurs in the inexperienced diver
after a change of pressure of five feet of water, but in the more experienced diver

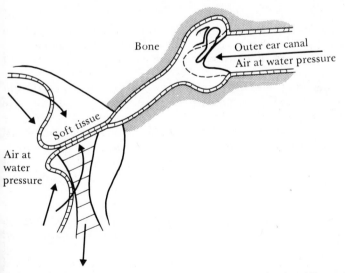

Fig. 21.4 Otitic or middle ear barotrauma as a result of a closed Eustachian tube preventing inflation or clearing of the middle ear.

the sensations are not so great, partly because of the fact that the eardrum has been stretched on many occasions, and partly because of the natural disinclination to take any notice of early warnings. As the eardrum does not stretch far enough to allow the pressure equalization, negative middle ear pressure extracts fluid from the blood vessels into the cavity of the middle ear (traumatic secretory otitis media). Bleeding into the middle ear then occurs. The small haemorrhages which occur into the substance of the drum are common in scuba divers and can be recognized up to two or three weeks later. They indicate poor technique of clearing the ears or diving with nasal congestion. If the pressure changes are great, or if there is any weakness in the drum, it may rupture. This occurs in pressure changes ranging from 9 to 90 ft (2·7–27 m) depending on the strength of the eardrum which may be atrophic from childhood secretory otitis media. If water enters the middle ear through the perforation, dizziness or vertigo occurs, and as such ruptures occur mostly in depths over 60 ft (18 m), it can be a danger to life.

Treatment
The diver, if underwater, needs only to return towards the surface when the pressure differential eases and clearing the ears will be easier. Auto-inflation of short duration may be attempted to fill the middle ear with air but if this is not enough, it may be necessary for the diver to come right back to the surface and even give up diving until he can inflate his ears easily. As free fluid or blood in the middle ear is removed, partly down the Eustachian tube and partly by being re-absorbed back through the mucous membrane lining, decongestant treatment to clear the nose and Eustachian tube is given. Recovery from such a bleed should be confirmed by the return of the hearing to normal. Only after a period would a myringotomy and suction removal of the blood be indicated.

Prevention
As the diver descends, he should normally inflate his ears starting on the surface and then every 2 or 3 ft (0·6–0·9 m), by the method which he has found easiest. If any discomfort develops, he should stop descending or ascend a few feet until he can clear his ears.

As the pressure differential develops, the soft tissue of the inner end of the Eustachian tube acts as a valve and closes more firmly causing 'locking', so that early rather than late inflation is indicated. The technique of inflating or clearing the ears should be practised repeatedly out of the water so that it can be performed easily and frequently when descending, without much concentration or effort.

Inner ear barotrauma

Scuba divers commonly have a temporary conductive deafness, but sensorineural deafness is rare and due to micro-emboli of the 'bends', sudden shock waves as occur in underwater explosions, noise exposure, and rupture of the round window membrane.

Another sport specific barotrauma of a rather different kind is that connected with shooting.[5] For such a condition, prevention by provision of suitable ear pads is effective, but such treatment is not effective underwater (Fig. 21.5). A similar

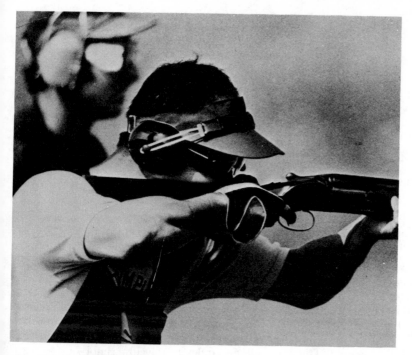

Fig. 21.5 Ear pads worn by competitor in trap shooting. (Photo: E. D. Lacey).

injury can also be caused by a direct blow over the ear in body contact sports but this is rare.

Rupture of the round window membrane

Prolonged or forceful performance of Valsalva's manœuvre causes a transient rise in blood pressure but a more persistent rise in the pressure of the cerebrospinal fluid.[6] The aqueduct of the cochlea connects the subarachnoid space to the cochlea, and in some people this canal is larger allowing a free flow of cerebrospinal fluid into the scala tympani of the cochlea, the opening of the aqueduct being adjacent to the round window. With a forceful auto-inflation or Valsalva's manœuvre, the transmitted cerebrospinal fluid pressure increase is sufficient to rupture the thin round window membrane separating the inner and the middle ears, allowing the perilymph to escape and causing loss of function of the hair cells.

Symptoms
The onset is a unilateral loud ringing or hissing noise in the ear with deafness (which may not be noted immediately, because underwater hearing is negligible). Vertigo, or loss of balance, may or may not occur showing involvement of the vestibular apparatus and may be present for up to three months. If questioned,

most patients will admit to having had more difficulty than usual in clearing their ears. The ear itself has a blocked or dead feeling, giving a sensation of fullness or of pressure building up in the ear.

Signs
Hearing loss is the cardinal sign, especially in the high tones, but sometimes in the whole frequency range of hearing. The patient at first, if the vestibular apparatus is affected, will have a spontaneous nystagmus and a staggering gait with a tendency to move or fall to the side of the deranged ear. In severe cases, vomiting may occur. (It is needless to say how this may threaten survival under-water.) The eardrum usually appears the same as in the unaffected ear, and any other signs would be coincidental and due to an actual dive or to possible otitic barotrauma.

Differential diagnosis
The condition is often diagnosed as a virus infection of the inner ear or as Meniére's disease. (The latter rarely affects a person with the mental stability required of an underwater devotee.)

Treatment
High concentrations of inspired oxygen should be given over a period of several days with a minimum one hour twice daily. At the same time, drugs to dilate the cochlear blood vessels can be given, although the effect on these vessels is not well documented. These include cyclandelate (Cyclospasmol), up to 3 g a day, or nicotinic acid (50 mg as often as necessary to produce flushing). The ad-ministration of steroids appears to be of use. In addition to treating the deafness, antiemetic drugs may be necessary for the vertigo. Because of the disability that deafness causes, it is obvious that specialist treatment is needed and it is required within the first week if there is to be any chance of complete recovery. Rupture of the round window membrane can be repaired by a relatively simple operation with recovery of the hearing loss.[7]

Prevention
The diver should have a wide margin of safety in his decompression staging to prevent 'bends' from developing. The occurrence of sudden sensorineural deaf-ness is another reason for not diving when there is any cause to suspect that the Eustachian tube will require prolonged or forceful Valsalva's manoeuvre.

Vertigo

There are various forms of dizziness which occur underwater. Over breathing lead-ing to lowered blood carbon dioxide can cause dizziness by reducing the blood supply to the balancing centre, by way of the intracranial vasoconstriction caused. Any anxiety state or mental tension can develop into a feeling of insecurity in the hostile underwater environment, giving a vague sense of imbalance or light headedness. True vertigo and loss of orientation can occur with some divers when they cannot see the bottom or when they are in a 'whiteout' state. This is a visual disorder, due to there being nothing to fix the eyes on. Under such circumstances, the diver should look for his bubbles and follow them up or close his eyes, as in searching for non-existent visual information, he will tend to disregard other postural cues.[8] Vertigo, mild to severe, can occur along with any of the disorders of the hearing mechanism leading to deafness already described.

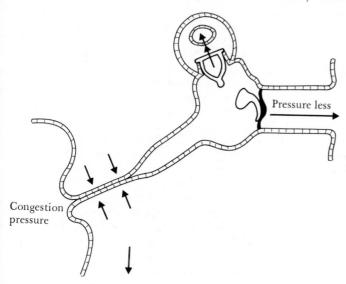

Fig. 21.6 Alternobaric vertigo. The loose ossicular ligaments allow the stapes to be depressed into the vestibule where it directly stimulates the utriculosaccular complex.

Alternobaric vertigo

This occurs during a diving ascent, as Eustachian tube blockage causes a build-up of pressure in the middle ear, the 'reverse squeeze' (Fig. 21.6), in which the eardrum sometimes ruptures.

Symptoms

As the pressure builds up in the middle ear before the onset of vertigo, the diver is aware of it and can slow down or stop his ascent until the air comes through the Eustachian tube, reducing the middle ear pressure. If not, then there is a severe loss of orientation with a rotary vertigo. The feeling of disorientation produces feelings of panic in the diver but usually the surface is reached. In some cases, the diver, if he can see his colleague, will notice a shimmer effect with his colleague seeming to be moving up and down due to a vertical nystagmus.

Treatment

As the vertigo is usually overcome, the diver survives, and ensures that his future ascents are not rapid and that he takes care not to dive when his Eustachian tubes are difficult to clear. If there is any warning that the dizziness is coming on, to descend prevents the onset. However, most sufferers are keen to get out of the water and so continue upwards. Treatment can be given to increase the patency of the Eustachian tubes to allow air to escape easily from the middle ear on ascent, thus preventing the 'reverse squeeze'. If one ear is becoming blocked then the surface diver can bend his head away from the affected ear and the pull of the tissues on that side of the neck allows the Eustachian tube to open more readily.

The nose and sinuses

As far as safe and pleasant swimming and diving is concerned, the state of the nose plays an important part. Any defect of the nose is liable to affect the Eustachian tube, and make clearing the ears by inflating the middle ear less easy or even impossible. Accordingly, the commonest medical aid used by swimmers and divers is some form of nasal decongestant and the commonest cause of trouble is the common cold. Any of the usual conditions causing nasal obstruction such as a deviated nasal septum, allergic rhinitis, vasomotor rhinitis ('sinus') or true sinusitis will need attention. Sometimes the persistence of adenoids in adults will require surgery. One of the causes of nose bleeds in scuba divers is poor pressure equalization in the sinuses causing the 'sinus squeeze'. Facial pains occur, and non-frothy blood coming from the nose or mouth may be coming from the sinuses.

Prevention of many disorders arising from water sports is based on having a healthy nose or, when there is nasal congestion, by the use of nasal decongestants either as drops, sprays, or oral preparations. For short-term use, local treatment is useful, but for long-term treatment specialist advice should be sought on simple surgical methods of permanently clearing nasal obstruction.

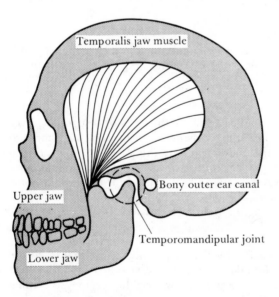

Fig. 21.7 The temporalis muscle reaches from the orbital margin in front, to the occiput, surrounding the outer ear canal except below. The pterygoid muscles are under the orbit and out to the angle of the jaw.

The jaws and earache

A common cause of earache in adults is referred pain in the ears from disorder of the temporomandibular joint which also results in 'blocked' ears, itchy ears and pains around the ears.

The prime cause is forceful clenching of the teeth in underwater swimmers on the mouthpiece of their snorkel or their regulator. The onset of symptoms is probably due to the presence of several factors working together, including a tendency in affected subjects to grind or clench their teeth. If there is faulty dentition due to lack of teeth or their malposition, or if dentures are unsatisfactory, this causes subconscious irritation leading to faulty habits of moving the jaws. Rarely is the joint physically affected, but the many muscles (Fig. 21.7) which move the joint tend to develop contractions to protect it, even to the point of spasm, causing aches and pains similar to backache and -pain. Pain can arise at the site where the muscles are attached to the bone of the skull, the jaw, or in the muscle itself and is referred to the face, forehead or the temples.[9]

N.R.

References

1. Jones, E. (1965) *External Otitis*. Springfield, Ill.: Charles C. Thomas.
2. Harrison, D. F. N. (1962) The relationship of osteomata of the external auditory meatus to swimming. *Annals. R. Coll Surg.*, **31,** 187.
3. Coles, R. R. A. (1963) 'Ears' and their after effects. *R. N. Diving Magazine*, **10,** 2:3.
4. Grigor, R. R., Hall, C. D. and Roydhouse, N. (1970) Report of Committee on swimming. *Sport Med. Bull. N.Z.F.S.M.*, **2,** 27.
5. Odess, J. S. (1974) The hearing hazard of firearms. *Physn Sports Med.*, October, 65.
6. Simmons, F. B. (1968) Theory of membrane breaks in sudden hearing loss. *Arch Otolar.* **88,** 41.
7. Pullen, F. W. (1971) Round window membrane rupture: a cause of sudden deafness. *Trans. Am. Acad. Ophthal. Oto-lar.*, **75,** 1421.
8. Ross, H. E., Crickmar, S. D., Sills, N. V. and Owen, E. P. (1967) Orientation to the vertical in free diving. *Aerospace Med.*, **40,** 728.
9. Roydhouse, R. H. and Horan, J. D. (in preparation) Temperomandibular dysfunction, a review.

22

Neck and back injuries

Introduction

In everyday life, the back and neck are subject to recurring strains leading to complaints of pain and stiffness. Most sports put stress on the spine and so such symptoms are found also in sportsmen. Since degenerative changes start in intervertebral discs from the age of about 20 years, it is to be expected that sportsmen will present pathological processes and clinical syndromes similar to those of their non-sporting friends. Such injuries range from minor self-limiting trauma to dislocation and paraplegia.

In most series,[1-3] back and neck lesions form from 10 to 20 per cent of sports injuries. The peak age incidence is in the third decade with 90 per cent occurring in males. Any body build may be affected.

Functional anatomy

Vertebrae consist of an anterior body and a posterior neural arch. The neural arch has pedicles and laminae and where these meet, superior and inferior articular processes arise. The processes of contiguous vertebrae articulate to form synovial joints known as apophyseal, posterior, or facetal joints. Two lateral transverse processes, and one posterior spinous process complete the bony ring and serve for muscular and ligamentous attachments. Vertebral bodies are bound together by firm cartilaginous discs composed of three parts—an outer casing (the annulus fibrosus), and an inner core (the nucleus pulposus), bounded above and below by the cartilaginous vertebral end plates.

In the period of active involvement in sport, the nucleus pulposus is mostly gelatinous fluid. This incompressible gel acts as a ball bearing so that in flexion and extension, the vertebral bodies roll over this nucleus. The action of the annulus may be compared to that of a coiled spring which, operating between two vertebral bodies, pulls them together.

The spine has many functions.[4,5] The bony elements are needed to support the head and ribs, and protect the spinal cord. Not only is stability needed to allow body weight to be transmitted, but also flexibility to allow movement of the spine as a whole and also between individual segments. Movement occurs in both the anterior cartilaginious joint and in the posterior synovial joints. The function of the disc is special. It acts both as a shock absorber and as a fulcrum of movement between vertebrae, thus allowing stresses acting on the spine to be transmitted equally in all directions. The spring-like action of the annulus makes for stability, and also prevents excessive movements in flexion and extension. There is no blood supply to the disc but fluid easily enters from the vertebrae through the vertebral end plates.

Classification of injuries

These may be divided into:

(1) Soft tissue, muscles, ligaments, or nerves.
(2) Bone.
(3) Discs.
(4) Other causes of back pain.

As in other areas, injuries may be direct or indirect, and the latter may involve overuse of the part.

(1) Soft tissues:

(a) *Muscles and ligaments*[6]

Direct injuries following a kick or blow occur usually in contact sports and form an important group of sports injuries. They range from trivial trauma to haematoma formation. In the lower lumbar region this may at times result in a localized subcutaneous collection of serosanguineous fluid which may require drainage.

Indirect injuries to muscles or ligaments are common. Muscle injuries particularly involve the erector spinae group in the lumbar region. The typical story is one of a sudden or poorly co-ordinated movement followed by pain and tenderness usually well localized in one area. Moving this affected part either by stretching or resisting extension will reproduce the patient's pain. Muscle injuries are particularly common in some types of sportsmen, including weight-lifters, field event athletes who have to hurl missiles and, in cricket, fast bowlers. Treatment of these injuries is standard as in muscle injuries elsewhere in the body (Chapter 17). The vast majority will heal completely. However a small proportion of patients are left with fibrous thickening in the muscle tissue, and these people are subject to recurring tears and disability. The treatment then is injection of the tender area with local anaesthetic and corticosteroid followed by exercises to stretch the affected part.

Although back ligaments are quite strong, they may, nevertheless, be acutely overstretched and so sprained. This occurs in a few typical sites, e.g. the lumbosacral joint and in the interspinous ligament ('sprung-back').[7] Ligaments are particularly likely to be sprained in injuries involving a fall in which there is a rotational strain to the lower spine, or on bending and lifting.[8,9] Ligamentous pain also occurs in sports that involve long periods of standing or crouching in a flexed position. The 'whip-lash' type of injury is not seen commonly in sporting injuries, though hyperextension strains do occur for example in diving.[10]

(b) *Nerves*

Injuries to the brachial plexus or its roots are not common but may occur following traction injuries. Such injuries are seen when the sportsmen falls on to the shoulder, or in falls in which the neck is forcibly side-flexed while traction is applied to the arm, as in riding accidents (Fig. 22.1). Damage to the spinal cord is almost invariably associated with spinal fracture or dislocation (see below).

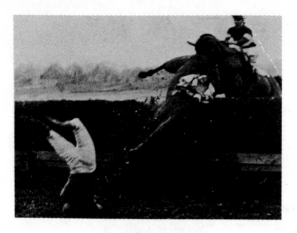

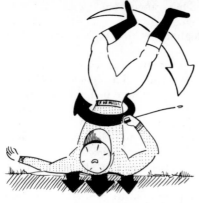

Fig. 22.1 A riding accident and the mechanism by which it gives rise to brachial plexus or spinal cord damage.

(2) Bone

(a) Fracture

Vertebral body fracture is relatively uncommon in sport. The mechanism is usually one of hyperflexion and compression producing an anterior wedging of the vertebral body (Fig. 22.2). This may occur anywhere in the spine but is most common at the thoracolumbar junction. Since the spinal cord ends at the level of the second lumbar vertebra, cord damage is seen only in fractures above this level. In the lower spine, the diagnosis is usually made on the type of injury and the degree of pain and disability, and is confirmed by X-ray. In the neck, X-ray views in flexion are necessary in addition to standard radiographs (Fig. 22.3). Injuries of C7 are notoriously difficult to see because of overlying structures, and expert radiography to eliminate the shoulder shadow may be needed to be certain of the presence of a fracture-dislocation. The well known situations causing broken necks include diving into shallow water, collapse of a rugby scrum or ruck, and faulty execution on a trampoline. However fracture dislocation can

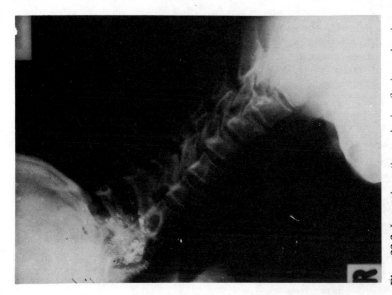

Fig. 22.3 Lateral radiograph in flexion showing rigidity of cervical spine due to muscle spasm and subluxation of C4 on C5.

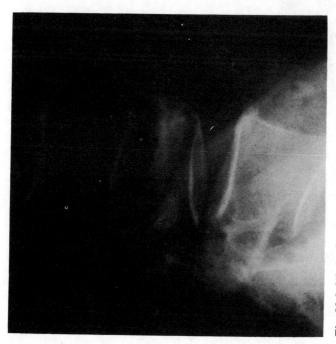

Fig. 22.2 Wedge fracture of the body of L3 following a compression injury.

follow apparently trivial injuries and one unfortunate football referee suffered a fractured cervical vertebral body when he tripped over a player. Paraplegia or death may follow, so the survival and future well-being of the sportsman with such an injury may therefore depend on proper first aid management.[11,12]

Fracture dislocation of the cervical spine necessitates admission to hospital where accurate reduction by specialist management can be obtained (Fig. 22.4). Fractures of the vertebral body usually heal well but there is occasional instability due to associated injury to the posterior structures and fusion may be necessary.

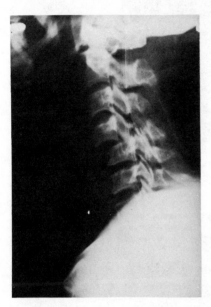

Fig. 22.4 Fracture dislocation of cervical spine with locked facets requiring specialist management.

Fractures of the spinous process occur usually in the cervical spine at C6 or C7. This follows an acute flexion injury and is associated with avulsion of the ligament. It has also been described when the flexed neck is given a direct blow. Pain is felt localized over the spinous process, and is made worse by flexion. The diagnosis is confirmed by X-ray (Fig. 22.5). Healing is usually by firm fibrous union.

Transverse process fracture is common in the lumbar spine (Fig. 22.6). There are two mechanisms which produce this injury, and they usually act simultaneously. These are a direct blow and an indirect forceful muscular contraction producing avulsion of the processes. The associated muscular tear produces most disability, and side-bending movements particularly are painful. Treatment consists of immobilization until healing allows pain-free movement, usually in about three weeks. Immobilization may be obtained by the use of a lumbosacral corset. Isometric and stretching exercises of the muscles are then performed to allow full mobility and strength to be regained. The ultimate prognosis is excellent.

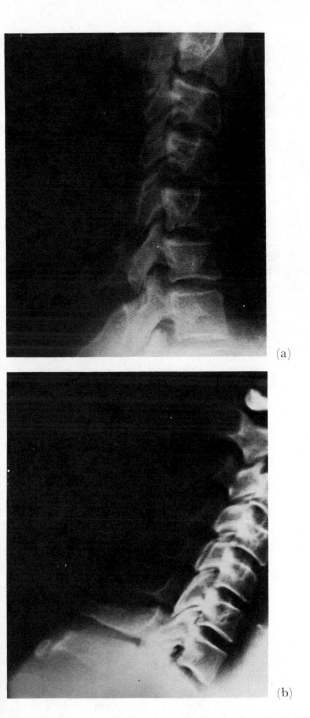

(a)

(b)

Fig. 22.5 Fractures of spinous processes. (a) C6, and (b) D1.

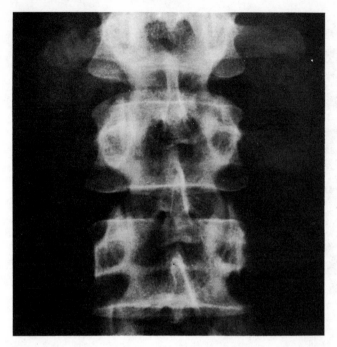

Fig. 22.6 Anterior radiograph showing fractures of *right* transverse processes of 2nd and 3rd lumbar vertebrae.

(b) Spondylolysis

Spondylolysis is a solution of continuity of the pars interarticularis of the lamina (Fig. 22.7). Previously considered to be a congenital defect, it is now believed to be a stress fracture since:

(a) this is not the site of fusion of ossification centres;
(b) it has not been found to occur at birth;
(c) there is an increasing incidence with age.

One suggested mechanism is that movement between adjacent articular facets produces a pincer effect on this area.

It is not an uncommon injury in fast bowlers, and in right-hand bowlers affects the left side, and conversely, in left-hand fast bowlers is more likely to affect the right side. It is also a major problem in weight-lifters, oarsmen and weight trainers.[13]

It may be asymptomatic or produce localised pain in the back. However, if there is nerve root pressure, it is much more likely that there is an associated disc protrusion rather than nerve pressure from the fibrocartilaginous mass that binds this fracture together. Treatment consists of rest, if necessary in plaster or corset, and avoidance of the particular strain involved in the sport. Unilateral lesions usually respond well to conservative treatment and the sport can then usually be resumed. When the condition is bilateral, there is a risk of

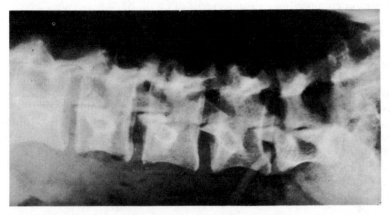

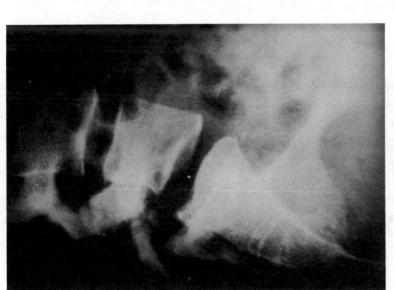

Fig. 22.7 Spondylolysis. (a) Tennis player (L5/S1). (b) A pole vaulter (L5/S1).

spondylolisthesis i.e. the upper vertebra slipping forward on the one below it. Other causes of spondylolisthesis include laxity of posterior structures without bony defect.

(c) Spondylolisthesis

It is seen most commonly as a slip forward of L5 on S1.[14] Symptoms may vary, the commonest being backache made worse by exercise and then felt not only in the back but radiating out towards the buttocks. It may also be associated with sciatica and in 5 per cent of cases there is associated intervertebral disc protrusion. Spondylolisthesis may also be symptomless, and thus sometimes is a chance radiological finding.[15]

Two signs are of importance: one is a dimpling of a skin above the level of the spondylolisthesis, the other presence of extra skin folds visible because of the altered spinal alignment (Fig. 22.8). The presence of spondylolisthesis is not necessarily a bar to active sports, as one of England's greatest fast bowlers can well testify. However an unstable lumbar vertebra is easily subjected to strains causing recurrent disabilities, and may constitute a great problem in the sport. At times interbody fusion will be indicated and one Olympic rower had such a fusion prior to becoming a medal winner.

(3) Intervertebral disc lesions

Intervertebral discs are large avascular structures. When they degenerate repair is not possible. This degeneration affects primarily the mucopolysaccharide com-

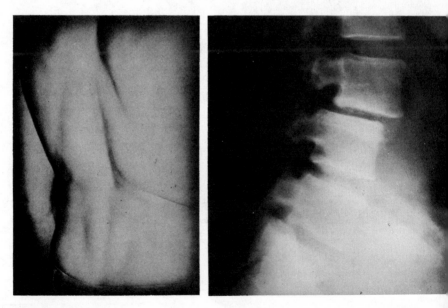

Fig. 22.8 Spondylolisthesis (L3/4) in an international oarsman. (a) Clinical appearance. (b) Radiological appearance.

ponents and follows wear and tear due to repeated mechanical stresses or trauma. After a time a tear is liable to appear in the degenerated annulus through which the nucleus bulges out. If this occurs forwards, upwards or downwards, no particular harm results. However, if this material bulges posteriorly or posterolaterally, it results in two complications:

(a) nerve root pressure;
(b) derangement of spinal mechanics.

Cervical disc protrusions are rare, possibly due to the added protection of the

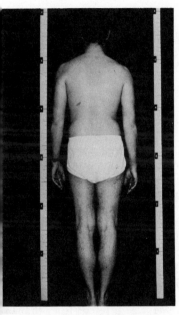

Fig. 22.9 'Spastic scoliosis' due to muscle spasm in disc derangement.

neurocentral joint in the cervical spine. Since the most common sites for disc protrusions in athletes are at the L4–5 and L5–S1 levels, the nerve roots involved may be L4, L5 or S1. Pain is felt in the leg usually spreading to below the knee, and is associated with paraesthesiae in the appropriate dermatome. Reflex changes occur with L4 or S1 lesions and appropriate muscle weakness or wasting may also be present. Straight leg raising is diminished. Derangement of spinal mechanics inevitably involves both disc and apophyseal joints. There are three main signs:

(a) loss of normal movement particularly forward flexion;
(b) scoliosis to avoid further nerve impingement (Fig. 22.9);
(c) an accompanying protective muscle spasm with loss of normal lumbar lordosis.

Protrusion occurs relatively late in the course of disc disease, and at an earlier stage of disc degeneration there may be an instability of the intervertebral joint as normal internal pressure is lost. Abnormal movement of the segment then occurs as a result of this instability.[16] This allows the posterior facetal joints to be easily sprained and may be accompanied by effusion in the apophyseal joints.[17] So patients with early disc degeneration may have attacks of acute back pain and stiffness.

The problem is one of diagnosis, and in the absence of neurological signs, the use of the label 'disc protrusion' is best avoided if it cannot be substantiated, for patients may present with the signs of an acute mechanical derangement, with pain, loss of movement, and spasm from causes other than disc protrusion.

The only accurate diagnosis that can be made in such cases is that the patient has an internal derangement of the intervertebral joint complex—the cartilaginous disc in front and the two apophyseal joints behind. Since the pathology in such cases is speculative, it would be better if only a descriptive title such as intervertebral joint derangement were used.

Intervertebral joint derangement
Attacks may occur in the neck ('torticollis') or in the lumbar region ('lumbago') and are common in younger age groups. They vary in intensity from being minor and lasting only a few days to sudden intense pain such that movement is virtually impossible and the patient is bedridden for several days. The prognosis for an attack is excellent but repeated attacks are liable to occur.

There has been much speculation (and dogmatism) about the pathology, and most of the intevertebral joint structures have been implicated at some time. In the disc itself it has been attributed to tears in the annulus, minor protrusions of the nucleus, acute hydrops of the disc, hypertrophy of the ligamentum flavum, changes in the facetal joints and finally, muscular lesions ('fibrositis'). Some cases of sciatica in athletes may present as complaints of a 'hamstring tear'.

Management
The management of intervertebral joint derangement is different from that of definite intervertebral disc protrusion. The former is traditionally treated with heat, rest and analgesics. However this group usually responds well to manipulative techniques and these produce the quickest results. The athlete needs to avoid the type of stresses that hurt his back, particularly forward flexion, until pain is completely gone.

Cases of intervertebral disc protrusions with nerve root pressure are best treated by complete rest, preferably in hospital, where they are nursed flat on a firm mattress and fracture boards. The patient must be impressed with the need for immobilization to effect adequate resolution. It may help to keep the patient immobile with continuous traction on the legs or pelvis. Analgesics and anti-inflammatory agents are of value, but there is no evidence of the value of muscle relaxants. As symptoms regress, exercises under supervision are commenced. There is no agreement about the best system of exercising, but isometric abdominal and spinal exercises have proved of value. Manipulation at this stage may help to reduce pain and increase mobilization. The indications for surgery are

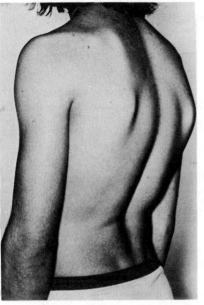

(a)

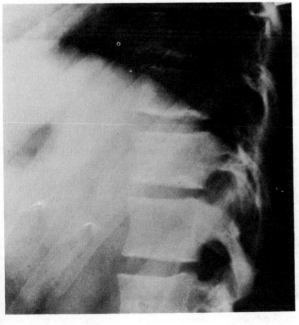

(b)

Fig. 22.10 Scheuermann's disease. (a) Clinical appearance. (b) Radiological appearance.

the usually accepted ones—the failure of an adequate conservative programme of management and/or persistent neurological signs.

(4) Other causes of back pain

(a) Scheuermann's disease

This follows a growth disturbance in adolescence of the vertebral epiphyseal ring. It results in deformity of the vertebral end plate with formation of Schmorl's nodes, vertebral body wedging and a smooth kyphosis (Fig. 22.10). This is seen usually in the thoracic region, especially on forward flexion. Although it can be asymptomatic, pain does tend to come on after active sport. Treatment with active back exercises is usually sufficient and sport should still be played. It is only with severe symptoms that pain may limit the degree of active sport participation—in such cases local spasm may respond well to manipulation and dorsal 'bouncing'. This condition may be associated with tight hamstring muscles.

(b) Perthe–Legge–Calves's disease

Though less common than Scheuermann's disease this form of spinal osteochondritis can be troublesome in the younger sportsman, and when diagnosed must be carefully followed up until resolution is complete. Any tendency to produce a secondary kyphosis may have to be prevented by the use of a spinal brace. Otherwise treatment is symptomatic with reduction in activity below the level at which pain is produced. Both osteochondritides can cause deformation of the vertebrae which leads to secondary backache in later adult life.

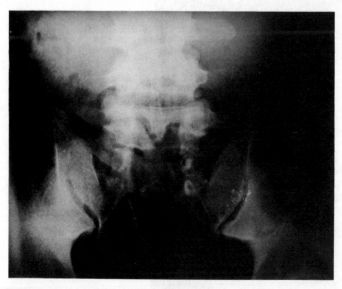

Fig. 22.11 Spina bifida occulta. Radiological appearance in an international oarsman complaining of low back pain.

(c) *Ankylosing spondylitis*

Persistent low back pain in the young male sportsman should always give rise to a suspicion of ankylosing spondylitis. Diagnosis rests on a raised sedimentation rate and typical changes of sacro-iliitis on X-ray. Treatment is according to accepted practice. This condition is not necessarily incompatible with sports activity.

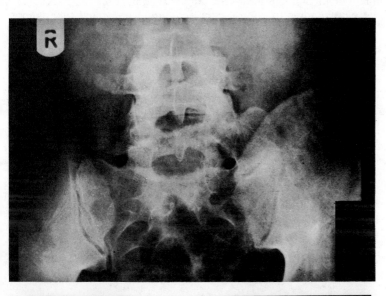

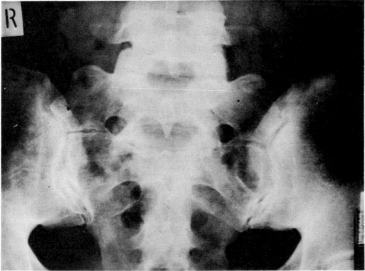

Fig. 22.12 Lumbosacral anomalies. (a) Incomplete (hemi); and (b) complete sacralization of L5.

Rare causes of low back pain

Various other causes of back pain may present in athletes from time to time. Spina bifida occulta is often silent but may be brought to light as a result of vigorous sports activity, particularly heavy weight-training (Fig. 22.11). Treatment is according to the needs of the case and sporting activity may have to be curtailed. Symptoms may also be experienced due to lumbosacral anomalies such as complete or incomplete lumbarization or sacralization (Fig. 22.12).

Although very uncommon in most Western communities, spinal tuberculosis does occur from time to time and should not be forgotten as a possible cause of low back pain: tumours, including osteoid osteoma and meningioma should also be born in mind in the obscure case.

Prevention of injury

Although it is impossible completely to prevent spinal injuries, it is nevertheless possible, with due regard to spinal mechanics, to limit them. It is necessary to teach correct lifting methods and techniques both at work and in sport, e.g. in weight-training. If particular strains are known to produce injury, it may be possible to avoid them. Proper postural control as in sleeping on a firm mattress, correct seating in cars, or the correction of a short leg, can all be of value. Muscles should be examined and a system of back, abdominal, or leg exercises, including hamstring stretching, instituted if necessary.

Finally there will be a group of spinal defects such as disc degeneration, spondylolisthesis or Scheuermann's disease in which sporting activity may need to be curtailed if there is recurring disability.

A.B.C.

References

1. Anonymous (1954) Hazards in competitive athletics. *Statist. Bull. Metropolitan Life Insur. Co.*, **35**, 1.
2. Williams, J. G. P. (1973) Sports injuries. *Folia Traumatologica*. Basle: CIBA–Geigy.
3. Thorndike, A. (1959) Frequency and nature of sports injuries. *Am. J. Surg.*, **98**, 316.
4. Newman, P. H. (1971) Muscle action of the vertebral column. *Br. J. sports Med.*, **5**, 34.
5. Troup, J. D. G. (1976) Biomechanics of the spine. In *Advance in Orthotics*, ed. Murdoch, G., London: Edward Arnold.
6. Ryan, A. J. (1976) Determining the causes of low back pain in athletes. In *Proceedings XX World Congress of Sports Medicine*.
7. Newman, P. H. (1952) Sprung back. *J. Bone Jt Surg.*, **34B**, 30.
8. Corrigan, A. B. (1968) Sports injuries. *Hosp. Med.*, **1**, 1328.
9. Roaf, R. (1960) A study of the mechanics of spinal injury. *J. Bone Jt Surg.*, **42B**, 810.
10. Southwich, W. O. (1973) Soft tissue consideration of cervical spine injuries. In *Sport in the Modern World*. Berlin: Springer Verlag.
11. Berlin, W. (1969) Cervical spine injuries: immediate first aid. *J. NATA* **4**, 13.
12. Murphy, O. B. (1971) In *Encyclopedia of Sport Sciences and Medicine*, ed. Larson, L. A., London: Collier-Macmillan.
13. Kotani, P. T., Ichikawa, N., Wakabayashi, W., Yoshii, T. and Koshimune, M. (1971) Studies of spondylolysis found among weight lifters. *Br. J. sports Med.*, **6**, 4.

14. Wiltse, L. (1970) Spondylolisthesis: Classification and aetiology. In *Symposium on the Spine*. St. Louis: C. V. Mosby.
15. Newman, P. H. (1963) The aetiology of spondylolisthesis. *J. Bone Jt. Surg.*, **45B,** 36.
16. Morgan, F. and King, T. (1957) Primary instability of the lumbar vertebrae as a cause of low back pain. *J. Bone Jt Surg.*, **39B,** 6.
17. Wiltse, L. (1970) Lumbosacral strain and instability. In *Symposium on the Spine*. St. Louis: C. V. Mosby.

23

Thoracic, abdominal and perineal injuries

Introduction

Injuries to the thorax, abdomen and perineum occur usually in the contact sports, as a result of direct trauma. Fortunately, on most occasions the injury is only a minor one and can be dealt with easily. In some instances, however, it may be of greater significance—Aristotle[1] himself describing how 'even the slightest blow could rupture an intestine without sign of injury to skin'. Sports injuries can therefore lead to serious problems and they can even be fatal. All attending physicians should be aware of these possibilities and they must be on guard constantly for their detection, early diagnosis and subsequent treatment.

Thoracic injuries

The chest consists basically of a bony cage designed for the protection of underlying major organs—the heart and lungs. This leads to the convenient classification of injuries of this region into superficial and deep.

Superficial injuries

Soft tissue
External injuries to the chest are common. Bruising and haematomas are frequently experienced. For these, immediate ice-packing is invaluable. Muscle strain, especially to the pectoral muscle group, is a disabling condition. Usually it results from direct muscular effort, when a characteristic tearing pain is experienced. This is followed by local tenderness and swelling. Again early ice-packing is important. This is maintained for 48 hours and followed by specialized physiotherapy. Progressive return to active function is encouraged. Operative suturing[2] of a complete rupture of the pectoralis major has been described with encouraging results.

Breast
Breast injuries are not common although with the introduction of equality of sexes, feminine participation in the contact sports will result in many more examples being seen. Such trauma may lead to a localized haematoma with damage to breast tissue, producing an area of fat necrosis.[3] This presents as a painless hard lump in the breast some weeks or even months after the traumatic incident. It is indistinguishable from a breast cancer and a surgical excision-biopsy is recommended for the correct diagnosis to be established.

Bony injuries

As a result of a direct blow or rotational strain, rib fractures are a common problem. Stress fractures[4] have also been described. They present with pain, associated with local tenderness, at the site of the fracture. Usually this is minor, being of the crack variety. If the injury is more serious, the fracture may be more obvious. Then, on examination, as well as severe local pain, crepitus may be felt at the fracture site. In all cases of rib injury a chest X-ray is advisable to eliminate underlying lung damage. On the X-ray plate the fracture site may not always be demonstrated, especially when it is of the minor variety. The diagnosis is then a clinical one confirmed by the period of four to six weeks it takes for the athlete's discomfort to settle enough for him to return to his full sporting activities. Treatment of rib fractures is symptomatic. Mild analgesics and encouragement are all that are generally required. If the pain is more severe, restricting plaster strips may be applied round the side of the chest. This then limits the movement of the fracture site, though it can result in such limitation of chest movement that underlying lung function can be embarrassed. Coughing may then be prevented and subsequent lung atelectasis with secondary infection can develop. Should the pain be more severe, intercostal nerve blocks with a long-acting local anaesthetic may be helpful. In the more violent sports, cases may present with multiple rib fractures and even a flail segment. Then more aggressive treatment will be required. The patient may be in severe respiratory distress and even require ventilatory support. In such cases where paradoxical breathing is due to the flail segment, a pad should be bandaged firmly over the area which is unstable. Emergency oxygen should always be available where chest injuries are likely. In extreme cases 'Ambu' bag ventilation or even intubation and assisted respiration may be life-saving. Such cases then need urgent hospitalization, when full control of the thoracic injury can be effected by surgical manoeuvre or by the establishment of positive pressure respiration.[5]

Along with rib injuries, a more specific type of injury involving the chest wall occurs when abnormal forces have been applied to the costochondral junction. This is an injury experienced in the front row of rugby scrums when the prop forward is buckled or lifted—a manoeuvre commonly practised by opposing teams. The costochondral junctions of the anterior aspect of the lower rib cage are sprung and can be completely avulsed. This lesion is a particularly painful one and complete recovery may take several months. Similarly, the sternum in somersaulting gynmasts can be subjected to such extreme stresses that complete separation of the manubrium from the body occurs.[6]

Deep injuries

Lungs

These, as the result of a direct blow, may suffer a contusion—showing on a chest X-ray as an area of consolidation. Usually it results in haemoptysis, and although this usually clears quickly it needs a period of clinical observation. Other cases of haemoptysis are found in those sports demanding forceful pulmonary exertion. This is thought to result from vascular engorgement leading to the rupture of small subendothelial blood vessels. All cases of haemoptysis require a full pulmonary investigation including chest X-rays, sputum cultures, and perhaps bronchoscopy to eliminate a more serious underlying cause.

Pleura

Injuries here are potentially serious, the commonest being a pneumothorax.[7] This results from a puncture of the lung by a fractured rib. It also may result spontaneously during exertion due to the rupture of a lung at a site of unsuspected pathology. Often this is due to an emphysematous bulla, but a fatal case of rupture of a tuberculous focus in a scuba diver has been documented.[8] The pneumothorax may result in an insidious presentation or it can become apparent as a dramatic episode of extreme and severe shortness of breath. All cases of thoracic trauma should have their chests examined carefully. By percussion and auscultation the presence of a pneumothorax should be detected, and can be confirmed by radiology. In cases where there is no respiratory difficulty, treatment can be delayed until the patient is admitted to hospital. When tension develops, the increase of an expanding pneumothorax is occurring with every breath. This must be treated immediately by the insertion of a chest drain. This usually is of the underwater type, but more recently the availability of a flutter valve type with an intercostal trocar set (Fig. 23.1) has made the emergency treatment of such conditions much easier. In extreme cases, an ordinary syringe needle size 18 can be inserted anteriorly through the second intercostal space

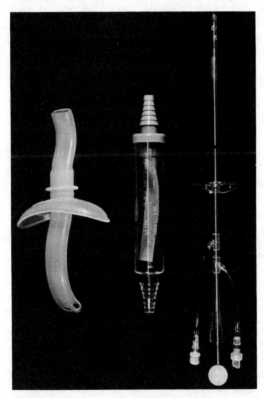

Fig. 23.1 Resusitube (Johnson and Johnson); intercostal trocar and cannula (Argyle 12 Fr.); one way flutter valve drain (Heimlich)—useful instruments in emergency chest trauma.

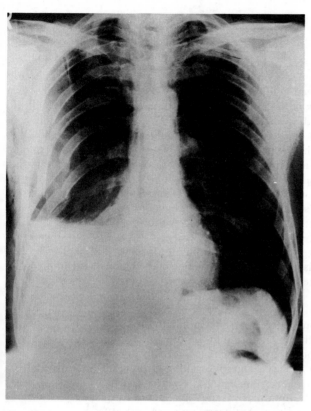

Fig. 23.2 Chest injury; right-sided fractured ribs, pneumothorax, and haemopneumothorax.

to relieve the pressure. A bilateral pneumothorax may also occur. This is an extremely serious condition and needs immediate bilateral chest drainage on the above lines. In association with a pneumothorax, a haemopneumothorax (Fig. 23.2) may occur as a result of lung damage or laceration to an intercostal vessel. On such occasions the volume of blood lost may be quite appreciable. The athlete will show many of the signs of shock; sweating, pallor, and tachycardia are then added to the signs of the pneumothorax. Such a condition requires chest drainage; for the haemothorax by the insertion of a lower chest intercostal drain laterally in the 8th space, and for the pneumothorax by an upper chest drain. In cases where extravasation of air has occurred from a lung laceration, surgical emphysema will be noted. This may be localized to a small area or be of wide distribution. No active treatment for this is required.

Airway obstruction
This is a serious respiratory problem.[9] It can occur as a result of a direct blow to the larynx. This then results in laryngeal haemorrhage and oedema with increasing respiratory distress. The blow may be severe enough to fracture the laryngeal cartilage. If the respiratory obstruction is complete, it is necessary to

carry out an emergency tracheotomy. Under other circumstances the obstruction may be further down the bronchial tree. This includes the all-too-common habit of chewing gum while participating in active sport. This foolishness is particularly common in football players, although it was ironic that in a recent fatal case, asphyxia was due to the impaction of chewing gum in the trachea of the referee.[10] Airway obstruction is seen commonly in unconscious patients, when asphyxia is due to the falling back of the tongue if the sportsman is left lying on his back. This in lay terms is called 'swallowing of the tongue'. The situation is easily controlled by turning the sportsman on his side then pulling the tongue or the angle of the jaw forward. Such a manoeuvre is well known in anaesthetics. The most common cause of airway obstruction is water. Drowning is usually due to ignorance or foolishness, but even the most experienced can be trapped. Expert treatment of these cases is of great importance. Clearance of the airway is essential. Mouth-to-mouth resuscitation is then the most valuable method of providing oxygen to the anoxic victim. A double-ended Resusitube (Fig. 23.1) is a valuable piece of first aid equipment to assist in this. In cases of cardiac arrest, external cardiac massage must be commenced immediately. If successful, further resuscitation by respiratory assistance with the correction of electrolytes and other vascular osmotic abnormalities can be important for satisfactory long-term survival.

Cardiac Injury

Heart or great vessel injury can result from trauma to the chest. Such a condition, if due to a direct penetrating lesion, may be obvious while others result from contusion.[11] This may be asymptomatic and not easily diagnosed. The development of precordial pain is very suggestive. This can be confirmed by an ECG recording. In cases of cardiac damage, ST segment depression with T wave eversion is diagnostic. Arrhythmias are not uncommon, but usually transient. Treatment is complete bed rest. Anticoagulants are best avoided.

Abdominal injuries

The position of the abdomen with its contained viscera makes it vulnerable to a direct blow during most sporting activities.

Abdominal wall

Many of the injuries here are superficial and may lead to conditions such as contusion of the abdominal wall. Generally this is of no consequence and can be controlled by the application of ice-packs. If the contusion is larger, it may be associated with muscular damage[12]—rupture of the rectus abdominis being the most common type. This results in severe pain and disability, and associated with this condition, there may also be a tear of the inferior epigastric artery. Then quite profuse bleeding can occur in the lower abdominal wall, shock results and a large tender mass can be palpated. Usually such injuries can be treated conservatively though bleeding, if severe, (and if the diagnosis is in doubt) makes a surgical exploration advisable. At times, muscular injuries may result from indirect trauma, e.g. avulsion of the anterior superior iliac spine as experienced in adolescents.[13] If the separation is complete, it may need surgical reduction

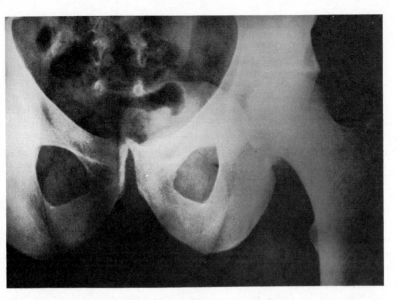

Fig. 23.3 Sclerosis and abnormal calcification at the symphysis in rectus abdominus traction injury.

Traction injuries of the rectus abdominis can cause a painful lesion localized at the os pubis where persistent pain and tenderness result in considerable functional disability. An X-ray examination will often show bony sclerosis (Fig. 23.3). This condition can respond to a local injection of cortisone.

Visceral injuries

More serious abdominal injuries result from trauma to underlying viscera.[14] Even the most minor knock may at times cause enough damage to lead to a serious abdominal emergency and perhaps death. It is important for any attending physician to be able to diagnose the clinical findings of such an abdominal injury. He should be always on guard for the development of a serious complication. The commonest injury from an abdominal blow is acute winding. This results in neurogenic shock due to stimulation of the solar plexus. The athlete doubles up with severe pain, finding difficulty in breathing. The abdominal wall then becomes rigid and the diaphragm undergoes spasm as well. He feels faint and is pale and clammy. Immediate treatment is to loosen any restrictive clothing. The manœuvre of pumping the athlete's legs into his abdomen is popular: it may lead to relaxation of the abdominal muscles and assist in circulatory return, but usually he recovers quickly without any residual symptoms. In the situation where symptoms or signs persist, serious injury must be kept in mind and the athlete kept under observation until a diagnosis is made. Also, and of more significance, the athlete may appear to recover but presents later with increasing abdominal pain or even collapse. This may be due to a delayed haemorrhage or even intestinal damage. Any case receiving an abdominal injury must be kept under observation and re-examined at frequent intervals[15] to detect any change in the patient's condition. The greater the delay in diagnosis of visceral injury the higher the eventual mortality becomes.[16]

The commonly injured organs are the following:

Spleen

The spleen is a soft haemopoietic organ situated posteriorly under the left diaphragm. It is very susceptible to direct trauma,[17] and is often associated with fractures of the 9th and 10th ribs which lie behind it. Trauma results in a rupture of the splenic capsule with haemorrhage. Such rupture may occur with the most minor injury or even spontaneously, e.g. when the athlete has been suffering from an unsuspected infectious mononucleosis. All the signs and symptoms are those of a haemoperitoneum. Initially, the athlete feels abdominal pain in his left upper quadrant. Of more significance, is pain felt behind the left shoulder tip, from referred diaphragmatic irritation. The haemorrhage, if increasing, then results in spreading generalized abdominal pain and increasing abdominal rigidity. Signs of bleeding are present, becoming more obvious with increasing blood loss. Initially, the athlete will develop pallor and tachycardia. Any drop in blood pressure may be a late phenomenon. Most athletes' cardiovascular systems are highly efficiently trained units, hence circulatory collapse, as shown by hypotension, may be a late manifestation. When there is significant shock, urgent resusctitation is necessary. This is then followed by immediate surgical splenectomy. Occasionally the injury is not sufficient to cause a complete disruption of the splenic capsule and a splenic haematoma may develop. This can be a dangerous situation leading to delayed abdominal haemorrhage.[18] Because this can occur at any time from one to two weeks after the injury, in all cases where damage to the spleen is suspected the athlete should be kept under hospital observation until this danger period is past. The diagnosis can be assisted by an abdominal X-ray film when a large splenic shadow can be demonstrated, or, when available, selective angiography[19] gives an even more rapid and accurate diagnosis.

Liver

Direct trauma to the upper aspect of the right side of the abdomen can, in sporting injuries, lead to hepatic damage. In most cases the injury is minor—a haematoma or small laceration—but damage to the liver may be more serious, the symptoms being similar to those from ruptured spleen except that the initial pain and tenderness is referred to the right side of the abdomen and the right shoulder tip. Subsequently the extent of the peritoneal haemorrhage again determines the general state of the injured person. In cases of sever haemorrhage, urgent resuscitation followed by surgical exploration[20] is needed. With minor injury a conservative policy can be followed, though when the site and extent of the injury is in doubt, a laparotomy should be performed. For minor lacerations suturing is all that is required. In more serious cases where a portion of the liver is devitalized, resection of part of the liver may be the treatment of choice.

Intestines

All organs of the peritoneal cavity have at some stage or other been involved in a sporting injury. In cases of pure gut injury the presentation is important as it tends to be delayed. Early peritoneal contamination with intestinal contents is prevented by mucosal pouting[21] through the intestinal wall tear. Significant abdominal pain, guarding and rigidity may therefore take some 8–12 hours before becoming severe enough for a firm diagnosis to be made. On clinical examination it is helpful to note that there are absent bowel sounds. An erect abdominal X-ray can be diagnostic if it shows free gas under the diaphragm (Fig. 23.4). In cases of doubt, peritoneal taps[22] have been advocated. Once a diagnosis is apparent, resuscitation and urgent laparotomy is required to confirm the organ injury and carry out any necessary repair. The site most commonly damaged is the region of the duodenum. This is probably because it is a closed loop between pylorus and duodenojejunal flexure. Then on compression an explosive force causes the injury.

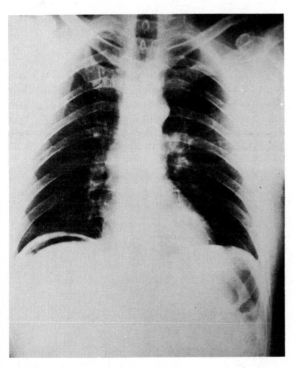

Fig. 23.4 Pneumoperitoneum; gas under the right diaphragm from a ruptured viscus.

In other cases the presentation of abdominal symptoms may be even more delayed. Then there may be only a vague abdominal pain followed by a gradual deterioration in the athlete's condition, taking several days to demonstrate an abdominal emergency. This also frequently occurs with a lesion involving the duodenum, but in this instance, to the retroperitoneal surface. There is no intraperitoneal contamination, and therefore minimal initial clinical signs. This is a particularly lethal condition[23] because of the enforced lateness of the diagnosis. In all cases where this condition is suspected, laparotomy is essential with careful inspection of the posterior surface of the duodenum.[24]

Pancreas

On rare occasions, pancreatic injury has occurred. This may be extensive with laceration and even transection. Here the end diagnosis is obvious and an early laparotomy confirms the damage. On other occasions the symptomatology may be less obvious. Again, it presents with vague abdominal pains, progressing to secondary complications. Usually this is by the presentation of a pseudocyst indicating the initial pancreatic damage. Such a condition then requires a specialized surgical drainage procedure. Usually the pseudocyst occupies the lesser sac and a cystogastrostomy is all that is necessary. Occasionally, the lesion is a true intrapancreatic cyst,[25] when a cystoenterostomy by Roux-en-Y jejunal loop is required for the drainage procedure. Initially, if pancreatic damage is suspected, a raised serum amylase is diagnostic. In cases where a pseudocyst has developed, barium meal and pancreatic scan are useful in confirming the diagnosis.

Inguinal hernia

The development of a hernia is a common condition. The indirect type is a result of a congenital weakness in the region of the internal abdominal ring and can present at any age. It consists of a sac of peritoneum protruding through the internal abdominal ring into which intestinal contents protrude. In this situation the neck is always narrow and therefore is a potential site for intestinal gut strangulation. The presence of a hernia in a sportsman, especially those competing in strenuous events, is a potentially dangerous situation. Strangulation and serious complications can occur at any time, for instance in scuba diving.[8] Here an increase in intra-abdominal pressure from underwater pressure changes results in an especially dangerous situation. Any such hernia should be repaired surgically before the athlete is allowed to compete. Sometimes, peculiarly enough, athletes are not aware that they have a hernia. This diagnosis should be made during the routine medical examination, a procedure which is recommended for all athletes at least once a year. Surgery then is recommended and the sportsman, once having had it carried out, is allowed to return to his sporting activities as soon as the repair has consolidated. This usually takes about six weeks.

Renal injury

Both kidneys are situated high in a retroperitoneal position on the posterior abdominal wall. They are both prone to damage from direct blows sustained in the loins. These injuries are variable[26]—they may be minor with bruising only, or they may result in actual rupture of the kidney substance (Fig. 23.5). The presenting sign of such trauma is pain occurring over the region of the kidney, followed by haematuria. Any such case requires observation and urological investigation. Usually, cases of kidney damage can be treated conservatively with confidence.[27] Most settle quickly, although on occasions, significant complications can develop. In extreme cases such severe haemorrhage may occur as to require an emergency nephrectomy. In the investigation of cases of traumatic haematuria, a significant number of congenital abnormalities of the renal tract[28] are discovered. Such a condition, usually hydronephrosis, requires less trauma to result in renal damage than a normal kidney. The incidence of microscopic haematuria in sports participants is remarkably high. In some sports, such as the contact sports, repeated episodes of microtrauma may be the obvious reason.

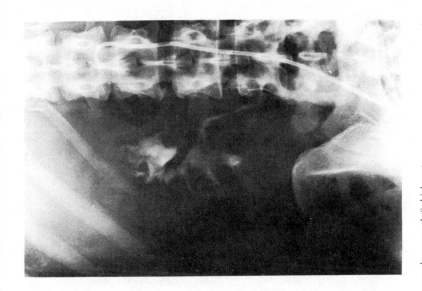

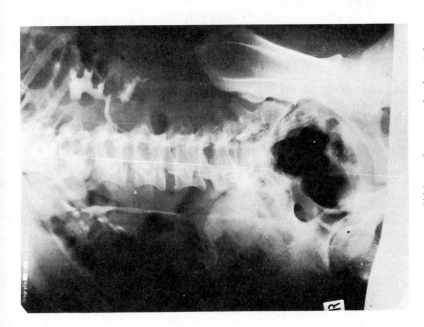

Fig. 23.5 Rupture of kidney; demonstration by (a) intravenous pyelogram (left kidney), (b) selective aortography (right kidney).

Such sportsmen presenting with recurrent haematuria[29] may develop a progressive structural abnormality usually involving the right upper major calyx (athlete's kidney).[30] These cases need close follow-up and if deterioration occurs, the athlete should be advised to give up the particular sport involved, e.g. boxing. Even in the non-contact sports the incidence of haematuria is common.[31] The cause of this is not obvious, but it may be due to a retrograde extravasation of red blood cells from an increase in renal vein pressure resulting from the renal vein kinking at its junction with the inferior vena cava during physical activity.[32] It is important to remember that in all cases of haematuria, a complete urological investigation should be carried out. Until a renal tumour has been excluded as a cause of the condition, a benign sporting cause cannot be accepted.

The effect of athletic exertion on kidney function in general may result in abnormalities other than haematuria. Proteinuria, myoglobinuria, and haemoglobinuria have all been noted. Proteinuria[33] immediately after exertion occurs frequently. It appears to be related to the intensity and duration of physical exertion and there is a decrease with the training effect. Haemoglobinuria[34] has been attributed to the development of intravascular haemolysis. Mechanical trauma to red blood cells flowing in the blood vessels through the soles of a runner's feet and through the hands of karate exponents[35] has been described as a cause of this condition—initially known as 'march haematuria'. Severe muscular exertion has been described as a cause of myoglobinuria,[36] especially when it is involved with the use of untrained muscle groups. Occasionally this condition has been severe enough to cause acute tubular necrosis.[37] In all situations where renal problems are liable to occur, a high fluid intake is recommended to promote a good urine output.

Perineal injuries

Skin
A very common condition which causes a lot of discomfort in sports is pruritis ani. This basically is a consequence of poor hygiene associated with excessive sweating. It leads to a perianal, reddened, eczematous-like lesion with intense itching. The treatment for this is to keep the perineal skin as dry as possible together with scrupulous attention to hygiene. The skin lesion itself can be brought under control quickly with corticosteroid creams. To this may be added clioquinol if bacterial or fungal infection is present. A condition experienced in cyclists in this region is known as 'saddle sore'. It is an acute lesion resulting from excessive friction between saddle and skin and is basically a paniculitis progressing to a localized area of fat necrosis. The immediate treatment is puncture of the lesion with a sterile needle to release a certain amount of oedema fluid. Afterwards the condition will settle quickly. If allowed to become chronic, it will cause a great deal of discomfort due to subsequent necrosis, ulceration, and chronic infection.

Anal canal
Injuries here are not common. Occasionally, lacerations and even penetrating rectal injuries have been experienced.[38] These need to be treated seriously and

require full investigation in the way of proctoscopy and sigmoidoscopy followed by specialized surgical treatment. Excessive straining may lead to an attack of 'piles' due to prolapse followed by strangulation of an internal haemorrhoid. If such a condition is treated quickly by returning the haemorrhoid through the anal canal, any further deterioration is prevented. Usually the condition has been present for too long and it can be treated only by the application of astringent lotions together with ice. Gradually the strangulated haemorrhoid will resolve. On occasions, thrombosis of an external haemorrhoid occurs, resulting in a painful perianal lump. Incision under local anaesthetic releases the tense clot and gives immediate relief.

Most of the conditions experienced in this region are due to exacerbations of existing anal pathology. It is recommended that, when athletes have their regular annual check, such conditions should be diagnosed and then corrected, so preventing further trouble. Pilonidal sinus, chronic fissures, haemorrhoids, and fistula-in-ano are all common problems which, if neglected, can lead to a considerable decrease at crucial times in an athlete's performance.

Urethra

Injuries here are experienced in cycling and gymnastics due to injury of the bulbous urethra from a direct astride blow to the perineum. As a result, a partial or complete rupture of the urethra occurs. This presents as a painful swelling in the area of trauma. Signs of internal damage become evident with the appearance of some urethral bleeding or the passage of blood-stained urine. These injuries are serious and need immediate investigation with athlete being instructed not to try to pass his urine until the nature of his injury has been decided. Full urological investigations by urethral instrumentation and urethrography are needed. In cases where the urethra is just bruised, normal micturition can be established. In cases, where more serious disruptive damage has occurred, supra-pubic cystotomy and even suturing of the ruptured urethra may be indicated.

Male genital organs

Penis

Injuries here are not common. Priapism[39] (persistent painful erection) occurs in racing cyclists. This is due to pressure on the pudendal nerve from a badly fitting saddle pushing up against the perineum. The treatment consists of sedation in the first instance then replacement of the saddle by one of a more comfortable shape.

Testicle

Here damage is sustained often from a direct blow resulting in a haematoma or even laceration. It is associated with the development of a large painful swelling, usually a haematocoele. If this condition is minor, it can be treated with ice-packs and rest, when gradual resolution will occur. If the condition is more severe, immediate surgical exploration is recommended.[40] Then if testicular lacerations are debrided and sutured, with haematomas evacuated, testicular viability can be preserved. Owing to the exposed position of these organs, injuries can be avoided when, in specific sports, suitable genital guards or boxes are worn. This is important in sports such as cricket and hockey.

When severe pain occurs in a testicle of an adolescent after a sporting activity, torsion of the testis, described as early as 1893 by Gifford-Nash in a boy after a boxing match, should be kept in mind.[41] Often, on early examination, all that can be detected is a slight irregularity of the cord above the testis. This is deceptive as reactionary swelling will develop later. It is of extreme importance to make this diagnosis as soon as possible as irreversible testicular infarction can occur within a few hours. It is possible to relieve the condition by manual rotation of the testis.[42] The direction in which the testis needs to be twisted is that which will relieve the athlete of his pain. Otherwise, immediate surgical exploration is required.

Female genital organs

Injuries here are usually vulval haematomas and lacerations resulting from direct trauma. These are commonly experienced in vaulters and in other sports involving jumping. Ice-packs are useful in preventing excessive haemorrhage. Water-skiers, in particular, are prone to gynaecological injuries. Forceful retrograde vaginal douching occurs, mainly in inexperienced skiers due to their having difficulty in standing up after starting their run.[43] This is especially noticeable in multiparas. Vaginal lacerations of sufficient severity to cause serious haemorrhage requiring surgical control have been described.[44] Similarly, early abortions, salpingitis, infertility, peritonitis, and the development of pelvic abscesses can be a result. The wearing of suitable rubber pants is a simple way to prevent this

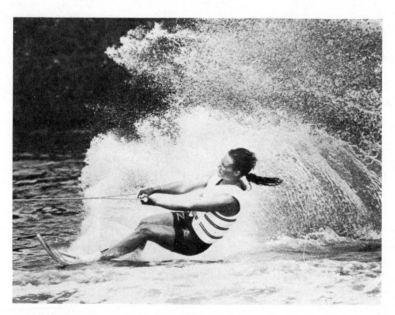

Fig. 23.6 Protective rubber clothing—as recommended in water skiing. (Photo: courtesy *New Zealand Herald.*)

type of injury (Fig. 23.6). This illustrates again the principle of the importance of wearing protective clothing thereby avoiding unnecessary sporting injuries.

G.D.C.

References

1. Poeur, D. H. and Wolliver, E. (1942) Intestinal and mesenteric injury due to non-penetrating abdominal trauma. *J. Am. med. Ass.*, **118**, 11.
2. Buck, J. E. (1973) Bilateral rupture of pectoralis major. Proceedings XVIII World Congress of Sports Medicine. *Br. J. sports Med.*, **7**, 70.
3. Bailey, H. and Love, McN. (1959) Fat necrosis of the breast. *A Short Practice of Surgery.* 11th Edn. London: H. K. Lewis.
4. Devas, M. B. (1969) Stress fracture of the rib. *Proc. R. Soc. Med.*, **62**, 936.
5. Lloyd, J. W. and Rucklidge, M.A. (1969) Management of closed chest injuries. *Br. J. Surg.*, **56**, 721.
6. Bozdech, Z. (1971) Gymnastics—fracture of the sternum. In *Encyclopaedia of Sports Sciences and Medicine*, ed. Larson, L. A., London: Collier–Macmillan.
7. Hinrichson, K. W. (1963) Fractured ribs and tension pneumothorax, injuries in football. *Med. J. Aust.*, **1**, 608.
8. Bickmore, G. H. (1971) Subaqua diving. *Practitioner*, **206**, 651.
9. Howaat, D. D. C. (1970) Upper respiratory tract obstructions. *Annals R. Coll Surg.*, **47**, 162.
10. Moncur, J. (1973) Inhalation of chewing gum: fatality during rugby. Proceedings XVIII World Congress of Sports Medicine. *Br. J. sports Med.*, **7**, 162.
11. Rose, K. D., Stone, F. and Fuenning, S. I. (1966) Cardiac contusion resulting from 'spearing' in football. *Archs Intern. Med.*, **118**, 129.
12. Fraser-Moodie, A. and Cox, S. (1974) Haematoma of rectus abdominis from the use of an exercise wheel. *Br. J. Surg.*, **61**, 577.
13. Godshall, R. W. and Hansen, C. A. (1973) Incomplete avulsion of a portion of the iliac epiphysis. *J. Bone Jt Surg.*, **55A**, 1301.
14. Bolton, P. M., Wood, C. B., Quarley-Papafio, J. B. and Blumgart, L. H. (1973) Blunt abdominal injury: a review of 59 consecutive cases undergoing surgery. *Br. J. Surg.*, **60**, 657.
15. Petty, A. H. (1973) Abdominal injuries. *Annals R. Coll. Surg.*, **53**, 169.
16. Evans, I. P. (1973) Traumatic rupture of ileum. *Br. J. Surg.*, **60**, 121.
17. Zakopoulos, K. S. (1973) Rupture of the spleen—a football injury. *Br. J. sports Med.*, **7**, 165.
18. Khanna, H. G., Hayes, B. R. and McKeown, K. C. (1967) Delayed rupture of the spleen. *Ann. Surg.*, **165**, 478
19. Redman, H. C., Reuter, S. R. and Brookstein, J. J. (1969) Delayed rupture of spleen diagnosed by splenic arteriography. *Ann. Surg.*, **169**, 57.
20. Hanna, W. D., Bell, D. H. and Cochran, W. (1965) Liver injuries in Northern Ireland. *Br. J. Surg.*, **52**, 99.
21. Jordan, J. S. and McAfee, D. K. (1963) Traumatic rupture of intestines. *Am. J. Surg.*, **29**, 630.
22. Perry, J. F., Demeules, J. E. and Root, H. D. (1970) Diagnostic peritoneal tap in blunt abdominal trauma. *Surg. Gynaec. Obstet.*, **131**, 742.
23. Moncur, J. (1973) Fatal football injury—ruptured duodenal diverticulum. Proceedings XVIII World Congress of Sports Medicine. *Br. J. sports Med.*, **7**, 162.
24. Cohn, J. (1952) Duodenal injuries. *Am. J. Surg.*, **84**, 293.
25. Campbell, G. D. and Campero, A. A. (1974) Intrapancreatic pseudocyst—rugby injury. *N.Z. med. J.*, **79**, 1068.

26. Kleiman, A. H. (1971) in *Encyclopedia of Sport Sciences and Medicine*, Ed. Larson, L. A., London: Collier Macmillan.
27. Slade, N. (1971) Management of closed renal injuries. *Br. J. Urol.*, **43**, 639.
28. Priestly, J. T. and Pilcher, F. (1938) Traumatic lesions of the kidney. *Am. J. Surg.*, **40**, 347.
29. Boone, A. W., Haltiwanger, E. and Chambers, R. L. (1955) Football haematuria. *J. Am. med. Ass.*, **158**, 1516.
30. Kleiman, A. H. (1960) Athlete's kidney. *J. Urol.*, **80**, 321.
31. Alyea, E. F. and Parish, H. H. (1958) Renal response to exercise. *J. Am. med. Ass.*, **167**, 807.
32. Bruce, P. T. (1972) Stress haematuria. *Br. J. Urol.*, **44**, 724.
33. Taylor, A. (1960) Characteristics of exercise proteinuria. *Chem. Science*, **19**, 209.
34. Spiler, A. J. (1970) March haemoglobineuria. *Br. med. J.*, **i**, 155.
35. Streeton, J. A. (1967) Haemoglobinuria in karate. *Lancet*, **ii**, 191.
36. Howenstine, J. A. (1960) Exercise induced myoglobinuria and haemoglobinuria. *J. Am. med. Ass.*, **173**, 493.
37. Hamilton, R. W., Gardner, L. P. and Penn, A. S. (1972) Acute tubular necrosis caused by exercise. *Ann. Intern. Med.*, **77**, 77.
38. Blankenship, J. R. (1971) Board surfing—unusual injuries. In *Encyclopaedia of Sports Sciences and Medicine*, ed., Larson, L. A., London: Collier-Macmillan.
39. Delle Sadie, P. F. (1956) Priapism of traumatic origin in bicycle racers. *Minerva Med. J.*, **47**, **1334.**
40. Preston, P. R. (1970) Traumatic rupture of testis. *Br. J. Surg.*, **57**, 71.
41. Gifford-Nash, J. (1893) Testicular pain in a boy after a boxing match. *Br. med. J.*, **i**, 742.
42. Sparks, J. P. (1971) Torsion of testis. *Annals R. Coll. Surg.*, **49**, 77.
43. Tweedale, P. G. (1973) Vaginal laceration in water skiers. *Canad. med Ass. J.*, **108**, 20.
44. Morton, B. C. (1970) Gynaecological complications of water skiing. *Med. J. Aust.*, **II**, 1256.

24

Injuries of the upper limbs

Although injuries to the upper limb form less than 20 per cent of all those received on the field of sport,[1,2] they are important for two main reasons:

(1) They tend to interrupt completely the patient's sporting activities.
(2) They are more likely to result in time off work.

Clavicle

Injuries to the clavicle include fractures, subluxation at the acromioclavicular or sternoclavicular joints, and rarely rupture of the conoid or trapezoid ligaments.

Fractures of the clavicle

The clavicle generally fractures across the middle third (Fig. 24.1), which results in a downward, forward and inward displacement of the outer fragment. Diagnosis is easily established by clinical examination, and is confirmed by X-ray.

Treatment is by the application of a 'figure of eight' bandage or padded rings which brace the shoulders back, and these are worn for three to four weeks. When symptoms are not severe, as in greenstick fractures, a simple webbing sling may be all that is required. Active shoulder movements are encouraged from the outset. Although these methods produce an excellent functional result there will frequently remain an ugly lump of callus at the fracture site.

When a good cosmetic result is important, for example in an adolescent girl who will want to be able to wear 'off the shoulder' dresses, the fracture may be treated either by formal reduction and the application of a moulded plaster of Paris 'cuirasse', or by keeping the patient in bed for three weeks lying supine with a high pillow between the shoulder blades. The cosmetic results of open operation in this area are poor as the scar tends to form keloid, but trimming of the callus or bone end may be necessary to prevent secondary ulceration through the skin.

Fractures of the outer third seldom result in much displacement (Fig. 24.2). All that is necessary is to provide a suitable sling to support the shoulder until it is pain free. Active movements are encouraged.

Complications
Clavicular fractures nearly always heal rapidly and non-union is rare. Occasionally anaesthesia follows damage to a supraclavicular nerve—it is seldom of any significance.

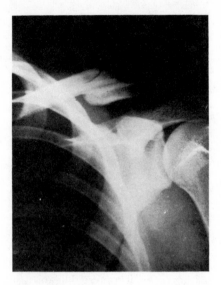

Fig. 24.1 Fractured clavicle in the middle third showing 'greenstick' refractive due to too early return to sport judo .

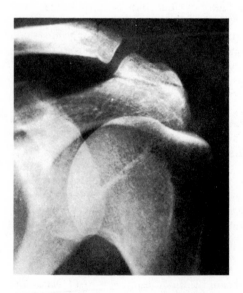

Fig. 24.2 Fractured clavicle in outer third (and also fractured acromion) from a shoulder charge in football.

Dislocations and subluxations

Dislocation or subluxation at the acromioclavicular joint is quite common.[3] The patient complains of pain well localized to the joint, with loss of function in the arm as a result. On examination the joint is tender, and when dislocation is complete there is a palpable and visible step (Fig. 24.3).

Treatment

Although the long-term functional results are uniformly good, the ugly step will persist unless treated vigorously and early. Treatment consists of elevating the shoulder while the acromion is pressed down. This may be achieved by the application of a webbing harness which is kept in place for at least six weeks. If a good cosmetic result is especially desirable a moulded plaster of Paris spica is substituted for the webbing harness.

The results of operative treatment are on the whole encouraging, a suitable technique being screwing the outer end of the clavicle to the coracoid. Recently Bearden, Hughston and Whatley have advocated coracoclavicular fixation by wire loop.[4]

In cases of subluxation, and for old dislocations, treatment is by vigorous mobilization. If pain persists, local injection of hydrocortisone may prove beneficial.

Sternoclavicular dislocation is rare,[5, 6] and the long-term cosmetic results very poor. Treatment should therefore be directed to relieving immediate discomfort (sling) and promoting functional recovery (exercises). Intra-articular hydrocortisone injections are usually successful for relief of pain.

Clavicular injuries are usually due to a fall or blow on the point of the shoulder, and are most common in Association and Rugby footballers and jockeys. They may also occur in gymnasts, cyclists, and wrestlers.

Prevention is virtually impossible other than in the avoidance of foolhardiness.

Shoulder joint

Apart from fractures of the upper humerus and scapula, and dislocation or subluxation, the shoulder joint[7] and its intimate structures are the site of a wide variety of painful conditions, all closely related, which may be included in the term 'painful shoulder syndrome'.

Fractures of the shoulder joint

Fractures involving the shoulder joint are relatively uncommon in sport. They include fractures of the surgical neck and greater tuberosity of the humerus, and of the scapula. Such injuries will invariably require treatment in accordance with generally accepted orthopaedic practice. Early and energetic mobilization is the only specific necessity in athletes.

In children, damage of the upper humeral epiphysis may occur, usually as a result of throwing. In the U.S.A. it is known as 'little league shoulder'.[8, 9] Treatment is according to accepted orthopaedic practice.

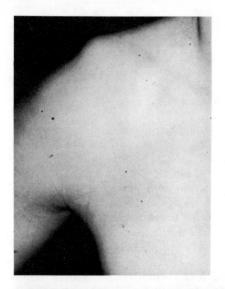

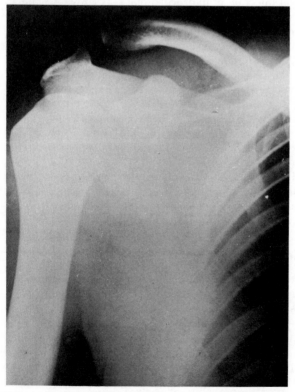

Fig. 24.3 Typical 'step' deformity of acromioclavicular subluxation. (a) Clinical appearance. (b) Radiological appearance.

Dislocations of the shoulder joint

Dislocations of the shoulder joint occur frequently in the body-contact sports, and are also seen in high jumpers, pole vaulters, water polo players and riders.[10] They occur typically when an extension force is applied to the abducted externally rotated arm. Diagnosis is established clinically, there being an obvious hollow under the deltoid where the humeral head normally lies. If possible diagnosis should be confirmed by X-ray, but this is not really necessary, and if there is likely to be much delay before X-rays can be taken it is better to get straight on with reduction, since the muscle spasm that develops so often after dislocation can, when established, make reduction technically difficult.

Prior to reduction, fracture should if possible be excluded, and the integrity of the circumflex nerve established by testing out the fifth cervical dermatome with a pin or other sharply pointed object.

Various techniques are available of which the Kocher or one of its variations is the most popular. It is carried out as follows: gentle downward traction is applied to the elbow while the upper arm is abducted about 15° and eased into full external rotation. The elbow is then carried forward and medially across the chest and when adduction is complete the arm is internally rotated. Reduction usually takes place as adduction is completed (Fig. 24.4).

This method is almost always successful in cases of recent dislocation if carried out slowly and gently. Any jerking or roughness will provoke spasm in the shoulder muscles and make reduction possible.

Alternatively the Stimson method may be used. This is a simple and *gentle* method. The patient lies face down on a plinth or table with the affected arm hanging over the edge towards the floor. A moderate weight (5–10 lb (2·25–4·5 kg); for example two bricks) is fixed to the wrist (*not* held by the patient), and under this gentle pull the dislocation usually reduces within about twenty minutes.

Reduction of the dislocated shoulder requires no anaesthetic as a rule, but in the more apprehensive patient, or when previous attempts have been unsuccessful for any reason, a light anaesthetic is necessary. Of particular value is the 'two and one' technique. The patient (whose co-operation must be secured!) breathes pure oxygen for two minutes, followed by pure nitrous oxide for a further minute. At the end of this time he is sufficiently anaesthetized to permit satisfactory reduction of the dislocation, or indeed any procedure in which painful stimuli are applied for only a limited period of time. The chief merits of this anaesthetic technique lie in its simplicity, the smoothness of induction and the absence of vomiting, coughing, etc. since the gases are non-irritant and cerebral anoxia does not occur. Recovery is rapid and not unpleasant, as it may be after pentothal.

Following satisfactory reduction (confirmed as soon as possible by X-ray) the shoulder should be immobilized for at least three weeks, prior to starting rehabilitation exercises. If mobilization is started too soon the risk of recurrence is high. Subsequently, no limitation need be placed on the patient's activities.

Complicated cases, where the mechanism or nature of the dislocation are unclear or there is associated bony/nerve damage or simple reduction fails, must always be referred for expert orthopaedic management.

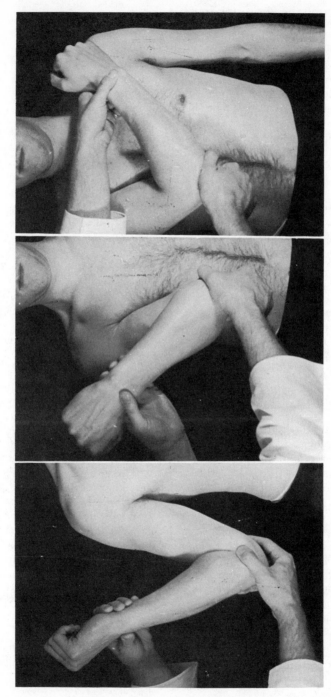

Fig. 24.4 The three stages in carrying out Kocher's manœuvre for reduction of a dislocated shoulder. For description see text.

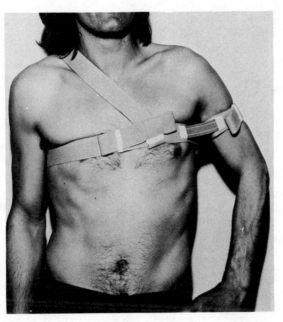

Fig. 24.5 Harness to prevent abduction of the shoulder and redislocation.

Recurrent dislocation

Recurrent dislocation of the shoulder is a particular bugbear to the sportsman, and is the result of too energetic early mobilization following an initial acute dislocation. Once a recurrent pattern of dislocation is established, surgical treatment is required if the patient is to return to full normal sporting activity, although an alternative, for example for the jockey or motor-cycle rider, is the wearing of a suitable harness and check rein which allow flexion and extension

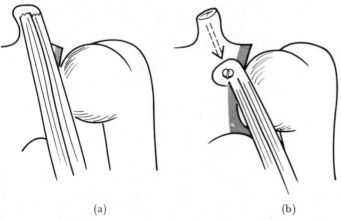

(a)   (b)

Fig. 24.6 Transposition of tip of coracoid; diagrammatic representation. (a) Pre-operative. (b) Post-operative.

of the elbow in adduction but make forced abduction difficult.[11] The cuff of the harness must be worn sufficiently loosely to allow it to slide if strong abduction forces are applied, otherwise there is a risk of fracturing the shaft of the humerus with the potential complication of nerve and blood vessel damage. If surgery is chosen, various well-proven techniques are available, including the Bankart[12] and Putti Platt techniques. Other variations include the transposition of the corocoid process to the anterior aspect of the glenoid, in order to strengthen the anterior capsule of the shoulder joint with the tendons of coracobrachialis and the short head of biceps (Fig. 24.6).[13]

Painful shoulder syndromes

This group of conditions includes various injuries and degenerative conditions, all of which are characterized by pain which is exacerbated by movement, and which may provoke a remarkable degree of functional disability.[14]

The shoulder joint is peculiar in that its stability is derived entirely from the surrounding soft tissues, capsule, ligaments, and muscles. It must serve as a firm yet highly mobile base for all the various activities of hand and arm. Any injury, therefore, which involves one of the supporting structures of the shoulder joint will invariably interfere with the mobility and efficiency of that joint.

Capsulitis

Capsulitis of the shoulder results from a sprain in which the degree of violence is not sufficient to provoke more than a transitory subluxation.

It may also follow excessive or unaccustomed use of the shoulder, particularly in implemental sports (when the handle of the implement is of an inappropriate size and the patient is therefore having to use an excess of muscular activity to control it), and in throwing sports.[15,16]

The joint is painful, particularly on movement, and in some instances limitation of movement is considerable (frozen shoulder). Symptoms are referable to

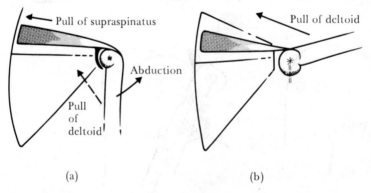

(a)   (b)

Fig. 24.7 Diagrammatic representation of the role of the supraspinatus in initiating abduction of the shoulder. In (a) the supraspinatus being inserted *above* the axis of the shoulder joint, can act as abductor; the line of pull of the deltoid in this position is below the axis and it therefore acts as adductor. In (b) the supraspinatus holds the humeral head in place against the pull of the deltoid which tends to displace it.

the whole of the joint area, and signs, particularly tenderness, are not well localized.

Supraspinatus syndromes

In these cases the lesion involves the supraspinatus 'unit' whose function is to initiate abduction at the shoulder through the first 10° to 15° of arc, and subsequently to stabilize the head of the humerus against the pull of the deltoid muscle which tends to displace it during full abduction (Fig. 24.7).

The supraspinatus tendon may be the site of partial or complete rupture, ectopic calcification, or peritendonitis.

Supraspinatus rupture
This presents with pain (a dull ache) at rest and inability smoothly to abduct the upper arm (supraspinatus 'hitch'), the patient producing abduction by elevating the shoulder joint which whips the arm laterally sufficiently to allow the deltoid to act as the abductor.

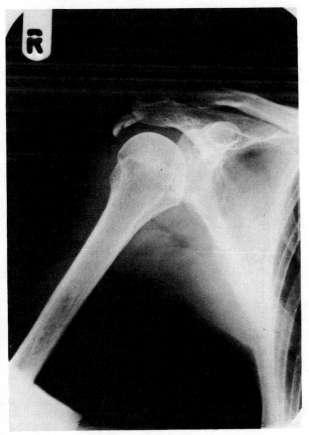

Fig. 24.8 X-ray photograph showing radio-opaque calcium deposits in supraspinatus tendon (rotator cuff).

Partial rupture is more common than complete, and usually takes the form of a tear of the common tendinous insertion or rotator cuff, rather than a tear localized to the tendon itself.

These injuries occur when a sudden abduction strain is applied to the upper arm while it is abducted. Such a strain is often applied in body-contact sports or in a fall, but may occur when the patient is asleep in bed, probably due to his rolling over on to the shoulder with the upper arm slightly abducted and the elbow fully flexed.

Ectopic calcification

Although more common in older age groups this condition is occasionally found in youth athletes. Pain is generally very severe, tenderness well localized, and any movement of the shoulder joint may be quite agonizing. Symptoms appear suddenly, but there is no history of injury. X-ray changes are typical (Fig. 24.8).

'Supraspinatus tendonitis'

This is a form of inflammation of the paratendinous tissues and is probably a form of subacromial or subdeltoid bursitis. Pain may be present at rest, but is typically felt on abduction of the arm, being confined to movements only within certain limits of arc. Its other name is the 'painful arc syndrome' (Fig. 24.9).

The limitation of pain to a certain part of the arc is explained by the fact that the acromion process overlies the affected area of tendon only during part of its excursion. The painful arc may also be demonstrable in cases of ectopic calcification where symptoms are less severe and movements are better tolerated.

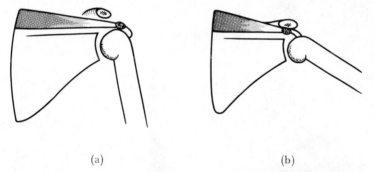

(a)   (b)

Fig. 24.9 Diagrammatic representation of the mechanism of the painful arc. In (a) the lesion is clear of the acromion and no pain is felt. In (b) the lesion is now rubbing the under surface of the acromion process and pain is felt.

Bicipital tendonitis.

Peritendonitis also occurs in the synovia of the bicipital groove. Pain is felt particularly on extension and abduction of the shoulder. Tenderness is well localized. It may occasionally be complicated by rupture of the tendon of long head of biceps, especially in the older patient. In some cases the tendon itself subluxes.[17]

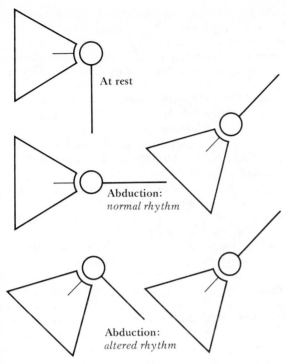

At rest

Abduction:
normal rhythm

Abduction:
altered rhythm

Fig. 24.10 Breakdown in scapulohumeral rhythm (by courtesy of *Medicine*).

Periarthritis

Contrary to popular belief, true osteoarthrosis of the shoulder is uncommon. When degenerative changes occur it is the soft tissues which are involved, and the term periarthritis is to be preferred.

In all cases there is a tendency for the shoulder to stiffen and extreme range of movement, particularly in abduction and internal rotation, is lost early. Apart from the subjective symptoms the main feature is breakdown in the scapulo-humeral rhythm, which is easily seen when the patient is viewed from behind, and which is present before limitation of movement can be demonstrated by goniometry (Fig. 24.10).

Treatment of painful shoulder syndromes

The majority of painful shoulder syndromes yield to a combination of topical injections of hydrocortisone with local anaesthetic, and mobilization. When a localized tender spot is found, e.g. the bicipital groove in bicipital tendinitis, 50 mg of hydrocortisone acetate in 2 per cent lignocaine (Xylocaine) is injected directly. Where no such spot is palpable, as in painful arc syndrome, the steroid is instilled into the subacromial bursa. Sometimes injection at more than one site is needed. Following injection immediate relief of pain may be felt together with an increase in pain-free active movement. After successful injection a programme of progressive mobilization is instituted.

In frozen shoulder stiffness is marked, being associated with subscapularis spasm. If no gain in range of movement follows injection, a formal mobilization under general anaesthetic may be required and this must be carried out firmly but gently.

Other forms of treatment available for stubborn cases include various modalities of heat, diathermy, ultrasound, and the exhibition of anti-inflammatory drugs such as phenylbutazone or indomethacin, which may be deployed as appropriate.

Ectopic calcification is usually so painful that attempts at mobilization are stubbornly resisted by the patient. In such cases dramatic relief may be obtained either by evacuation of the calcareous deposits by formal surgery, or by the injection of hydrocortisone, though whether in the latter case it is the drug itself or decompression of the tendon by the concomitant needling which is effective cannot be stated with certainty, since percutaneous 'aspiration' of the deposit with a large bone needle is sometimes equally effective.

In selected cases frozen shoulder responds dramatically to hypnosis (posthypnotic suggestion) but the specialized technique required and difficulty in selecting suitable patients limit its usefulness.

Of occasional value for resistant cases of supraspinatus syndrome and ectopic calcification is radiation therapy—a 200 kV machine is used with a hard filter and doses of 100 rad are administered daily for up to five days, although one or two doses only may be needed. Relief in many cases may be quite dramatic. This method of treatment may be regarded as perfectly safe, being productive of no post-irradiation phenomena.

Postural defects

Many cases of pain in the region of the shoulder (rather than in the joint itself) are due to postural defects, either spinal, or due to imbalanced action of the suspensory muscles of the shoulder girdle, for example cases of mild serratus palsy. Diagnosis is established if the patient is stripped to the waist and viewed from behind. Even mild degrees of asymmetry are obvious, and alteration in scapulo-humeral rhythm is detected by watching as the arms are abducted in unison. Serratus palsy is shown up by 'winging' of the scapula as the patient pushes himself away from a wall or undertakes 'press-ups'. Postural defects must be differentiated from unilateral muscular hypertrophy such as occurs in athletes and sportsmen with a 'one-arm' action, for example shot putters, tennis players and oarsmen who row on one side of the boat only.

Treatment

Treatment consists of correcting the defect if it is mobile (in spinal defects) (Fig. 24.11) and initiating a vigorous course of shoulder girdle elevation exercises, such as:

(1) Shoulder shrugging—against resistance.
(2) Progressive overhead weight-lifting and spring work.
(3) Press-ups.

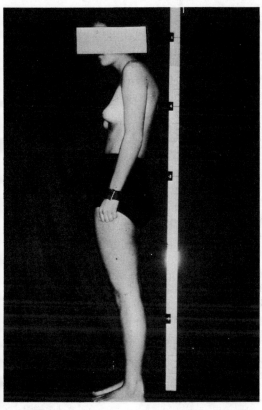

Fig. 24.11 Postural defect in a young sportswoman giving rise to shoulder girdle pain.

Fibrositis

Although this term does not meet with wholesale approval, the type of lesion to which it is applied is widely enough recognized to render its use acceptable. In these cases there is pain in one or more muscles of the shoulder girdle, typically the trapezius or rhomboids, with some degree of spasm. This pain is present at rest, as a dull ache, with acute exacerbations on exercise, and the patient frequently complains of 'stiffness' although the range of movement at the shoulder is not diminished. The affected muscle groups are tender to the touch—often the tenderness is well localized into 'myofascial tender spots'—and some degree of irregularity or 'nodule' formation is palpable.

Treatment
Treatment consists of heat and massage followed by exercise. Occasionally these cases tend to chronicity in which case local hydrocortisone injections may be given to any 'trigger spots' with effect. In recurrent cases search must be made for an underlying primary pathology such as a dorsal disc lesion or postural defect which will require appropriate treatment.

Nerve injuries

Injuries to the components of the brachial plexus and the nerves of the arm are happily uncommon, and generally take the form of a neuropraxia. However, when more severe damage occurs the resulting disability may be great. Early recognition of these injuries is demanded if their effects are to be in any way mitigated. Even quite severe degrees of nerve damage are amenable to rehabilitation. Jokl[18] cites the case of Harold Connolly who won the 1956 Olympic Gold Medal for throwing the hammer after having received an injury at birth resulting in an Erb-Duchenne/Klumpke combined upper and lower plexus lesion of the left arm. Circumflex palsy following shoulder dislocations has already been noted above.

Other Injury

Occasionally the major vessels may be damaged—haemorrhage is obvious but thrombosis may cause diagnostic difficulty.[19]

The arm

Injuries to the upper arm consists of bruises, muscle tears (partial or complete), and fractures of the humerus. Both bruises and fractures may be complicated by nerve injury, particularly to the musculospiral nerve.

Bruises

These may be quite painful and result in temporary functional weakness. Treatment consists of providing a sling for a day or two and teaching the patient static exercises. If symptoms persist for more than two days formal physiotherapy (short wave diathermy, ultrasound or massage) may be desirable. The risk of myositis ossificans should be borne in mind.

Subperiosteal haematoma
Once diagnosed, treatment is by short wave diathermy or ultrasound.

Muscle tears

Muscle tears are not so common in the upper limb.[20] Occasionally complete rupture of the long head of biceps occurs (Fig. 24.12). This is usually associated with pathological changes in the bicipital groove and shoulder joint. Operative repair is not usually successful, and functional disability is minimal. Treatment is by short wave diathermy, ultrasound and exercises.

Injury to muscle attachments is not uncommon and such conditions as avulsion of the bicipital tubercle or stress fracture of the olecranon[21] may be met as a result of sudden or sustained stress at muscle origin or insertion. The nature of the lesion will dictate the treatment.

When the damage occurs to the tendon attachment itself (usually on the olecranon) granulation tissue may form at the site and erode the bone,[22] or ectopic calcification may occur (Fig. 24.13). In such cases operative intervention and decompression may be necessary.

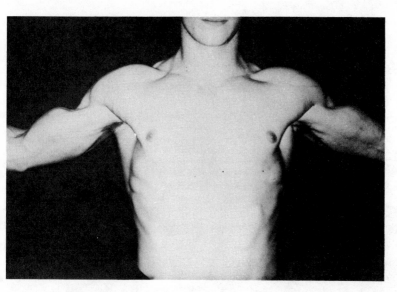

Fig. 24.12 Complete rupture of long heads of *both* biceps brachii in a gymnast.

Fractures

Fractures of the humerus do not present any peculiar problems in athletes and sportsmen. They are treated according to standard orthopaedic practice. The possibility of associated nerve injury should always be remembered and excluded, for in most cases delay in diagnosis may render late operative decompression valueless. Occasionally fracture may follow severe muscular violence, being unrelated to any extrinsic cause of injury,[23, 24]

J.G.P.W.

The elbow

Fractures and dislocations

These injuries are important because so often inadequate treatment will lead to permanent functional disability.

Fractures

Fracture of the olecranon can be caused by a fall on to the tip of the elbow or by excessive action of the triceps muscle. Occasionally a stress fracture[21] of the olecranon (Fig. 24.14) is produced by overuse injuries of baseball or javelin throwing, and this fracture can be easily treated by rest in a split plaster for three to four weeks. However, in most olecranon fractures, the strong pull of triceps is a factor in determining a wide separation between the fragments and operative intervention with internal screw fixation is necessary. During periods of plaster immobilization (three to five weeks) the elbow can be subjected to isometric

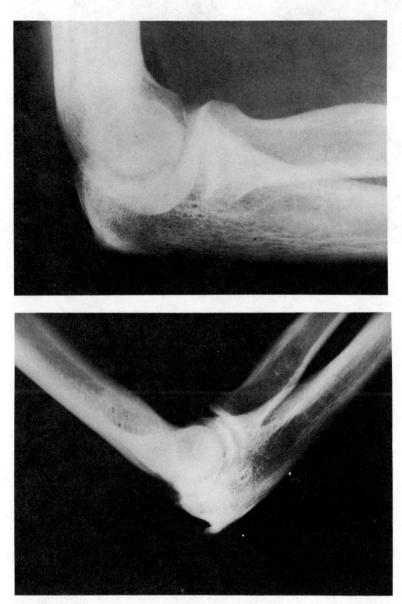

Fig. 24.13 Lesions of attachments of triceps to olecranon. (a) Erosion in a fencer. (b) Ectopic calcification in a squash player.

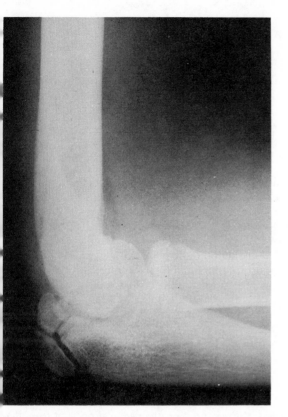

Fig. 24.14 Stress fracture of the olecranon in a young tennis player.

exercises while at a later stage active elbow movements, followed by increasing exercises are instituted.

Supracondylar fractures may extend in a Y- or T-shaped manner into the joint, and because of displacement require internal fixation with wires or screws. Early mobilization, with gentle assisted movements, is needed to prevent intra-articular adhesions.

Fractures of the lateral condyle and medial epicondyle (common in children), need accurate reduction and often internal fixation with wires to prevent any disturbance in growth and subsequent angulation of the forearm.

Fractures of the radial head are produced by a fall on to the outstretched hand that forces the forearm into the extreme lateral position so that the radial head is knocked against the capitellum, splitting the radial head or chipping off a piece. At the same time the cartilage of the capitellum is damaged and may form a loose body in the elbow joint. Usually the injury responds to rest in a sling for three weeks with contrast hot/cold baths to facilitate movement. However, even after slight damage to the radial head there may be some limitation in joint excursion. Severe damage to the radial head necessitates excision.

Fractures around the elbow joint may be complicated by joint stiffness, loss of normal carrying angle, myositis ossificans, ulnar nerve damage and Volkmann's ischaemic contracture.

Dislocations

Dislocations of the elbow usually occur as the result of a hyperextension injury so that the olecranon and head of the radius are displaced backwards and laterally, although forward dislocation of the forearm bones has been described. The severe soft tissue disruption produces a subperiosteal haematoma, and if reduction is delayed, or early passive movement or stretching performed, a mass of heterotopic bone may be formed. Immediate reduction is mandatory, with three weeks' rest in a sling. Active exercises can be instituted during the third week if symptoms are subsiding and activity is not accompanied by a recurrence of swelling.

In addition to ulnar nerve damage and the vascular disturbances which can occur with severe elbow injuries, a dislocation may be complicated by a variety of fractures. These are often forgotten! In young athletes the most important associated injury is a fracture of the medial epicondyle which may be trapped in the joint leading to incomplete reduction shown by restricted flexion. Anterior dislocation, although rare, may be accompanied by a fracture of the olecranon, which requires internal fixation to ensure stability. Marginal or comminuted fractures of the radial head are sometimes found with dislocations, and the comminuted fragments may block the normal range of elbow movements.

Complications of fractures and dislocations

Fracture dislocations

Not uncommonly when dislocation takes place a fracture also occurs, and the fragment, if intra-articular, may prevent reduction. This fragment may be the capitellum, part of the trochlea or the coronoid or olecranon process of the ulna. Open reduction is then necessary with replacement of the fragment which may require internal fixation.

Brachial artery compression

This is most common in supracondylar fractures in children with posterior displacement, and is sometimes seen in posterior dislocations.

Usually pulsation returns to the radial artery at the wrist if initial immobilization after reduction is established in some degree of extension, although occasionally operative decompression of the brachial artery is necessary. In all cases of severe elbow injury the possibility of brachial artery occlusion must be borne in mind, and when found referred for *immediate* surgical treatment, if possible with the elbow *extended*.

Nerve injury

The ulnar nerve, where it lies in relation to the joint behind the medial epicondyle, is especially vulnerable.

In cases of dislocation with rupture of the medial ligament it may become trapped within the joint, or it may be involved in fractures of the medial epicondyle.

Ulnar neuritis

Ulnar neuritis also occurs secondary to cubitis valgus in inadequately treated supracondylar fractures. The integrity of the nerve is established by testing for sensation in the medial border of the hand and fifth digit, and by demonstrating active opposition of thumb and little finger. The degree of interference may be established by comparing nerve conduction time with that in the contralateral side.

Operative decompression with or without transposition may be required when ulnar nerve lesions are detected.

Myositis ossificans

This condition is most commonly seen after elbow injuries, particularly dislocations. There can be no doubt that too early or too vigorous mobilization plays a large part in its development. Murray[25] suggests also that badly timed operative intervention is also provocative.

Treatment is reduction of activity until such time as active calcification has ceased.

Residual disability always persists, and may be quite severe in a large proportion of cases.

Stiffness

Stiffness and limitation of movement almost invariably follow elbow injuries in which there is damage to the capsule or formation of periarticular haematoma. Extension is the movement most usually involved.

The complication is to some extent preventable if steps are taken early to limit haematoma formation, namely by the application of cold compresses and immobilization. Aspiration of any haemarthrosis also seems to diminish the likelihood of permanent restriction of joint range.

When mobilization is started attempts at improving range of movement by passive methods, including manipulation, must *not* be made, as experience shows that they tend if anything to exaggerate the degree of limitation.

Mobilization by energetic *active* movement is most likely to prove successful. At the same time any tendency on the patient's part to counteract his disability by the introduction of 'trick movements', especially at the shoulder joint, must be heartily discouraged. Residual stiffness after elbow injury is not *per se* a contraindication to further participation in sport.

Loose bodies

Occasionally loose bodies may be found in the elbow joint (Fig. 24.15). They give rise to symptoms of locking, or may be asymptomatic, being found incidentally on radiography for trauma. When they produce symptoms they may be removed surgically. As some degree of stiffness almost invariably results from arthrotomy of the elbow joint, the procedure should be avoided unless symptoms are really troublesome.

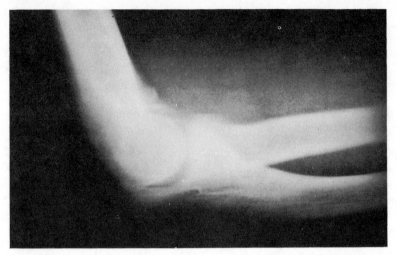

Fig. 24.15   Loose bodies in the elbow joint of a young oarsman (tomograph).

Degenerative changes

Osteoarthrosis of the elbow joint is not uncommon in games players and is not confined to those in the older age group (Fig. 24.16). Usually it presents as pain and sometimes tenderness around the joint, often ill-defined. On examination there is usually some restriction of extension and often a small effusion. Short wave diathermy and gentle active exercise will frequently help as will anti-inflammatory drugs, but the most dramatic relief may be obtained from a small dose of intra-articular steroid.

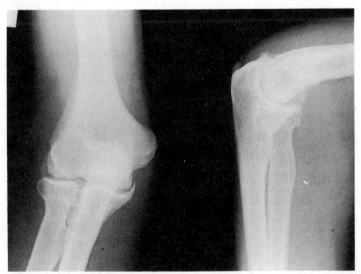

Fig. 24.16   Degenerative joint disease (osteoarthrosis) of the elbow in a 39-year-old squash player.

Sprains

As in any other joint, the application of stresses insufficient to cause fracture, dislocation or complete ligament tear, may yet be enough to provoke a transitory subluxation or sprain, which may be complicated by haemarthrosis. The elbow is painful, especially on movement, and there is some restriction of extreme joint range. The capsule is tender and may be felt to be distended with blood. Treatment consists of aspirating the effusion and applying a firm supporting bandage and sling. Early gentle exercises are encouraged, and are increased in severity as symptoms subside.

During the period when the joint is irritable no exercises with weights should be undertaken outside the middle range. Inner and outer range exercise against resistance tend to overstretch the capsule of the joint and prolong the recovery phase.

'*Pulled elbow*'

A special type of sprain that may be found in children, not uncommonly after judo, is 'pulled elbow' in which the radial head is pulled out of the annular ligament. The history is typical: symptoms are pain and tenderness over the radial head associated with limited movement, particularly pronation and supination.

Treatment is by a simple manipulation that seldom requires an anaesthetic. The hand is firmly grasped and the wrist extended while the operator supports the back of the elbow with his other hand. The patient's elbow is held at a right angle and reduction accomplished by firmly and alternately pronating and supinating the forearm with a screwing movement while maintaining compression along the axis of the radius. The head of the radius slips back into place with a satisfactory click.

Bruises of the elbow

Bruises of the extracapsular tissues are quite common and are treated along the usual lines with cold compress. Occasionally they are complicated by neuropraxia of the ulnar nerve ('funny bone') which is quite alarming for the patient but which recovers spontaneously and rapidly as a rule. Should paraesthesia or other sensory phenomena persist, decompression or transposition of the nerve may become necessary.

Effusion into the olecranon bursa may also follow bruising.[26] Treatment by aspiration and the application of pressure with a sorbo or gamgee pad and elastic bandage may be successful, but if the bursa refills, excision may be required. Alternatively the response to short wave diathermy is usually excellent with absorption of the effusion complete after about six daily treatments.

Secondary infection may convert an olecranon bursa into an abscess. In these cases drainage is all that is required together with a course of systemic antibiotic, as the walls of the bursal cavity will adhere to each other and so obliterate it. Incisions over the olecranon bursa should be sited in such a way as to avoid the development of an adherent scar over the point of the olecranon process.

Tennis elbow

This is a group of conditions characterized by pain and tenderness over the common extensor origin on the lateral epicondyle.[27] Pain may also be felt along the course of the extensors in the forearm. It includes periostitis[28] and subperiosteal haematoma of the lateral epicondyle, strain of the extensor origin, calcification in the extensor origin, and strain of the lateral ligament of the elbow joint.

There does not seem to be a single predisposing cause, as it is commonly found not only in athletes but also in women in early middle age (usually after wringing out the washing!) and is sometimes associated with cervical spondylosis. Some cases are clearly due to entrapment of the radial nerve.[29]

There has been considerable discussion regarding the cause of sports-specific tennis elbow and an incorrect size of grip can now be incriminated as a cause in most cases, particularly in badminton and golf. As far as tennis is concerned the picture is still obscure since most racket handles are close to the ideal circumference. In some cases a change from wood or steel racket without associated change of technique may be a cause. In high class players the situation is most complex[30, 32] and recurrence after treatment can only be prevented by close study and co-operation between player, coach and clinician.

In every case the cause and exact lesion should be accurately identified if treatment is to be lastingly effective.

There is a wide variety of forms of treatment available for tennis elbow, though none is absolutely reliable because of the variety of local pathology:

(1) Hydrocortisone by injection in doses of 25 to 50 mg directly into the tender spot.
(2) Mills' manipulation. The fingers and wrist are fully flexed and the forearm pronated. Held thus the elbow is quickly brought into full extension.
(3) Short wave diathermy and deep frictions.
(4) Ultraviolet light (counter irritant). A third degree erythema is produced using the Kromayer with pressure applied for 70 to 90 seconds directly on the tender spot.
(5) Immobilization for three weeks in a plaster of Paris cylinder which holds the elbow in 90° flexion but allows pronation and supination at the wrist.
(6) Tenotomy. This may be carried out 'blind' using a wide bore hypodermic needle and combined with infiltration with local anaesthetic and hydrocortisone. The needle is held tranversely across the epicondylar ridge with the cutting edge of the bevel laid flat and the needle is then advanced down the epicondylar ridge with a 'sawing' movement pausing at intervals to inject a little of the anaesthetic steroid mixture.

   Alternatively formal open decompression may be carried out. In cases of chronic epicondylitis with damage to the extensor origin, the histology shows a typical pattern of disordered scar formation (Fig. 24.17).
(7) Radial nerve compression must be treated by appropriate release procedures.[29]

The type of treatment selected in the first instance will depend to a considerable extent on available facilities. As a rule hydrocortisone should be used, followed by physiotherapy if injection is unsuccessful or only partly successful. Manipula-

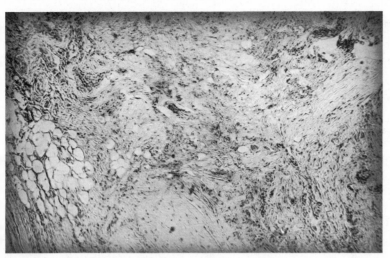

Fig. 24.17 Histological changes in 'tennis elbow' (low power), showing disordered old and new scar formation, areas of haemorrhage, and fatty infiltration (by courtesy of *Rheumatology and Rehabilitation*).

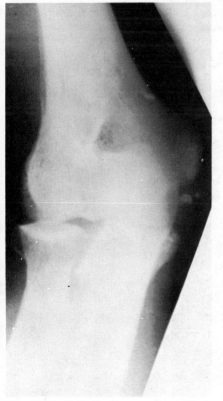

Fig. 24.18 Golfer's elbow; radiograph showing ectopic calcification.

tion should be used only by those with experience in this manœuvre. Immobilization should be reserved for those occasional stubborn cases which do not respond to more active treatment. In chronic cases, surgery gives good results if progressive and effective rehabilitation follows the operation.

Following successful treatment for tennis elbow the sportsman should have his technique thoroughly examined to eliminate faults which might lead to recurrence.

Golfer's elbow

This condition is the opposite of tennis elbow in that it affects the common flexor origin on the medial side of the elbow. It includes periostitis and subperiosteal haematoma, common flexor origin strains, and sprains of the medial ligament. Ectopic calcification is not uncommon and is quite often seen in top class tennis players (Fig. 24.18).

In golfers it seems to be most common on the right side and is thought to be due to taking too big a divot in the chip shots.

Treatment is the same as for tennis elbow, though the manipulation is exactly the reverse, that is, extension of the elbow with the wrist and fingers fully extended

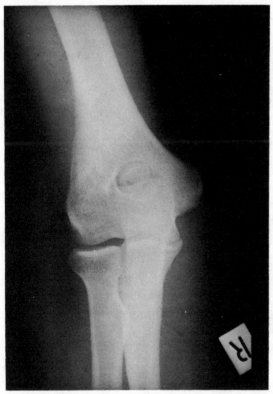

Fig. 24.19 Bony anomaly in olecranon fossa causing pain and disability in a fast bowler (cricket) (by courtesy of *British Journal of Sports Medicine*).

and the forearm supinated. This manipulation is not generally as successful as Mills' manœuvre.

At the same time any detectable technical faults should be corrected.

Thrower's elbow[33]

Elbow injuries in throwers are typically of the whiplash type and are due to hyperextension at the elbow joint, as a result of which the olecranon process impinges on the floor of its fossa in the lower end of the humerus. As a result there may be a fracture, stress fracture or, in adolescents, a traumatic epiphysitis. Where there is a bony anomaly in this region symptoms may be provoked by less violent exercise (Fig. 24.19).[34]

Treatment consists of temporarily limiting the excursion of the joint by means of a check rein. Should symptoms persist, or recur when full activity is resumed, either complete rest must be prescribed, or the bone fragment removed at open operation.

Cases of epiphysitis settle down very satisfactorily with rest which is best enforced at the outset with three to four weeks' immobilization in plaster.

Javelin thrower's elbow

Miller points out that whereas the expert javelin thrower is most likely to suffer the olecranon lesion, the tyro gets a medial ligament strain from 'round arm' throwing (Fig. 24.20).[35]

Such cases respond well to exercise and hydrocortisone injections, but will inevitably recur unless the throwing technique is revised. Occasionally in javelin throwers the true golfer's elbow is encountered, that is, the common flexor origin strain.

Cubitus recurvatus

Hyperextension of the elbow joint may occur in isolation or as part of the condition 'hypermobile joint disease' (Fig. 24.21).[36] If symptoms persist in the face of energetic modification of throwing or hitting technique, the provoking sport may have to be abandoned.

Baseball elbow

The commonest elbow injuries in baseball are due to the repeated trauma of forced, rapid extension causing cartilage flaking, leading to development of loose bodies or cartilaginous outgrowths.[37, 38] Later osteophytes occur, especially on the inner aspect of the trochlea, and if troublesome may require excision. Small ossicles may develop in the medial ligament and cause symptoms by friction against the adjacent soft tissues or ulnar nerve. These ossicles require enucleation with repair of the ligamentous deficit. Sudden hyperextension by the triceps can produce a flake fracture of the tip of the olecranon. This injury usually responds to three to four weeks' rest in the extended position, although occasionally internal fixation is required.

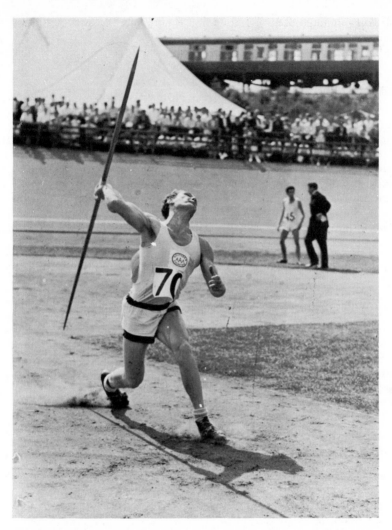

Fig. 24.20 An excellent example of the 'round-arm' throw. Medial ligament strain in such cases is hardly surprising!

Baseball pitchers especially can develop swelling of the muscles in the antecubital fossa because when trying to increase the amount of ball swerve they forcibly supinate the wrist at the termination of the throw. Such an action produces excessive loading on the biceps tendon and anterior forearm muscles. Although the swelling usually responds to rest and elevation, in gross tissue oedema division of the antecubital fascia may be necessary to prevent neurological and vascular complications.

Acute strain with swelling or haemorrhage in the body of triceps may occur in pitchers, and myositis ossificans may supervene. Complete rupture of the tri-

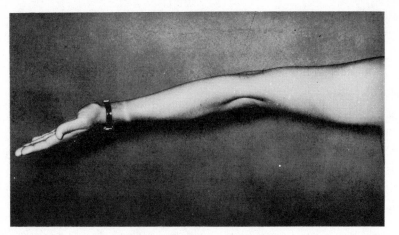

Fig. 24.21 Cubitus recurvatus in a female pentathlete.

ceps tendon requires surgical suture with plaster immobilization for four to six weeks, followed by graduated flexion exercises at the elbow.

Young boys (8–12 years), who have unfused epiphyses in their elbows, may produce significant displacement and in certain instances permanent damage to the growing centres by repeated pitching (Fig. 24.22). Since many of the young

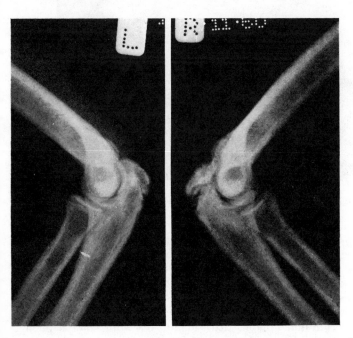

Fig. 24.22 X-ray photographs of the elbow showing traumatic epiphysitis of the olecranon after throwing a cricket ball.

players rely solely on the fast ball, intelligent adult coaching, with a restriction on fast balls and duration of throwing, will prevent this condition.

D.S.M.
J.G.P.W.

Forearm injuries

As in the upper arm, injuries consist of bruises, muscle tears (uncommon) and fractures. Treatment is as described above. In addition tenosynovitis may cause considerable trouble in management.

Tenosynovitis

Tenosynovitis affects most commonly the extensor group in the forearm in racket players and in oarsmen. It can slso been seen in canoeists. Previously, this condition has given rise to very severe disability in sport (Fig. 24.23). The features

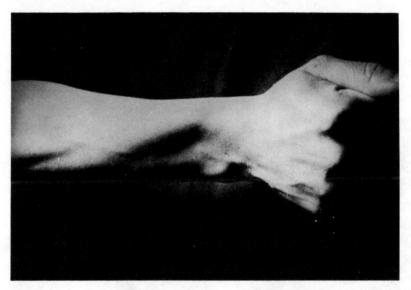

Fig. 24.23 Acute crepitating tenosynovitis of the extensors in the forearm showing typical swelling.

are typical; pain is experienced over the dorsum of the forearm, there is palpable and visible swelling, and crepitus may be felt around the long extensor tendons. To some extent, it seems that it is associated with hypertrophy of the bellies of the abductor longus and extensor brevis muscles of the thumb where they lie over the long extensor tendons. Conservative management includes rest, either full immobilization in plaster of Paris or in firm Elastoplast strapping, combined with the exhibition of antiinflammatory drugs in large doses, for example phenylbutazone (200 mg after meals three times a day). This condition responds particularly well to infiltration over a wide area with local anaesthetics and large doses of hyaluronidase, upwards of 6000 international units: hydrocortisone may also be included in this injection.[39] Recently pilot studies on the early surgical treatment of this condition have been most encouraging. Following fasciectomy and excision of the paratenon (which can be carried out under local anaesthetic), the patient is able to resume rowing within 48 hours and may be back virtually in full training before the sutures are removed from the arm. Certainly, with this procedure, the total disability period is greatly reduced and it offers a most satisfactory, if somewhat drastic means of early return to sport.

J.G.P.W.

Injuries of wrist, hand and fingers[40]

There are few sports in which the fingers, hands, and wrists are not exposed to injury. Injuries to the phalanges and the interphalangeal joints are apt to be regarded as trivial and as not requiring a great deal of attention. They may, however, be of great economic importance, and improperly treated may cause serious incapacity. There are certain guiding principles in the treatment of these injuries. Injured fingers must be immobilized preferably in flexion; the so-called tumbler grasping position of the hand will indicate the optimum position for each finger. Only the injured finger should be immobilized. All other fingers must be exercised from the beginning. If fingers and/or the hand are severely injured the hand must be kept elevated to reduce the oedema which will lead to stiffness. Fingers must only be immobilized for as short a time as possible; three weeks is the longest time a finger should be fixed in splintage before movements are commenced. Angulatory displacements of phalanges must be reduced properly, keeping in mind the fact that when the hand is closed to make a fist, the fingers all point to the thenar eminence.

Mallet finger

This common finger deformity is caused by a tear of the extensor expansion from its attachment to the base of the terminal phalanx. Sometimes there is an associated fracture caused by avulsion of a small triangular fragment of bone (Fig. 24.24). The terminal phalanx is flexed and there is loss of power of extension. Many methods of treatment have been described in the past, including moulded splints, plaster casts, transfixing the reduced finger by Kirschner wires which cross the terminal joint and so on, but experience shows that excellent functional results are obtained by strapping the terminal interphalanageal joint in neutral position. When this is done with Micropore, the end of the finger can be covered with a waterpoof finger cot which enables the hand to be used for every day chores. An intelligent patient can re-apply the strapping at weekly intervals for about five to six weeks. This treatment gives very satisfactory results. There may be a slight lag to extension when the strapping is finally removed, but this is never of any extent and gradually corrects itself over a few months provided the joint is not exposed to further injury during this time.

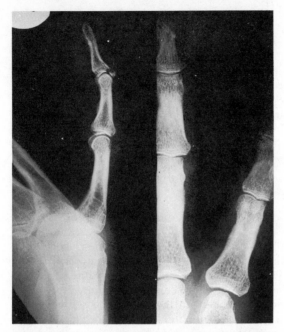

Fig. 24.24 Mallet finger injury; a small flake of bone has been pulled off the distal phalanx by the extensor tendon.

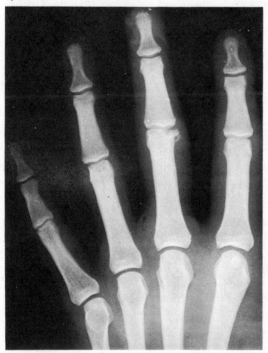

Fig. 24.25 Small condylar fracture of head of proximal phalanx.

Sprains and fractures

At the proximal interphalangeal joints, sprains and sprain fractures (where a small particle of bone is avulsed from the phalanx) are common (Fig. 24.25). These can be treated by immobilization in a splint which is moulded into the optimum position. An easier method is to bandage the affected finger to its neighbour for two weeks, and at the end of that time commence very gentle unsupported active movements in hot water, or wax baths if available.

Fractures of the proximal phalanges tend to displace with anterior angulation due to the pull of the lumbrical muscles, which come from the palm and pass round the phalanx to gain attachment to the extensor expansion on the dorsal aspect (Fig. 24.26). This angulation must be corrected otherwise there will be a loss of flexion of the finger and inability to grip properly (Fig. 24.27).

At the metacarpophalangeal joints, sprains and dislocations, after reduction, are treated for the first two weeks in the 'boxing glove' type of bandage. A thick pad of cotton wool is placed in the hand and the fingers bandaged over it. Gentle movements are encouraged within the limits of the bandage which is applied more loosely at the end of a week. At the end of two to three weeks, active movements are supervised by therapists.

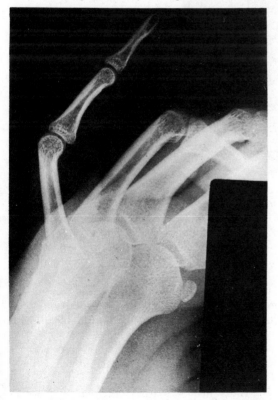

Fig. 24.26 Fracture of proximal phalanx of little finger with typical angulation due to lumbrical muscle pull. (See also Fig. 24.27.)

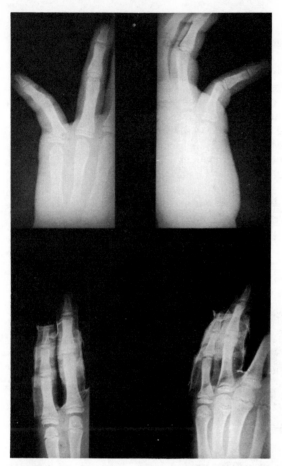

Fig. 24.27 Displacement reduced and finger treated by strapping to adjacent ring finger.

Severe sprains, sprain fractures and dislocations at the metacarpophalangeal joint of the thumb are common in rugby, skiing, wrestling and similar sports.[41] Failure to appreciate the nature of this injury will leave a thumb which is unstable and prevent a sportsman from holding a tennis racket, golf club or other athletic gear.

The ulnar collateral ligament is torn from its attachment at the base of the proximal phalanx and can be prevented from uniting by the interposition of the abductor aponeurosis (Fig. 24.28). Surgical exploration and fixation of this ligament will give a stable joint.

Fractures of the metacarpals are common in all sports where body contact takes place. Fractures of the shafts are seldom displaced as the adjacent bones act as splints. A dorsal plaster slab bound on the hand with soft bandages will protect the hand until union is firm. This takes from three to four weeks (Fig. 24.29). The fifth metacarpal is frequently broken at the neck. It lies exposed at the outer side of the hand where a blow on the knuckle will break the neck,

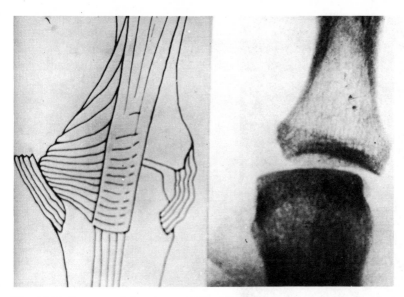

Fig. 24.28 Rupture of the ulnar collateral ligament of the thumb with interposition of adductor aponeurosis and instability.

hence the term 'punch' fracture (Fig. 24.30). The head and neck are displaced into the palm of the hand by the violence causing the break, and this is reduced by flexing the small finger to 90° at the metacarpophalangeal joint. Pressure is then applied to the proximal phalanx and thus to the displaced bone to correct it; a small dorsal slab of plaster will retain the reduction.

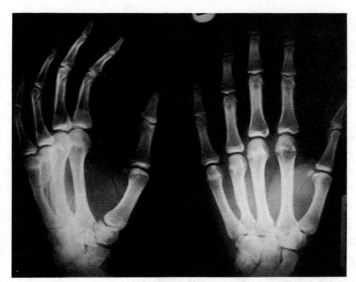

Fig. 24.29 Oblique fracture of shaft of 4th metacarpal. A stable fracture which does not require prolonged immobilization.

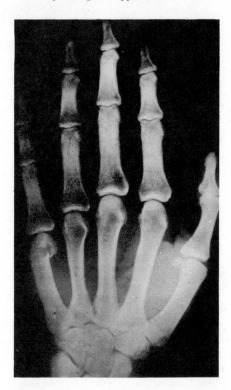

Fig. 24.30 'Punch fracture' of neck of 5th metacarpal.

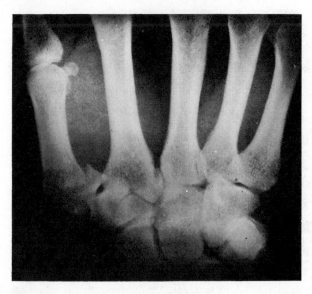

Fig. 24.31 Transverse fracture of base of thumb metacarpal—*not* a Bennett's fracture.

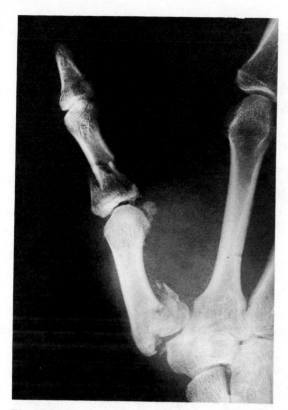

Fig. 24.32 Bennett's fracture dislocation; fracture *through* base of phalanx *into* joint causing displacement. Note also fracture of proximal phalanx.

The thumb metacarpal is frequently broken at the base; a distinction must be made between the simple transverse fracture across the shaft (Fig. 24.31) and the oblique fracture which enters the carpometacarpal joint (Fig. 24.32). This is an unstable fracture dislocation (Bennett's fracture). It must be reduced, the reduction maintained by traction or, if difficulty is experienced in doing this, open operation will enable the displacement to be corrected and fixed with a screw or small metal pin (Fig. 24.33). Some writers maintain that the end results are satisfactory even if the displacement is not reduced properly, but many athletes have stiffness, restricted movement, and arthritic changes because satisfactory reduction was not maintained.

Carpal bones

The problems associated with fractures of the scaphoid are now well known and there have been many publications on the subject.

A fall on the outstretched hand may fracture the scaphoid, but the fracture may not be visible in the initial X-ray. There is always the temptation to treat the injury as a sprain which it resembles.

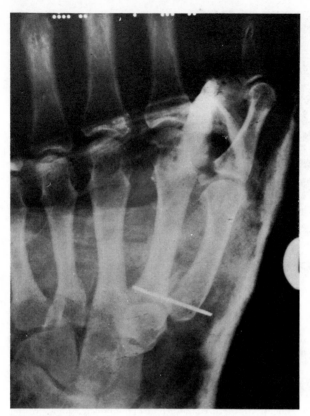

Fig. 24.33 X-ray photograph of a Bennett's fracture treated by internal fixation. In fractures of this type maintenance of reduction by more conservative measures is very uncertain.

If there is tenderness in the anatomical snuff-box of the thumb, and the space between the extensor tendons of the thumb is obliterated by swelling, then it must be assumed that the scaphoid is broken and treatment prescribed accordingly. A scaphoid plaster is applied. This is one that includes the thumb as far as the interphalangeal joint in a position of opposition. A second X-ray within 10 to 14 days will reveal the fracture as bone absorption occurs at the fracture line. In addition to the usual anteroposterior and lateral views, an oblique view must be taken because of the shape of the bone. Even when treatment is promptly undertaken there is no guarantee that union will take place; in about one-third of scaphoid bones the blood supply which enters it along the oblique ligamentous ridge does not reach the proximal third of the bone. If, therefore, the fracture is near the proximal pole in such a scaphoid, the proximal third will be deprived of its blood supply and undergo avascular necrosis (Fig. 24.34).

The problem that faces the surgeon with such proximal fractures is how long to immobilize the wrist in the hope of getting union. Watson-Jones[42] maintained that it was essential to immobilize the wrist for up to six or eight months if necessary. At the present time this is not considered ideal. A hand and wrist fixed

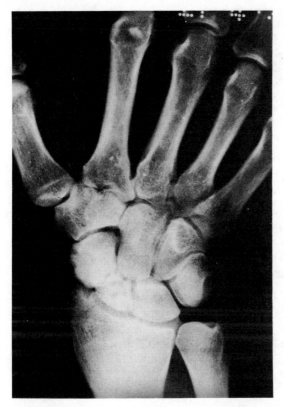

Fig. 24.34 Avascular necrosis of scaphoid due to proximal fracture line interfering with blood supply.

for that length of time can present other problems, muscular wasting, bone atrophy and other stigmata of disuse. This is a not uncommon fracture in a goal-keeper and fixation of his wrist for this length of time would certainly put an end to his active career. If after immobilization for about ten weeks, doubt exists as to the state of union, the better functional result will probably be obtained by removing the plaster, applying bandages to protect the wrist and encouraging gentle active movements. If established non-union is present after such a trial a decision can be made regarding bone grafts or excision of the small proximal fragment. Many patients are seen incidentally with non-union who have performed strenuous work for many years with nothing more than vague discomfort. Often the condition is discovered by chance when the patient presents having sustained another injury.

Dislocation of the semilunar

A fall on the outstretched hand can force the semilunar bone out of the pocket in which it lies on the articular surface of the radius. It comes to rest in the very

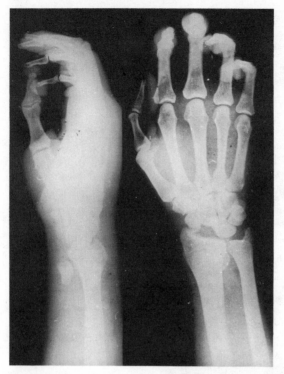

Fig. 24.35 Dislocation of the semilunar. Note gap in proximal carpal row and extruded bone lying anterior to the wrist.

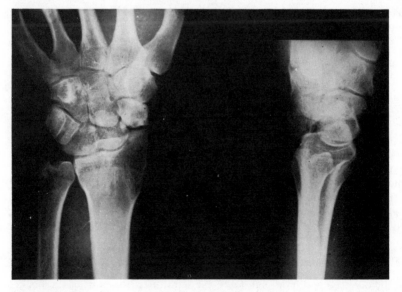

Fig. 24.36 Old transscapho-perilunar dislocation of wrist with osteoarthrotic changes.

restricted space deep to the annular ligament and there may damage or press on the median nerve (Fig. 24.35).

The picture presented, therefore, is a swollen wrist, the swelling lying anteriorly, stiffness of the fingers which are semiflexed, and some impairment of the median nerve. The X-ray is characteristic. Seen early the displaced bone can usually be reduced under general anaesthesia without much difficulty. Traction is applied longitudinally to the fingers and the bone is gently eased back into position. A well-padded plaster cast should be applied for two to three weeks. If this dislocation is missed, the median nerve may be damaged irreparably.

Occasionally the semilunar bone may remain in position, but the carpal bones surrounding it are dislocated posteriorly—this is a perilunar dislocation. Because of its situation in the wrist, the scaphoid usually breaks, one half remains in its normal position while the other half accompanies the posteriorly displaced carpus, the injury is then a transcapho-perilunar fracture dislocation (Fig. 24.36). This severe displacement can be reduced, by traction longitudinally on the fingers, followed by gentle manipulation of the displaced carpus.

Because of the extensive disruption of the wrist joint, prolonged immobilization is required, and often there is quite severe residual stiffness of the wrist.

Osteochondritis of the semilunar

This form of osteochondritis which affects the semilunar has been ascribed to repetitive injuries to the bone. It is a rare condition but can give rise to considerable disability.

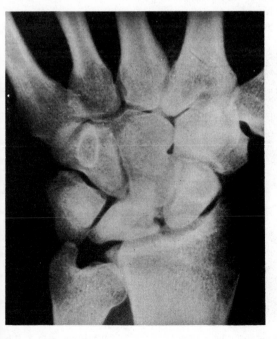

Fig. 24.37 Keinbock's osteochondritis of the semilunar.

The patient complains of gradual stiffness of the wrist occurring over a period, with pain on palmar and dorsiflexion. Swelling of a diffuse type is present. X-ray studies show the classical irregular collapse of the bone with fragmentation and flattening (Fig. 24.37).

Treatment is by immobilization in a cast until pain has subsided. Osteoarthrotic changes are liable to occur and surgical treatment may be necessary. Attempts have been made to replace the bone with a plastic-type one, but the results are not impressive. Occasionally, excision of the proximal row of the carpus or arthrodesis may be necessary.

Bony anomalies

Peculiarities of skeletal form may occur anywhere and can give rise to clinical problems in some sportsmen (Fig. 24.38). Treatment depends on the condition.

Soft tissues

Bruising
Soft tissue injuries of the fingers are common in virtually all sports. Bruising may produce disability out of all proportion to the actual tissue damage. Primary treatment consists of cold compress together with the encouragement of movement. If bruising is extensive, the possibility of more serious underlying injury must be excluded. Bruising at the tip of the finger may produce a *subungual haematoma* which can be intensely painful. Treatment is by trephining; a short bevel hypodermic needle may be used held with the point against the discoloured area

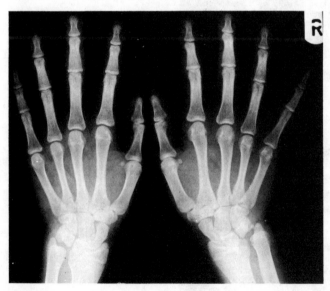

Fig. 24.38 Bony anomaly; familial overlong ulnar heads causing disability in a young hockey player.

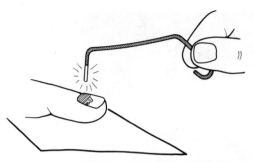

Fig. 24.39 Method of trephining nail with a red-hot paper clip to release a subungual haematoma.

of the nail and introduced with a gentle twisting motion. Alternatively, and more effectively if available, an unfolded paper clip heated to a dull red heat can be used for this trephining (Fig. 24.39). If the nail is badly lifted from its bed, and in particular if there is marginal detachment, removal of the nail by simple avulsion under local anaesthetic may be preferred. In such cases, a tulle dressing should be applied for a few days and thereafter the finger exposed to the air so that the nail bed can dry.

Lacerations

Lacerations of the fingers may be quite severe: whereas previously such injuries required suture, they can now be more effectively closed using sterile adhesive tape such as Micropore or Ethistrip. Once the wound is well closed, active movement may be started without undue delay.

Sprains

Sprains of the interphalangeal joints are common and Burry[43] has described a condition of 'Strine Rules Duke' peculiar to antipodean football. Other particular conditions are bowler's finger where the digits of the ten-pin bowler are injured due to mistimed release of the bowl.

Dislocations

Dislocations of the interphalangeal joints are not uncommon particularly in such sports as rugby and football. They may be reduced on the spot by simple traction provided that there is no evidence of bony damage or other injury (which is usually self evident). Following reduction, the digit may be lightly strapped to the most convenient adjacent finger and activity should be encouraged forthwith. Even where dislocation is accompanied by a rupture of a collateral ligament of an interphalangeal joint, early activity is usually preferable. Primary repair gives uncertain results, although in some cases where early mobilization is unsuccessful, secondary repair has to be considered.

Boxer's knuckle

Soft tissue injuries to the knuckle are not uncommon, particularly in boxers. A condition is described as boxer's knuckle which is in fact more than one pathology. A traumatic bursa may form over the metacarpal head which can become

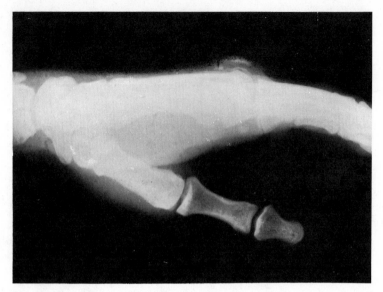

Fig. 24.40 Boxer's knuckle; 'bursagram' by Dr P. N. Sperryn.

chronically inflamed[44] (Fig. 24.40). The other form is distraction of the inter-metacarpal ligament. This can be a source of quite considerable deformity. The habit of bandaging the hands prior to a bout where the tapes are applied to the outstretched extended hand around the bases of the fingers, leads to this condi-tion. In extension the intermetacarpal ligaments are relatively slack allowing abduction of the fingers. As the hand goes into flexion, the slack is taken up in bringing the fingers into apposition. Any material inserted between the fingers will, under such circumstances, tend to cause distraction of the intermetacarpal ligaments. The treatment of these conditions is essentially symptomatic.

Tendon injuries

Tendon injuries, other than those associated with mallet finger, are not common although ruptures of the deep flexor tendons may occur as judo injuries due to the jodoka's grip on the clothing being forcibly broken. In such cases, expectant treatment is to be preferred. If lasting disability occurs, tenodesis may have to be performed. Rupture of the extensor expansion on the dorsum of the proximal interphalangeal joint may occur in some ball games, giving rise to the 'Bouton-niere' deformity. This is difficult to treat. The angulation should, if possible, be reduced and surgery may be required to prevent recurrence. Lesions of tendons in the hand are uncommon except in penetrating injuries. Inflammation of the sheaths does, however, occur. Trigger finger is an occupational hazard in fencing and de Quervain's disease is also seen in sportsmen, although it does not appear to be a sport-specific. Treatment is by infiltration with hydrocortisone and a local anaesthetic in the first instance. Where this is unsuccessful, surgical decompres-sion may be carried out and give a permanent cure.

Carpal tunnel syndrome

Carpal tunnel syndrome may present in sportsmen as in the population at large and can be particularly disabling for racket players. Treatment is infiltration of the carpal ligament with a local anaesthetic and hydrocortisone, which should give temporary relief and may provide a permanent cure, otherwise surgical decompression must be carried out. The median nerve should be visualized throughout its length beneath the ligament in this procedure, otherwise recurrence will occur if a distal band is left undivided.

Ganglia

Ganglia arising usually from the wrist joint but occasionally from the interphalangeal joints, metacarpophalangeal joints, or tendon sheaths can cause a degree of disability out of all proportion to their size. Treatment may be dispersal by pressure, injection and aspiration or, as may be necessary in some cases, surgical removal.

Rehabilitation of hand injuries

In virtually all cases of hand injury, whether involving soft tissue or bones and joints, the most effective rehabilitation is return to sport as soon as possible. Active movements are introduced into the programme as early as possible and swelling discouraged by elevation. In general, the principles laid down in *Rehabilitation of the Hand*[45] may be followed with confidence.

A. McD.
J. G. P. W.

References

1. Thorndike, A. (1959) Frequency and nature of sports injuries. *Am. J. Surg.*, **98,** 316.
2. Sperryn, P. N. and Williams, J. G. P. (1976) Why sports injuries clinics? *Br. med. J.*, **3,** 364.
3. Bateman, J. E. (1971) In *Encyclopedia of Sport Sciences and Medicine*, ed. Larson, L. A., London: Collier-Macmillan.
4. Bearden, J. M., Hughston, J. C. and Whatley, G. S. (1973) Acromioclavicular dislocation: method of treatment. *J. Sports Med.*, **1,** 4: 5.
5. Tyer, H. D., Sturrock, W. D. S. and Callow, F. McC. (1963) Retrosternal dislocation of the clavicle. *J. Bone Jt Surg.*, **45B,** 132.
6. Burrows, H. J. (1951) Tenodesis of subclavius in the treatment of recurrent dislocation of the sternoclavicular joint. *J. Bone Jt Surg.*, **33B,** 240
7. O'Donaghue, D. H. (1970) *Treatment of Injuries to Athletes.* 2nd Edn. Philadelphia: W. B. Saunders.
8. Cahil, B. R., Tullos, H. S. and Fain, R. H. (1974) Little league shoulder. *J. sports Med.*, **2,** 150.
9. Lipscombe, A. B. (1975) Baseball pitching injuries in growing athletes. *J. sports Med.*, **3,** 25.
10. De Palma, A. F. and Flannery, G. F. (1973) Acute anterior dislocation of the shoulder. *J. Sports Med.*, **1,** No. 2, 6.
11. Feagin, J. A. (1974) Elastic arm-torso harness. *J. sports Med.*, **2,** 99.
12. Naves, J. (1962) Results of the Bankart operation in recurrent dislocation of the shoulder in case of sportsmen. *J. sports Med. phys. Fitness.* **2,** 89.

13. Moskwa, J. Personal communication.
14. Weston, A. and Williams, J. G. P. (1972) Soft Tissue Rheumatism. In *Medicine 1 Rheumatic Diseases.*
15. Bateman, J. E. (1969) Shoulder injuries in the throwing sports. In *Symposium on Sports Medicine.* St. Louis: C. V. Mosby.
16. Brewn, B. J. (1969) The throwing arm-soft tissue injury. In *Symposium on Sports Medicine.* St. Louis: C. V. Mosby.
17. O'Donoghue, D. H. (1973) Subluxing biceps tendon in the athlete. *J. sports Med.,* **1,** 3: 20.
18. Jokl, E. (1958) *Clinical Physiology of Physical Fitness and Rehabilitation.* Springfield Ill.: Charles C. Thomas.
19. Wright, R. S. and Lipscomb, A. B. (1974) Acute occlusion of the subclavian vein in an athlete: diagnosis, etiology and surgical management. *J. sports Med.,* **2,** 343.
20. Buck, J. E. (1973) Bilateral rupture of pectoralis major—a unique experience, Proceedings XVIII World Congress of Sports Medicine. *Br. J. sports Med.,* **7,** 70.
21. Devas, M. B. (1969) Stress fractures in athletes. *Proc. R. Soc. Med.,* **62,** 932.
22. Williams, J. G. P. (1973) Lesions of tendon attachments. *Rheum. Rehabil.,* **XII,** 182.
23. Bingham, E. L. (1959) Fractures of the humerus from muscular violence. *U.S. Arm. Forces Med. J.,* **10,** 22.
24. Peltokallio, P., Peltokallio, V. and Vaalasti, T. (1968) Fractures of the humerus from muscular violence in sport. *J. sports Med., phys. Fitness,* **8,** 21.
25. Murray, C. R. (1941) The timing of the fracture healing process. *J. Bone Jt Surg.,* **23A,** 598.
26. Larson, R. L. and Osternig, L. R. (1974) Traumatic bursitis and artificial turf. *J. sports Med.,* **2,** 183.
27. Badgley, C. and Hayes, J. (1959) Athletic injuries to the elbow, forearm, wrist and hand. *Am. J. Surg.,* **98,** 432.
28. Mercer, W. (1950) Tennis elbow. *Practitioner,* **164,** 293.
29. Roles, N. C. and Maudsley, R. H. (1972) Radial tunnel syndrome: resistant tennis elbow as a nerve entrapment. *J. Bone Jt Surg.,* **54B,** 499.
30. Priest, J. D., Jones, H. H. and Nagel, D. A. (1974) Elbow injuries in highly skilled tennis players. *J. sports Med.,* **2,** 137.
31. Bernlang, A. M., Dehner, W. and Fogarty, C. (1974) Tennis elbow: a biomechanical approach. *J. sports Med.,* **2,** 235.
32. Nirschl, R. P. (1974) The etiology and treatment of tennis elbow. *J. sports Med.,* **2,** 308.
33. Woods, G. W., Tullos, H. S. and King, J. W. (1973) The throwing arm: elbow joint injuries. *J. sports Med.,* **1,** 4: 43.
34. Williams, J. G. P. (1972) A congenital abnormality of the olecranon fossa. *Br. J. Sports Med.,* **6,** 68.
35. Miller, J. E. (1960) Javelin thrower's elbow. *J. Bone Jt Surg.,* **42B,** 788.
36. Lichtor, J. (1972) The loose-jointed young athlete. *J. sports Med.,* **1,** 1: 22.
37. King, J. W., Bradsford, H. J. and Tullos, H. S. (1969) Epicondylitis and osteochondritis of the professional baseball pitcher's elbow. In *Symposium on Sports Medicine.* St. Louis: C. V. Mosby.
38. Brown, R., Blazina, M. E., Kerlan, R. K., Carter, V. S., Jobe, F. W. and Carlson, R. (1974) Osteochondritis of the capitellum. *J. sports Med.,* **2,** 27.
39. Williams, J. G. P. (1971) Acute overuse injury—a case of tenosynovitis. *Br. J. sports Med.,* **5,** 231.
40. McCue, F. C., Hakala, M. W., Andrews, J. R. and Gieck, J. H. (1974) Ulnar collateral ligament injuries of the thumb in athletes. *J. Sports Med.,* **2,** 70.
41. Flatt, A. E. (1969) Athletic injuries of the hand. In *Symposium on Sports Medicine.* St. Louis: C. V. Mosby.

42. Watson-Jones, R. (1955) *Fractures and Joint Injuries*, 4th Edn. Edinburgh: E. & S. Livingstone.
43. Burry, H. C. (1973) Strine Rules Duke. *Communication to British Association of Sport and Medicine*.
44. Sperryn, P. N. (1973) Traumatic bursitis in a boxer's hand, Proceedings XVIII World Congress of Sports Medicine. *Br. J. sports Med.*, **7**, 103.
45. Wynn-Parry, C. B. (1973) *Rehabilitation of the Hand*, 3rd Edn. London: Butterworth.

25

Injuries of the lower limbs

The incidence of leg injuries is as high as 60 per cent in some series of sports injuries, and the knee is most frequently affected as it is the one joint which carries the full weight of the body while having no inherent bony stability.[1] [3]

The pelvis

Fractures

Although pelvic fractures with solution of the pelvic ring and some degree of displacement occur in sport, they are very rare. They usually follow high-speed falls, as from a horse, bicycle or racing car, particularly if the vehicle rolls upon and crushes the patient (Fig. 25.1). They may also occur in the various codes of rugby football.

Such cases of fractured pelvis present the typical features and require management along the standard lines. The possibility of urethral damage must always be remembered where disruption of the symphysis or pubic arch is found.

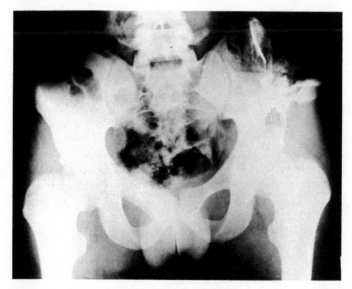

Fig. 25.1 X-ray photograph showing comminuted fracture of the iliac crest. This degree of severity is uncommon in sports injuries.

Isolated pelvic fractures, particularly of the iliac crest are relatively more common, due to direct violence, or as avulsion injuries due to violent contraction of the trunk muscles. A similar fracture involves the anterior superior iliac spine, when the origin of sartorius is avulsed.

In the young sportsman avulsion or epiphysitis of the epiphysis of the iliac crest may occur (Fig. 25.2). In these cases treatment is symptomatic. The application of cold and pressure in the early stages will prevent excessive haematoma formation. Later, heat and gentle exercise are introduced in a programme of

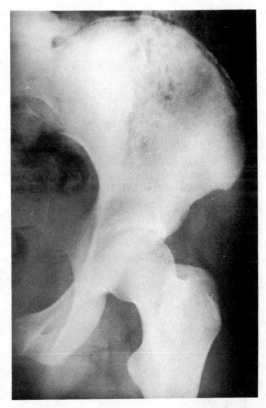

Fig. 25.2 Epiphysitis of the iliac crest in a young sprinter.

gradual mobilization. When pain is severe a few days' bed rest may be necessary. Operative replacement of the avulsed fragment is normally unnecessary and may lead to persistent post-operative symptoms, due to adherent scar tissue.

Progressive rehabilitation is the key to successful treatment, and return to full activity is permissible when pain and tenderness have completely disappeared (usually four to six weeks). In stubborn cases relief of symptoms may be achieved by local steroid injections.

Bruises and strains

Bruises and strains of the muscle origins on the iliac crest are common. Clinically they are similar to fractures in this region, but pain and tenderness are not so severe and X-ray shows no bony injury. Treatment is along similar lines and resolution may be expected within seven to ten days. Pain and tenderness will persist for long periods if rest alone is prescribed.

Ultrasonics are of value in these cases to encourage both early resolution and the localization of tenderness in chronic cases prior to local steroid injection.

Strains may also be found frequently at the other sites of muscle origin, particularly the ischial tuberosity and the inferior pubic ramus.

Hamstring origin strains are common among sprinters and footballers. The patient may present with a history of sudden severe pain in the lower part of the buttock during exercise, or the onset of symptoms may be insidious. On examination the ischial tuberosity is tender, as may be any of the attached tendons. Pain is felt when the hamstrings are stretched, for example by toe-touching with the knees straight, and there may be limitation of straight leg raising. Lassegue's sciatic stretch test is negative. Differential diagnosis is from sciatica which is generally also insidious in onset.

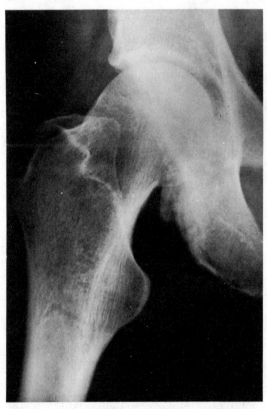

Fig. 25.3 Chronic hamstring origin strain with secondary calcification.

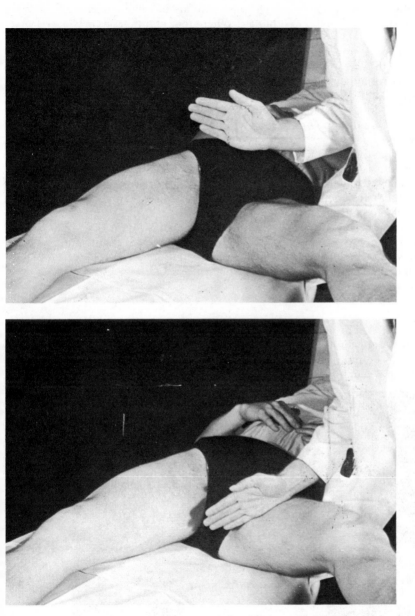

Fig. 25.4 The technique of adductor stretch for rider's strain. The affected leg is widely abducted and the ulnar border of the operator's extended hand is brought down forcibly on to the tendon.

Treatment consists of short wave diathermy, gentle stretching, and exercise to tolerance in the early stages. Deep frictions are of value if technically possible (i.e. the subject is not too well built!). Where the condition has become chronic, local injection of steroid is indicated and this may need to be repeated. In all cases the patient must be taught to keep doing stretching exercises for at least three months after injury. These are best incorporated in the limbering up process prior to training or competition. Secondary calcification may occur in chronic recurrent hamstring origin strain and is very difficult to treat (Fig. 25.3). Local steroid injections are often helpful, but the relief tends to be short lived. Results of surgery are disappointing and the victim may have to accept a lower level of activity.

Occasionally avulsion or stress fractures of the ischium are encountered, or the ischium is itself avulsed. These may be suspected when the local reaction is very marked or when the lesion does not respond to treatment. X-ray examination will not always show up these injuries. Treatment is modified activity with avoidance of pain-producing exercises.

Adductor origin (rider's) strain is most commonly seen in cyclists, horsemen, runners, fast bowlers and association footballers. Pain and 'stiffness' are felt high in the groin, there is local tenderness and pain on abduction. Treatment is by manipulation (i.e. adductor stretch under general anaesthetic; Fig. 25.4), steroid injections or massage.

Osteitis pubis

This is a most disabling condition which happily is not common. Footballers appear to be most often affected (indeed the condition is also known as 'inguinocrural pain of footballers''),[4] but runners and walkers may succumb.[5]

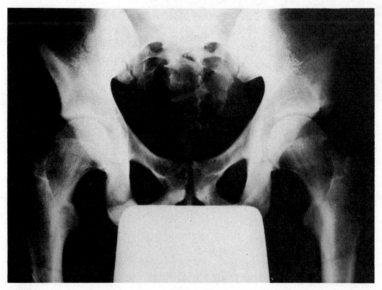

Fig. 25.5 Bilateral deformity of femoral heads in a case of traumatic osteitis pubis.

The patient complains of more or less severe pain in the groins with occasional radiation to hips, abdomen and external genitalia.[6] Onset is usually insidious but may be related to some specific sporting activity.

Symptoms are exacerbated by exercise and relieved by rest. Frequently the condition is chronic by first presentation, and the victim gives a history of alternating periods of rest and training with a monotonous cycle of recurrence.

The cardinal feature on examination is tenderness over the symphysis pubis accompanied by swelling. Pain may be aggravated by hip joint movement or by contraction of rectus abdominis as in 'sit ups'. Limitation of hip movement (especially rotation) often associated with deformity of the femoral head as after a slight epiphyseal slip is probably a causative factor (Fig. 25.5). Pain on pelvic compression is an inconstant finding. Pyrexia has been described in a number of cases and dysuria is occasionally a feature.

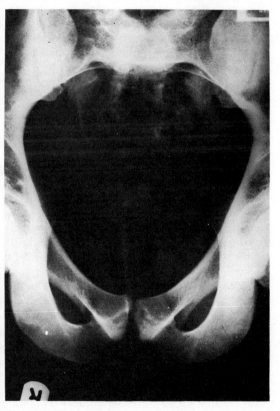

Fig. 25.6 Traumatic osteitis pubis; X-ray shows typical eroded appearance of symphysis.

X-rays reveal a typical 'eroded' appearance of the symphysis with some widening of the gap between the bone ends (Fig. 25.6).[8] In old cases abnormal calcification may be shown.

Laboratory investigations are unhelpful since a moderate leucocytosis and raised sedimentation rate are by no means constant. Urinalysis is usually normal.

Histological material displays varying appearances usually in keeping with a chronic inflammatory response, possibly due to local infection.

Differential diagnosis

It is essential to exclude not only other possible musculoskeletal causes of pain, e.g. adductor origin strain, but also disease of the genito-urinary tract, particularly prostatitis and Reiter's syndrome. Ankylosing spondylitis must also be remembered as a possible cause of inguinocrural pain.

Treatment

Opinions vary as to the treatment of choice in this condition, but it would appear that temporary reduction of physical activity, together with full doses of antiinflammatory drugs (e.g. phenylbutazone 200 mgm after meals thrice daily, for 3–4 weeks), has much to offer. Cochrane[9] advises concomitant treatment with short wave diathermy. Severe and chronic cases may demand surgical intervention, and fusion of the symphysis is advised although the results are by no means always good. When hip joint mobility is reduced remobilization is essential.

Following resolution of symptoms, by whatever means obtained, progress to resumption of full normal activity must be gradual.

The hip joint

Hip joint injuries are remarkably uncommon in sport.[10] That most frequently seen is the simple sprain with or without haemarthrosis (synovitis/capsulitis).

Sprain

There is usually a history of a 'wrench' or twist and the patient presents with a painful limp. Limitation of movement may be marked and if a haemarthrosis is present the hip is held in flexion and abduction. Especially in children, referred pain may be felt on the medial side of the knee.

Treatment consists of support with a suitable spica bandage, limited weight bearing (stick or crutches) and active unresisted exercises. On this regime symptoms rapidly subside and more vigorous exercise becomes possible. Competition should be discontinued for three weeks at least.

The chief importance of this injury is its similarity to intra-articular suppuration, early tuberculosis and injuries to the head of the femur. X-rays should always be taken in two planes, and aspiration of the joint may be undertaken as a diagnostic measure. (There is no uniform therapeutic need to aspirate a simple haemarthrosis.) In addition, further differentiation may be achieved by investigation of the leucocyte count and blood sedimentation rate. Generally it is as well to refer all cases of hip injury with limitation of movement and deformity for a specialist orthopaedic opinion. In this context mention may be made of the case of a professional footballer with a stiff painful hip treated by his club 'trainer' for ten days as a 'sprain' from whose hip joint was later aspirated 50 ml of pus.

Trochanteric bursitis

This condition is not common and is seen less in men than women. The bursa overlying the gluteal attachments and separating them from the iliotibial band may become inflamed either as a result of a direct blow or as an over-use injury due to recurrent 'snapping' of the band across the trochanter. In the latter case the patient will often have previously developed a trick movement which tends to make the condition worse.

Treatment is rest, short wave diathermy, and in chronic cases, local steroid injection. When trick movements have been developed, motor re-education may be necessary. Surgical intervention is seldom required.

Other trochanteric injuries, particularly fractures or avulsions, are treated by rest and appropriate analgesics followed by mobilization when it can be tolerated. More active treatment is not usually required.

Other injuries

More serious injury to the hip joint is very rare in sport, though fractures of the femoral neck are a recognized hazard in bicycling as a result of high-speed falls. In adolescents upper femoral epiphysiolysis may be precipitated by athletic activity, but complete slip is exceptionally rare. Most often there is progressive slip with increasing disability following a relatively minor degree of trauma.

Dislocation of the hip, central dislocation with fracture of the acetabulum, and fractures of the femoral head or acetabular rim occasionally occur (Fig. 25.7).[11] If serious injury is suspected the patient is removed from the field of play on a stretcher, and no attempt should be made to correct any displacement. Treatment is according to accepted orthopaedic practice.

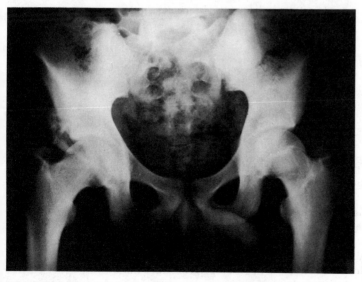

Fig. 25.7 Acetabular rim fracture in a young footballer with minimal symptoms; he first presented a month after injury 'because the discomfort persisted'.

Following successful rehabilitation comes the problem of return to sporting activity. It is widely held that secondary osteoarthritic changes are precipitated by further severe exercise, but the evidence that this is so is of the *post hoc ergo propter hoc* type, and severe osteoarthrosis is not infrequently seen even when vigorous exercise is avoided after such injuries. As a rule it is advisable to recommend that the patient should give up body-contact sports (Fig. 25.8).

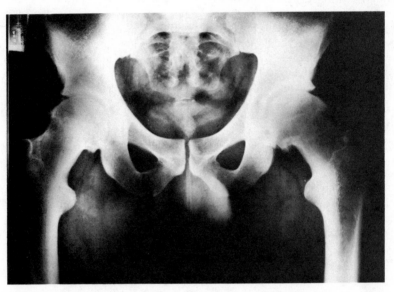

Fig. 25.8 Osteoarthrosis of the hip joint (primary cause uncertain) in a professional Rugby League footballer who was still playing.

The thigh

Injuries of the thigh include bruises, muscle strains, and very rarely, femoral fractures.[12]

Bruises

The classic injury is the 'charley-horse', the blow on the front of the thigh during active contraction of the main bulk of the quadriceps.[13] Even if complete rupture of rectus femoris does not occur muscle damage tends to be quite extensive with marked intramuscular bleeding. Treatment is along the lines set out in Chapter 17. Bed rest may well be required in the early stages, and the risk of developing a secondary myositis ossificans must always be born in mind (Fig. 25.9).

Occasionally bruising over the bony prominances (greater trochanter, lateral femoral condyle) is associated with grazing of the skin ('mat burn', 'grass burn'). In such cases healing may be delayed due to secondary infection which requires energetic treatment.

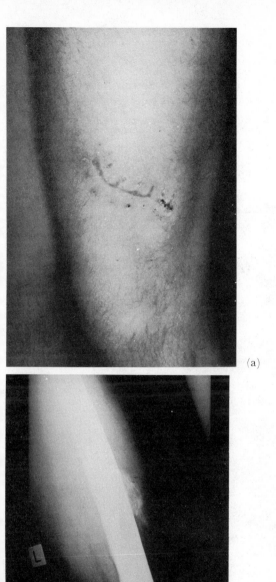

(a)

(b)

Fig. 25.9 (a) Lacerated bruise on front of thigh after an accident in a cycle race. (b) Secondary ectopic calcification which followed.

Muscle strain

Muscle strains in the thigh typically involve either the hamstrings or the quadriceps group. Their possible aetiology and the general principles of treatment have been set out in Chapter 17 (Fig. 25.10).

Psoas (or iliopsoas) strains are characterized by pain on exercise and deep tenderness in the groin. Discomfort may radiate to lower abdomen, upper thigh or genitalia. Pain is made worse by external rotation of the hip *in extension*. In chronic cases calcification may occur. Treatment involves ultrasound or dia-

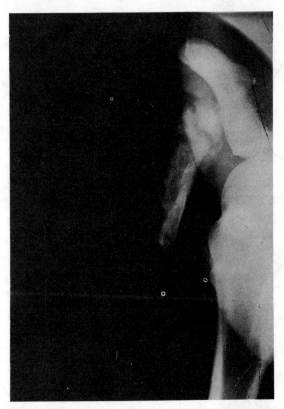

Fig. 25.10 Old rectus femoris origin strain; calcification at upper attachment.

thermy together with exercise—in more chronic cases injection of the psoas attachment to the lesser trochanter using local anaesthetic and hydrocortisone is usually effective.

Hamstring tears may involve semi-membranous, semitendinosus or biceps (long head) and although they are relatively simple to treat, recurrence is common; it is often possible to feel knotty fibrous thickening in the hamstrings of veteran sprinters. In those cases where early recurrence takes place following apparently effective treatment, very determined efforts must be made not only to maintain full extensibility in the affected muscle group but also to correct any biomechanical fault in the patient's technique or style which may be provoking the strain.

Bicipital tendonitis is occasionally seen and is sometimes difficult to differentiate from strains of the lowest muscle fibres or sprains of the lateral ligament of the knee.[14] Differentiation in the latter case can be made because pain is not reproduced by 'springing' the knee.

This condition, or its close relative biceps insertion strain can also frequently mimic lateral meniscus tear, particularly when the knee is not properly examined *in flexion*. The reason will be apparent from reference to the illustration (Fig. 25.11).

Treatment is by hydrocortisone injection backed up by graded exercise.

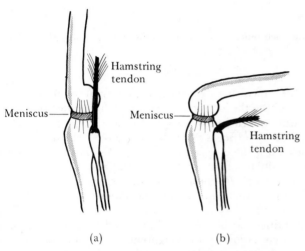

(a)   (b)

Fig. 25.11 Relationship of hamstring tendon to meniscus and collateral ligament. (a) Close in extension. (b) More widely separated in flexion.

Fractures

Femoral fractures need no specific comment in the present context. Treatment is along generally accepted lines. It is essential that any patient with an obvious or suspected femoral fracture should be moved with extreme care—bad handling may cause further severe damage to the soft tissue, particularly the muscles and vessels due to laceration by the mobile bone-ends.

The knee joint

The knee joint is the site of a wide variety of different injuries and disorders[3, 11, 15, 16, 17] which may best be understood if considered from an anatomical point of view (Fig. 25.12). It is, in addition, the site of referred pain from the hip.

The capsule of the knee joint is lined throughout on its 'non-weight-bearing' aspects by a delicate synovial membrane (see Chapter 15) thrown into folds beside the patella (the alar folds), and is reinforced at certain sites by more or less well-

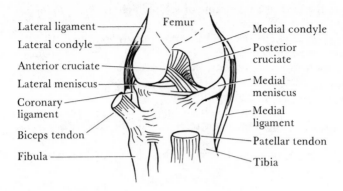

Lateral ligament
Lateral condyle
Anterior cruciate
Lateral meniscus
Coronary ligament
Biceps tendon
Fibula
Femur
Medial condyle
Posterior cruciate
Medial meniscus
Medial ligament
Patellar tendon
Tibia

Fig. 25.12 The anatomy of the knee joint; anterior aspect of the joint open with the patella removed.

differentiated ligaments, chief of which are the medial and lateral collateral ligaments. In addition, there lie within the joint in association with the intercondylar septum the anterior and posterior cruciate ligaments. In the anterior part of the capsule are the patella and the quadriceps and patella tendons, which together with the quadriceps muscle form the extensor apparatus. Within the joint and applied to the margins of the tibial condyles are the medial and lateral menisci (cartilages) tethered to the tibia by the coronary ligaments.

The weight-bearing surfaces of the femur, tibia, and patella are covered by articular cartilage.

Any of these anatomical entities may be the site of injury or disease. In addition, there are a number of other conditions in the neighbourhood of the knee joint which may be encountered among athletes.[14]

Capsule sprains ('Sprained knee')

Such injuries are due to the application of stresses to the knee joint resulting in movement outside the normal range, but which are not sufficiently violent to provoke fracture, dislocation or ligament tear. Normally the patient can pinpoint the time of the injury—the knee became painful but usually he was able to continue playing. The onset of swelling is delayed, often by some hours, and the patient frequently complains that his knee was stiff and swollen when he woke up on the morning after a game. On examination the knee joint will be tender all over, more markedly so at one particular site, and will be found to contain a small effusion. There is generally slight limitation of movement at extremes of joint range, the degree of limitation being directly proportional to the amount of effusion. Such an effusion need not be aspirated; any aspirate that may be removed by the overenthusiastic is usually clear or straw-coloured and glairy.

Treatment of simple capsular sprain consists of exercises, initially static or non-weight bearing but gradually increasing in scope and vigour. A crêpe bandage may be worn in the initial stages (but must be discarded as soon as possible) and if pain is very severe, the patient may require a stick. Generally, however, a simple capsular sprain is not unduly painful and when pain is severe some other injury should be suspected.

Stable instability

A particular complication of capsular sprain (usually hyperextension strain) as well as of more severe injury is loss of functional stability of the knee joint and repeated 'giving way' or 'letting down'. When such a situation presents in a knee (or other) joint which is clinically stable it is presumed that there has been damage to the proprioceptive feedback mechanism.[14] Treatment calls for proprioceptive rehabilitation of the joint and involves use of such appliances as the 'wobble board' together with controlled exercise with the joint stressed, e.g. the 'Groucho Marx Walk'.

Traumatic synovitis (haemarthrosis)

Sometimes the type of injury which provokes a sprain of the knee joint will produce a sudden, extremely painful swelling of the knee, and the player is unable to continue the game. In such cases damage to the synovia has occurred (perhaps by 'nipping' of the synovial fringes of the alar folds between the femoral and tibial condyles). In such cases the effusion is well marked (50 ml or more) and is deeply bloodstained. The knee is extremely painful and sometimes exquisitely tender, and is held in a position of about 20° flexion, which gives maximum capsular relaxation. Limitation of movement is much more marked than in capsular sprain.

When such cases present careful search must be made for associated injury of ligaments or joint surfaces, and the examination should include X-rays; examination under general anaesthesia may also be required. It is said that haemarthrosis with distension of the joint capsule is not seen in association with complete ligament rupture, as the contents of the joint are able to escape through the breach; though this is often true exceptions occur with sufficient regularity to suggest that such injuries should always be deliberately excluded in cases of haemarthrosis.

The presence of blood within the joint does not of itself demand evacuation, but if the haemarthrosis is very tense and is significantly inhibiting knee movement or quadriceps function (see below) it is advisable to aspirate. In the acute case intra-articular steroids should *not* be used.

When aspiration is carried out, and indeed in all cases of haemarthrosis, a pressure bandage should be applied. The classical type of pressure bandage is the 'Robert Jones', but it is cumbersome, and if carelessly applied readily comes loose.

A crêpe and cotton wool dressing is a very efficient and satisfactory method of applying pressure. Exercises within the limits of pain tolerance are instituted from the outset and even when aspiration has not been undertaken, early resolution of the haemarthrosis may be expected. Provided that quadriceps tone is maintained, return to sport is usually permissible within three to four weeks.

On no account should unqualified rest be prescribed in the treatment of these or any other forms of minor knee injury. The primary cause of delayed recovery in all cases of knee injury is wasting of the quadriceps group of muscles, particu-

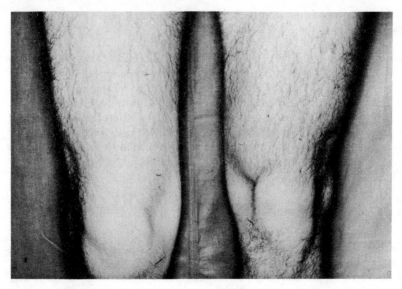

Fig. 25.13 Muscle wasting following injury to right knee joint.

larly the vastus medialis. The wasting becomes increasingly more marked as the time lag between the injury and the initiation of the active treatment lengthens, becoming at the same time increasingly more difficult to treat.

The degree of functional disability resulting from a knee injury is inversely proportional to the power of the quadriceps, and therefore the active restoration and maintenance of power in this muscle group is the key to early recovery from knee injuries.[18, 20] Ideally treatment should be started before the quadriceps has begun to waste, that is, at the latest, the day after injury (Fig. 25.13).

Chronic effusion ('water on the knee')

From time to time a sportsman presents complaining of a swollen knee with little if any pain and no *recent* history of trauma (although almost invariably there has been some injury in the past). In these cases an effusion is found, frequently quite large, together with loss of quadriceps bulk and tone. In the absence of some obvious abnormality such as clinical instability or a strongly positive McMurray's sign it may be inferred that this is due to failure of effective rehabilitation of some prior injury. Treatment is aspiration of the effusion (typically clear or faintly straw coloured and glairy) and instillation of hydrocortisone (25–50 mg). A firm pressure bandage is applied followed by a regime of quadriceps rehabilitation as for chondromalacia (p. 460). If stable instability is a feature of the history, the rehabilitation programme must also involve proprioceptive re-education.

Collateral ligament injuries

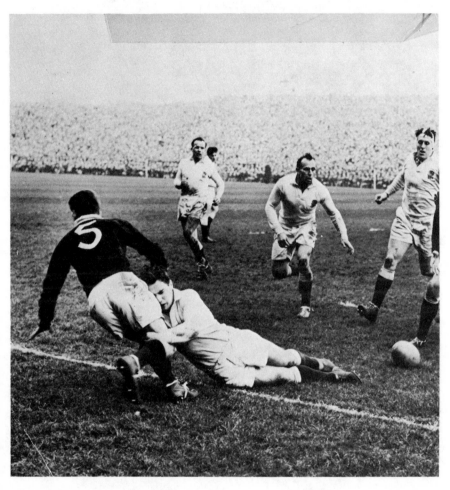

Fig. 25.14 These photographs illustrate how strains may be thrown on the collateral ligaments of the knee. In (a) the strain is thrown on the lateral ligament of the left knee of player No. 5.

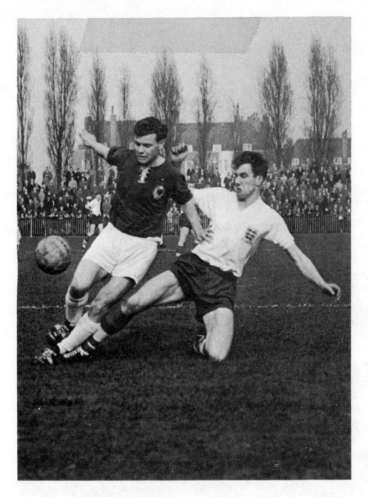

Fig. 25.14 (b) The strain is thrown on the medial ligament of the right knee of the white-shirted player. (Photo: Sport and General.)

These injuries follow severe abduction or adduction strains on the knee joint (Fig. 25.14).[21, 22] Simple sprain or partial or complete rupture may be seen, the latter associated with cruciate or meniscus injury if the damaging strain has any rotational component.[11]

In collateral ligament sprains the clinical picture is similar to that of capsular sprain, with pain, tenderness and occasionally swelling localized to one or other ligament (Fig. 25.15). Pain is also reproduced by 'springing' the knee, that is abducting or adducting the extended knee. (The collateral ligaments are attached eccentrically and are normally slightly lax when the knee is flexed.)

A more subtle test for medial collateral ligament damage has been described by Trickey.[23] The knee is flexed and the lower leg externally rotated. The tibia is then drawn forwards (as in eliciting the old style 'anterior drawer sign'; see cruciate ligaments below) and pain or laxity are indications of medial collateral ligament damage.

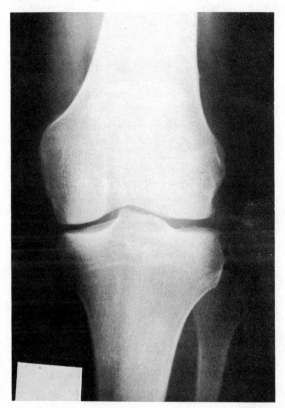

Fig. 25.15 Lateral ligament sprain; flake of bone pulled off tibial attachment of lateral ligament of the knee.

Treatment of collateral ligament sprains is by exercise, to which may be added ultrasonics, shortwave diathermy or injection of local anaesthetic with hyalase. If a local anaesthetic is used subsequent activity must be carried out under strict control.

Stubborn cases respond well to injection with steroids.

Partial ligamentous tears

In these cases symptoms are similar to those of sprain, but are more pronounced. In addition, there may be associated effusion or even haemarthrosis and some laxity of the ligaments may be demonstrated on 'springing'. There is, however, no frank instability of the joint.

Treatment consists of immobilizing the joint so as to prevent the application of abduction or adduction stresses to it, quadriceps tone being maintained with static exercises for a period of four to six weeks to allow healing to take place.

The degree of immobilization required will depend on the severity of the injury, and may be maintained by a plaster of Paris cylinder (bivalved in the later stages of treatment to allow removal of the limb for flexion exercises) or, better still, the short leg guard and hinge. The latter permits flexion exercises from the first, while preventing rotation and abduction or adduction at the joint.[24]

As in all cases, vigorous quadriceps drill is carried on throughout the period of treatment, and the patient is only allowed to return to his sport when his quadriceps on the injured side is as good as, or better, than that on the un-injured side.

Complete ligamentous tear

Complete rupture of a collateral ligament presents a knee that is swollen and unstable, showing well marked laxity on 'springing' and widening of one side of the joint gap on stress X-rays (Fig. 25.16). Local tenderness is marked, but surprisingly the patient often complains of little pain.

Treatment is by surgical repair of the torn ligament together with the associ-

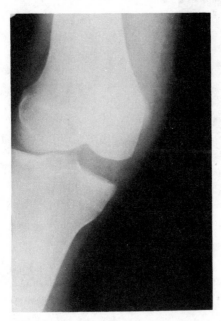

Fig. 25.16 X-ray photograph of the knee. Medial collateral ligament tear demonstrated by taking the X-ray while the tibia is abducted, thus opening up the unstable joint.

ated capsular defect. Frequently the meniscus is also detached (especially on the medial side, where the inner fasciculus of the ligament is attached to it) and the anterior cruciate may also be torn—the 'unhappy triad'.[16] In such cases meniscectomy is also undertaken, but there is generally no need to repair the anterior cruciate unless the tibial spine has been avulsed.

Post-operative immobilization for six weeks together with quadriceps drill, and vigorous rehabilitation at the end of immobilization, is required. It is unusual for a knee that has been the site of so severe an injury to become strong enough to enable resumption of body-contact sports unless a very dynamic policy of re-habilitation has been pursued as soon as immobilization is over.

Pellegrini-Stieda's disease
In this condition there is heterotopic calcification in the upper fibres of the medial collateral ligament.[25] The patient presents with a hard tender swelling over the medial aspect of the lower end of the femur, and a history of previous abduction strain on the knee joint may be elicited. There is local tenderness and pain may be felt on 'springing' the knee. Sometimes a small effusion is present, and quadriceps wasting may be marked. The X-ray appearances are typical (Fig. 25.17).

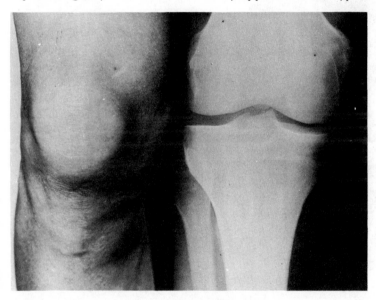

Fig. 25.17 The clinical and radiological appearances of Pellagrini–Stieda's disease.

Treatment is by restoration of quadriceps tone, together with local injection of hydrocortisone into the tender site. This is usually enough to effect relief from painful symptoms, through the lump will usually persist. In obstinate cases surgical excision of the deposit may be required, together with re-attachment of the upper end of the medial ligament.

The condition is probably due to faulty healing following partial avulsion of the upper attachment of the medial collateral ligament.

Posterior capsular tear
Posterior capsular tear is an uncommon injury in sport but may follow severe hyperextension strains. In the absence of damage to associated structures, the signs include painful swelling behind the knee with haemorrhage into the popliteal fossa. Instability in extension may be marked and is an indication for explora-

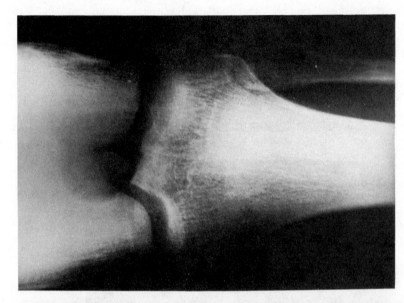

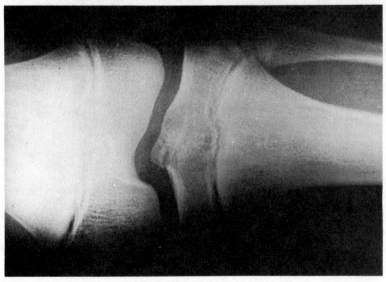

Fig. 25.18 Cruciate ligaments. (a) Fracture of anterior tibial spine (distal attachment of anterior cruciate ligament) in a young footballer causing (b) loose body at maturity.

tion and repair of the defect. After care is as for complete collateral ligament tear.

Cruciate ligaments

Anteroposterior shearing stress causing damage to the cruciate ligaments is relatively uncommon in sport except perhaps in the U.S.A., where the techniques of tackling in American Football make such injuries a recognized hazard. Complete rupture or avulsion of a cruciate, or fracture of its bony attachment (Fig. 25.18) do, however, occur with monotonous regularity, and are characterized by anteroposterior instability of the knee (Fig. 25.19). Clinically, posterior cruci-

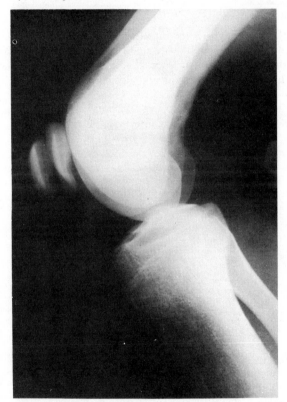

Fig. 25.19 Anteroposterior instability of the knee joint demonstrated by superimposition radiograph.

ate instability is demonstrated by the 'posterior drawer sign', but the anterior drawer sign for anterior cruciate laxity is only valid if the lower leg is *internally rotated*. Laxity of the cruciates, particularly the anterior, is very common; indeed, it is tempting to say that anterior cruciate laxity can be disregarded when a positive anterior drawer sign is elicited in all cases in which there is no evidence in the history nor any other clinical finding to suggest recent rupture.

When rupture is diagnosed the choice between surgical repair and conservative management must be made. Where there is definite evidence of bone damage (avulsion of the attachments) on X-ray, replacement and fixation with wire sutures or screws is indicated and is generally successful.

Various authors have techniques of repair chiefly remarkable for their diversity and ingenuity but repair of tears in the ligaments themselves is not generally indicated, for a perfectly sound knee may result from conservative management with the accent on development of the supporting musculature. Pes anserinus transplant is, however, worth considering for rotational instability[26, 27] and lateral pivot shift may require surgical repair.

Clinical laxity is relatively unimportant if the knee is functionally stable.

The menisci and coronary ligaments

There is a tendency to label the majority of knee injuries as 'cartilages', but in fact damage to the menisci is found in a remarkably small percentage of cases.

True cartilage tears are more common on the medial than lateral side, and are seen more often in men than women. The tear is really a split in the long axis of the cartilage which, when extensive, allows the free border to 'bowstring' across the joint into the intercondylar space. The other common variety of tear is the 'horn tag' or parrot beak tear usually found posteriorly (Fig. 25.20).

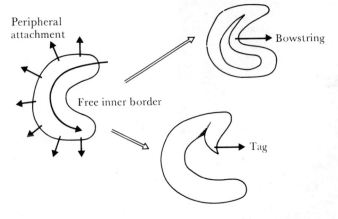

Fig. 25.20 As the free border is submitted to rotational stress it splits, either along the length of the meniscus to 'bowstring' or 'bucket handle' or onto the border to form a tag.

In some cases cartilage tear may be mimicked by an intact but excessively mobile meniscus due to laxity of the coronary ligaments or by a congenitally abnormal meniscus such as the discoid type. Classically the tear presents as pain on the inner or outer side of the joint line following a rotational strain on the flexed weight-bearing knee (Fig. 25.21).[28] This may be associated with locking of the knee or a block to full extension due to the interposition of the free border of the meniscus between the femoral and tibial condyles. The patient complains of a painful knee which may be the site of a small effusion. There is tenderness along the margin of the tibial condyle, and sometimes the meniscus can be palpated, moving in and out as the knee is gently flexed and extended in its middle range. If the knee is not locked extension is usually full, but there may be

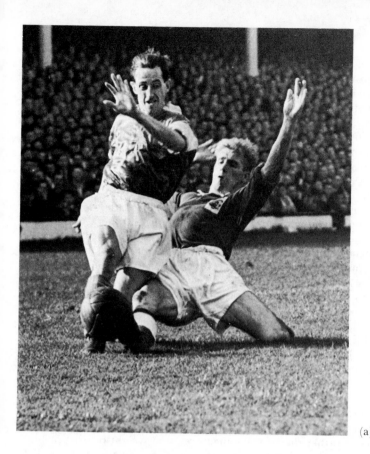

(a)

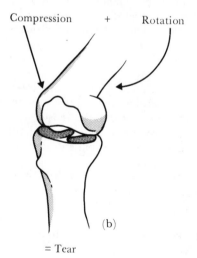

Compression   +   Rotation

(b)

= Tear

Fig. 25.21 '... following a rotational strain on the flexed weight-bearing knee'. In (a) just such tackles as that illustrated are severe rotational strains thrown on the knee. The mechanism is illustrated in (b). (Photo: Sport and General.)

some limitation of full flexion with pain felt at the side and back of the knee. McMurray's sign may be elicited, and will serve to strengthen the diagnosis, but it must be regarded with circumspection as false-positives and false-negatives are not uncommon.

When the knee is 'locked' there may be complete immobility, but much more often there is a block of full extension. The displaced meniscus may be reduced by McMurray's manœuvre which often requires general anaesthesia. In the absence of a clear history other causes of locking of the knee must be excluded (see p. 454).

The treatment of meniscus tears is meniscectomy, either with removal of the inner detached portion or with complete removal of the cartilage. The former is technically more simple and quite as effective if the peripheral part of the meniscus is not unduly mobile. There is much to be said for regarding classical tears as semi-emergencies and carrying out immediate operation, as quadriceps wasting may be prevented, with subsequent ease of rehabilitation. In doubtful cases conservative measures may be used at first *provided quadriceps tone is maintained*. The key to successful meniscectomy is adequate pre-operative exercise.

Following operation, a fairly vigorous programme of rehabilitation is required—there is no need to immobilize the knee joint. Some effusion may be expected, but this will subside within a few days, particularly if an effective pressure bandage is worn.

Usually a patient is fit to resume training within one month, and may compete again two weeks after this. On no account should a patient be pushed too hard within the first few weeks—overenthusiastic rehabilitation, with particular reference to weight-bearing exercises, may easily provoke chronic effusion and may lead to serious and prolonged disability. Limitation of movement must be overcome by active rather than passive measures, and weight-bearing or high-load exercises should only be instituted if the patient can accomplish them without pain (some degree of discomfort is inevitable). Competition should never be permitted while symptoms persist or there is any demonstrable quadriceps weakness.

Cysts of cartilages

The lateral meniscus is most commonly affected (Fig. 25.22). A firm, sometimes tender, swelling presents over (usually) the anterolateral aspect of the joint line. Fluctuation is seldom elicited as the contents of the cyst are under tension.

Symptoms are variable, and may be due to the cyst itself or to concomitant chondromalacia. Pain is sometimes felt, but most frequently patients present because of the presence of the lump.

Aspiration is generally valueless, and treatment is by operation with excision of the cyst together with the affected cartilage.

Coronary ligament strains

These are not uncommon and present much the same clinical picture as true meniscus injuries. Pain is not usually very severe and locking does not occur. Tenderness is related to the joint line and may be pronounced. Swelling is rare and there is seldom any effusion. McMurray's sign is negative.

Treatment consists of graduated exercises to which may be added short wave

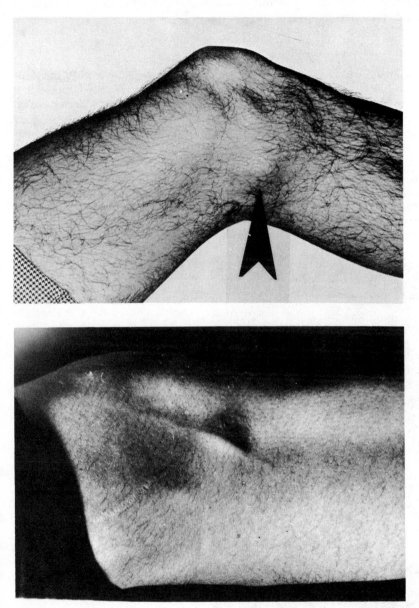

Fig. 25.22 Cystic meniscus. (a) Medial side in a middle distance runner. (b) Lateral side in a footballer.

diathermy or ultrasonics. Topical hydrocortisone in doses of 25 mg often produces a dramatic amelioration of symptoms, though even with the most vigorous treatment, pain may persist for three weeks or more.

Locking of the knee joint

Locking of the knee occurs when there is a mechanical defect within the joint which prohibits movement through its full normal range. It may occur within the same limits of arc (when it is due to a meniscus tear or chondromalacia) or in any position (when a loose body is usually the cause—such a loose body may be bony, cartilaginous or fibrous).

Transient 'locking' with subsequent acute haemarthrosis may be due to nipping of the alar folds. In recurrent cases pedunculated tags may form which require surgical removal. Investigation of the locked knee or the intermittently locking knee should include X-rays which may show the presence of a loose body.

In cases of difficulty, arthroscopy may be of great diagnostic value and may be carried out as an immediate prelude to arthrotomy if indicated.

The treatment of locked knee is the treatment of cause. As a temporary measure

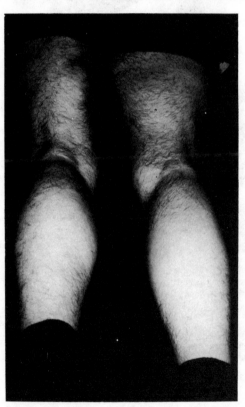

Fig. 25.23 Hamstring spasm secondary to an injury to the left knee joint. Note the visible knot of spastic medial hamstrings in the left leg.

the knee can frequently be 'unlocked' by manipulation, but subsequent meniscectomy or arthrotomy and removal of loose bodies is required.

Spontaneous healing of a torn meniscus seldom, if ever, occurs and the untreated knee progresses through a series of episodes of locking associated with quadriceps wasting and increasing disability until such time as either the patient is so discouraged that he gives up his sport, or he has to give it up through the onset of secondary degenerative changes.

Chondromalacia may present as 'locking' of the knee, but close questioning of the patient will usually reveal that what really happens is that as the knee is extended it stiffens up and becomes painful, but that if the patient persists in the movement there is a sudden painful giving way allowing completion of extension—in other words there is a 'painful arc' which inhibits but cannot prevent full movement. Sometimes true locking occurs when there has been desquamation of the patellar cartilage with loose body formation.

Osteochondritis dissecans[29] is a common cause of loose body formation in the younger patient and may present as locking of the knee. Replacement of the fragment is of dubious value and removal at arthrotomy probably offers the best hope of early functional recovery.

False locking

Not infrequently inability fully to extend the knee after trauma is erroneously described as 'locking'[14] and is attributed to meniscus tear. Care should be taken to exclude hamstring insertion strain (see above) or secondary hamstring spasm as the cause.

In some instances secondary hamstring spasm may be so marked and persistent that energetic measures must be taken for its suppression, i.e. with ice, massage and stretching, before the knee itself can be properly examined and treated (Fig. 25.23).

Functional and structural anomalies

The most important anomalies are valgus ('knock-knee') and varus ('bow-legged') deformities. The former is most common in women and girls and may be an element in the production of chondromalacia patellae. These deformities usually mitigate biomechanically against top class sports performance, but may be associated with ligament and capsular injuries at lower levels of sport.

Genu recurvatum is less common but is occasionally met (Fig. 25.24). It may exist by itself or be part of a generalized 'hypermobile joint disease' in which all the patient's joints are excessively mobile, tending particularly to hyperextend.[30] When the condition is marked, body-contact sports should be avoided as well as those involving severe take-off thrusts from the leg, for example high jumping.

Condylar anomalies are not common, but a low lateral or high medial condylar ridge may predispose to patellar subluxation or dislocation.[31]

Other anomalies such as discoid menisci are rare.

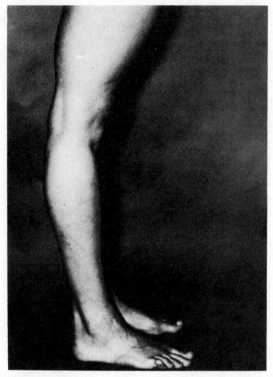

Fig. 25.24 Genu recurvatum; a cause of chondromalacia patellae in a young pentathlete with hypermobile joints.

Severe knee injury

Dislocation of the knee joint

Such a severe injury, associated as it is with extensive capsular and ligamentous damage, will generally preclude the possibility of further serious sport. Treatment is according to accepted practice. Rehabilitation in such cases is geared to the more modified requirements of the patient. Further sport is permissible only if the knee will meet its demands as demonstrated by a suitable 'fitness test'.

Fractures involving the knee joint

Fractures involving the knee joint (other than fractures of the patella) are not common in sport. Avulsion of the tibial spine (anterior cruciate ligament) has already been discussed. Tibial plateau fractures and fractures involving the condyles of the femur may be met, particularly after riding or driving accidents. Epiphysiolysis is sometimes seen in children and may follow relatively trivial injury.

There is no special problem in the management of these injuries which is according to usual orthopaedic practice—the type of subsequent rehabilitation and the possibility of return to sport will depend on the nature and severity of the injury.

Tumours

Occasionally in young patients, tumours, including giant cell tumours and sarcomata, may present in sports injuries clinics and in such cases the knee is a common site. This possibility must not be overlooked (Fig. 25.25).

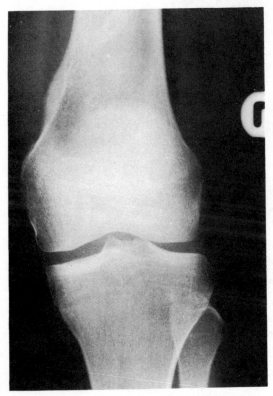

Fig. 25.25 Cautionary tale; osteosarcoma presenting as a netball injury.

Degenerative conditions

Osteoarthrosis is a common late sequel of knee injury, especially if the treatment at the time was inadequate; additional factors in the aetiology include obesity in the patient and congenital deformity of the knee joint.

It is typically a disease of middle age and senescence, and may not manifest itself until a specific incident of trauma 'triggers off' symptoms. It may, however, present in the younger subject with a long history of knee trouble (Fig. 25.26).

The essentials of treatment are maintenance of mobility and muscle tone, together with attention to diet in the overweight. Some cases may benefit by operation (removal of loose bodies, patellectomy, etc.), but conservative measures should be employed as far as possible: of these short wave diathermy and graduated exercises are the most valuable. Intra-articular hydrocortisone may also be helpful, but should not be repeated too frequently.

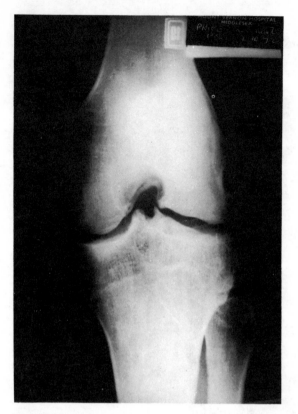

Fig. 25.26 Osteoarthrosis of the knee joint in a 29-year-old Olympic weight lifter.

Osgood–Schlatter's disease

Osgood–Schlatter's disease or anterior tibial osteochondritis is a condition in which the epiphysis of the anterior tibial tubercle becomes infarcted due to excessive pull from the patella tendon (Fig. 25.27). It is more common in boys than girls and the age range is from 10 to 16 years.

Treatment is a period (usually three months is enough) off sport. Although apparently contrary to the principle of 'active' treatment of sports injury, the prescription of rest here is frequently justified because the patient is often the victim of excessive parental pressure. In late cases, excision of the epiphyseal debris may be necessary.

Popliteal cysts

Fluctuant swellings in the popliteal fossa may be tuberculous in origin (Baker's cysts—rare), aneurysmal, or most commonly 'bursal'. This latter group includes gastrocnemius bursa and ganglions. They present as smooth, firm fluctuant swellings lying in the popliteal fossa. They seldom provoke symptoms, though occa-

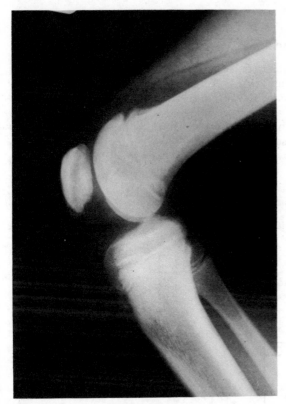

Fig. 25.27 Two birds with one stone! Osgood–Schlatter's disease and Sinding–Larsen–Johannson's disease in the same knee.

sionally pain, usually aching in quality, is attributed to them. When large they may embarrass full excursion of the knee joint. Generally, their only effect is the mental disquiet occasioned by their presence.

Aspiration is seldom successful and operative removal is indicated when their presence is a positive embarrassment.

Other bursae around the knee joint

Occasionally an athlete is troubled by the presence of a pre-patellar or infrapatellar bursa, which may become inflamed ('housemaid's knee') or the site of a chronic effusion.

Septic bursitis is treated by incision and drainage under antibiotic cover, chronic bursitis by excision of the bursa if symptoms warrant this procedure. Simple aspiration may be tried as a temporary measure, but is seldom productive of a permanent cure. When bursitis is due to surface friction in sport, some protective padding should be worn.[32]

The patella

Chondromalacia patellae

This is a condition in which the undersurface (articular cartilage) of the patella undergoes fibrillation and roughening.[33-35] There is no change in the underlying bone in early cases. It is a disease of youth rather than senescence (Fig. 25.28).[36]

Chondromalacia is a kind of clinical chameleon and may mimic practically all the other injuries and disabilities of the knee. In the classical case the clinical picture is definite. Pain or discomfort is felt in the knee after exercise, on going up or, more frequently, down stairs, or after sitting for a long time with the knee bent; when accompanied by the signs of retropatellar tenderness, compression

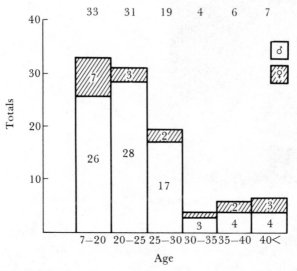

Fig. 25.28 Chondromalacia patellae; age and sex distribution in 100 cases in sportsmen.

pain and sometimes swelling of the knee, together with loss of quadriceps bulk and tone, the diagnosis is established.

Compression pain is now readily elicited by Clarke's sign by pressing distally on the upper pole of the patella as the patient lies relaxed with his knee extended (Fig. 25.29). The patient is then asked to contract his quadriceps while the patella is pressed upon the articular condyles of the lower end of the femur. If the patient can complete and maintain the contraction without pain the sign is negative. In chondromalacia patellae the contraction elicits sharp retropatellar pain and cannot be maintained—the sign is then positive.

Many accounts of the condition are available in the literature and there is remarkable conformity in clinical pictures described.[19, 33, 34, 35, 36, 37, 46] Few authors have, however, noted the apparent importance of vastus medialis

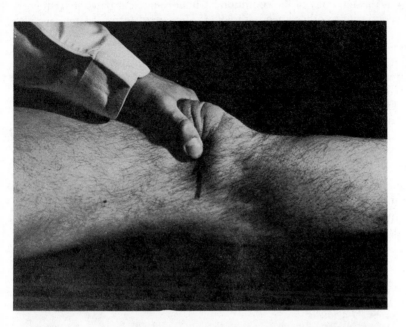

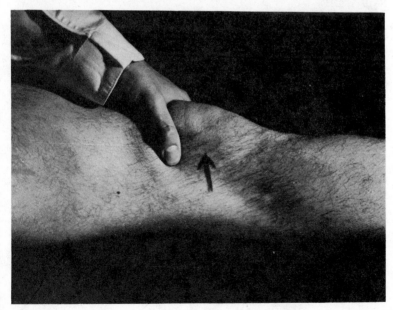

Fig. 25.29 Eliciting Clarke's sign. (a) The patella is pressed distally as the patient lies with his knee extended and his quadriceps relaxed. (b) The patient is now contracting his quadriceps and so pulling the patella proximally over its articulation with the femur.

function in the aetiology of the condition.[3] Chondromalacia patellae frequently occurs secondarily to other knee pathology[37] after quadriceps wasting (see also below).

Reference to the anatomy of the extensor apparatus of the knee[19] indicates immediately that vastus medialis has a function mechanically different from the other three components of the quadriceps muscle. Vastus medialis is inserted onto the medial side of the patella, whereas the quadriceps tendon is inserted superolaterally (Fig. 25.30). Furthermore, the fibres of vastus medialis (particularly in its more distal part where they lie more horizontally) are inserted directly onto

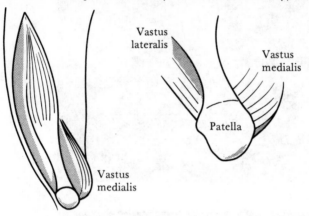

Fig. 25.30 Anatomy of elements of the quadriceps muscle as an expression of their function. Note axis of lower fibres of vastus medialis.

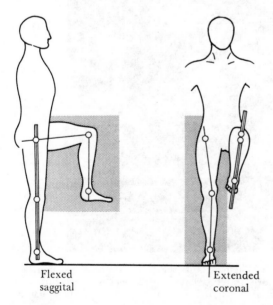

Fig. 25.31 Planes of the knee joint in flexion and extension.

the patella, while the rest of quadriceps is inserted by its more vertical and oblique tendon.

When the knee is flexed, the hip, knee joint and ankle together lie in the sagittal plane of the body. It is only during the last few degrees of extension that the plane of the knee joint rotates through almost a right angle and comes to lie coronally (Fig. 25.31).

In flexion the pull of the quadriceps tendon on the patella tends to press the patella more firmly on to the articular surface of the femur. (French[38] has suggested that in extreme flexion the pressure on the under surface of the patella may be equivalent to 20 times the body weight.) However, in the last few degrees

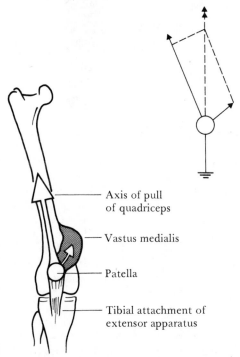

Axis of pull
of quadriceps

Vastus medialis

Patella

Tibial attachment of
extensor apparatus

Fig. 25.32 Mechanics of the extensor apparatus of the knee in extension (by courtesy of *Rheumatism*).

of extension, when the plane of the leg has turned through 90°, the quadriceps tendon tends to displace the patella laterally, in the same way that the bowstring displaces the arrow. Vastus medialis (which only functions in extension—though this is not universally agreed[39]) can now be observed restraining this tendency (Fig. 25.32).

The geometry of the situation is clearly demonstrated by the parallelogram of forces. Where there is any weakness or failure of vastus medialis, for example due to inhibition associated with painful limitation of extension after trauma, the displacing tendency of the quadriceps tendon pull can only be resisted by the relatively high lateral condylar ridge, and the situation is exacerbated by

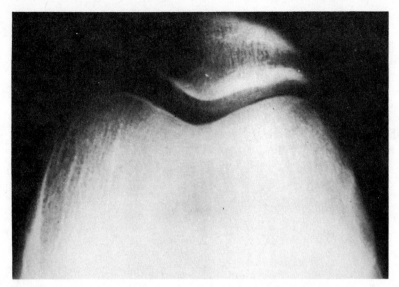

Fig. 25.33 Chondromalacia patellae; tipping of patella to lateral side on skyline view, sometimes called 'subluxation of the patella'.

local mechanical factors such as small or excessively large patella, patella alta, low condylar ridge or patellar instability.[40–42] Hughston's view that the patella actually *subluxates* is not entirely convincing, but the tipping of the patella (Fig. 25.33) he describes is certainly seen with wasting of vastus medialis.[41]

The relationship of the biomechanical effect of vastus medialis weakness to the pathological changes is difficult to evaluate but it does appear that concentration of the load on articular cartilage is of relatively little importance. Compression of the patella in extension against the medial femoral condyle[31] must be reduced when the vastus medialis is weakened. It seems that loss of normal compression of the articular cartilage rather than excessive weight-bearing triggers off the initial degeneration.[43]

Given such a biomechanical basis for the condition, treatment clearly involves restoration of normal vastus medialis function, and results of such a procedure involving specifically *straight leg* static quadriceps re-education (if necessary electrically assisted[44]; Fig. 25.34) are good[19] (Fig. 25.35).

A few cases fail to respond. Further management involves the positive exclusion of other pathology as well as direct confirmation of the diagnosis, preferably by arthroscopy. The choice of surgery is then lateral retinacular release[45] or anterior tibial tubercle transplant.[46] These procedures give better results than all others, probably because they are the most sound biomechanically.

Fractures of the patella

Such fractures are treated according to standard orthopaedic practice. Stress fractures of the patella[47] are sometimes met—treatment will depend on the degree of displacement (if any) and the severity of symptoms. They must be differentiated from unilateral bipartite patella[48] (Fig. 25.36).

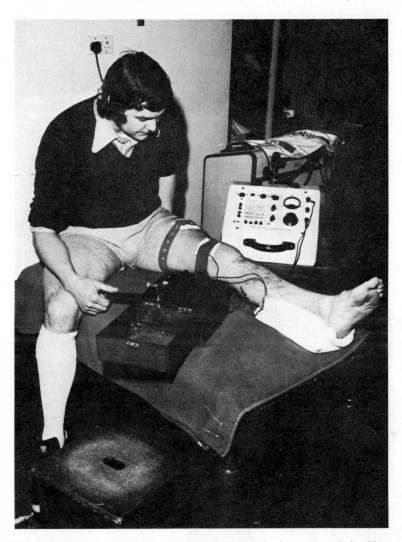

Fig. 25.34 Sequential Faradism for the re-education of vastus medialis. Vastus medialis is stimulated just before the main quadriceps mass.[44]

Bipartite patella

This congenital condition is occasionally a cause of pain in the knee and secondary chondromalacia, particularly if the smaller piece is misaligned. If symptoms persist in the face of energetic conservative management, excision of the piece is justified.

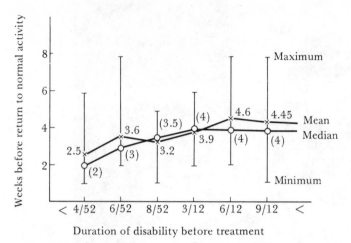

Fig. 25.35 Conservative management of chondromalacia patellae, recovery times for 97/100 cases responding to appropriate vastus medialis re-education.[19]

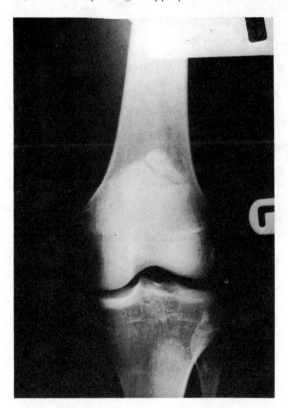

Fig. 25.36 Bipartite patella; not to be confused with a fracture.

Dislocations of the patella

Simple dislocation is clinically obvious as a rule. Treatment is by reduction and subsequent quadriceps rehabilitation. Sometimes the accompanying haemarthrosis will require aspiration. Recurrent dislocation is quite common in cases where the patella is small (the condition may be bilateral). Various methods of treatment are available, but operation is usually required, the type chosen depending on the views and experience of the individual surgeon.

Sinding–Larsen–Johannson disease

This is a rare disease, more common in adolescents, which is a form of osteochondritis of the ossification centre of the lower pole of the patella.[49] The clinical features are similar to chondromalacia, with tenderness and thickening of the lower pole of the patella and pain on kneeling. The X-ray changes are similar to those observed in other osteochondritides (Fig. 25.27). Choice of treatment depends on the age of the patient and the presence or absence of Osgood–Schlatter's disease; six weeks' to six months' rest from sport may be required, together with crêpe bandage support. In late adolescents or young adults, treatment is the same as for chondromalacia. Stubborn cases may require surgical removal of the lower pole of the patella.

The patellar tendon

Like other major tendons, this structure may be the site of peritendonitis, focal degeneration, and partial or complete rupture (see Chapter 16). Complete rupture is fortunately rare, occurring in the older subject. It is an orthopaedic emergency requiring referral for surgical repair.

Extensive incomplete rupture may occasionally pass incorrectly diagnosed as a patellar ligament strain. Pain is felt by the patient on forced extension of the knee, the tissues around the patellar tendon are thickened, and there is a well marked change in the patellar shadow on lateral soft tissue X-ray (Fig. 25.37). The patient frequently presents late with weak or incomplete extension. Treatment depends on the degree of disability, but exploration and plication of the patellar tendon may be necessary.

Chronic patellar tendon strain is a well-known condition observed in high jumpers, basketball players and runners.[50, 51] The main clinical feature is pain in the tendon on exertion. On examination a well localized tender spot is palpable. Histologically, the appearances are of focal or central degeneration with loss of the normal striated collagen, and areas of the tendon demonstrating a 'wet tissue-paper tearing effect'. Blood vessels are also found at the site of degeneration (Fig. 25.38). Treatment by hydrocortisone injection, ultrasonics, rest, short wave diathermy, and heel padding have all been tried and may produce relief in a number of cases. Recently, surgical decompression under local anaesthetic with accurate localization of the lesion has been practised (Fig. 25.39), and if this procedure is immediately followed up by an intensive programme of rehabilitation, return to full training, symptom-free, may be achieved within a period of fourteen days.

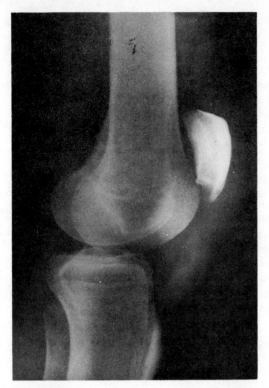

Fig. 25.37 Partial rupture of a patellar tendon; soft tissue radiograph showing character-istic appearances. (The apparent density of the patella is a technical artefact.)

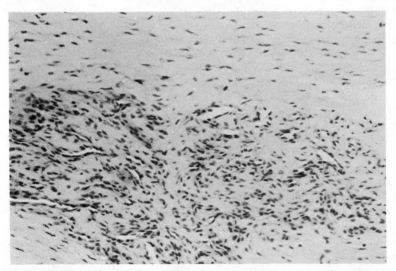

Fig. 25.38 Patellar tendon; focal degeneration—histology ($\times 225$) showing infiltration of tendon with granulation tissue and loss of normal collagen pattern. (Photomicrograph by Dr Leowi.)

This condition is frequently found and associated with chondromalacia patellae which is a particularly cogent reason for embarking on intensive post-operative rehabilitation.

Peritendonitis of the patellar tendon is quite common, frequently in association with focal degeneration, when adhesions between the site of the degeneration and the surrounding tissues may be demonstrated. Unlike other tendons such as the Achilles tendon, the patellar tendon has no well-formed paratenon so that the delineation of the adhesions between the tendon and the surrounding tissue

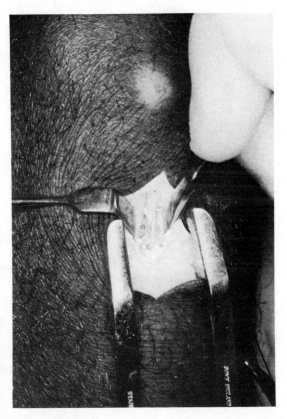

Fig. 25.39 Focal degeneration of the patellar tendon. Operative appearance showing extensive lesion.

is less well marked. The condition is almost impossible to differentiate clinically from chronic patellar tendon strain (focal degeneration), since its clinical findings are identical, but at operation it may be demonstrated when dense adhesions between the tendon and the surrounding structures can be cleared away leaving a clean tendon with no intratendonous lesion. In these cases of true peritendonitis, the post-operative regime is as for patellar decompression and the results are uniformly excellent.

The lower leg

Injuries of the lower leg include fractures of tibia and/or fibula, tibialis anterior and posterior compression syndromes, tendoperiostosis, muscle strains and bruises, and Achilles tendon lesions.[52]

Because of the general nature of sporting activities, especially the degree of running involved, the pattern of injury tends progressively from extrinsic to intrinsic as the site moves distally.[53] Thus whereas in the upper leg and thigh direct injury or acute strains occur, lower in the leg chronic over-use injury predominates.[54]

Fractures

Fractures may be due to direct violence as in the various football codes, or indirect violence (particularly rotational strains) as in skiing. Stress fractures are also common.

The treatment of major fractures is according to standard orthopaedic practice. The history of the mechanism of injury is important as it may suggest damage in other sites also, for example the knee joint in torsion fractures of tibia and fibula.

Minor fractures of the fibula may pass unnoticed at first, being labelled 'bruise' or 'sprain'. When recognized they may be treated by simple support and exercise, unless there is any evidence of associated joint derangement. Fractures of the distal third of the fibula are often associated with rupture of the medial ligament of the ankle joint, and this injury must be excluded before mobilization is undertaken (see p. 485). Occasionally the tibiofibular articulations may be damaged.[55]

Stress fractures[56]

Stress fractures of the tibia and fibula have already been discussed in Chapter 14.

They should always be suspected in the patient with a history of progressive pain in the leg associated with exercise, if an area of local bony tenderness is demonstrable. Sometimes a bony swelling may be palpable but this is uncommon.

Differential diagnosis is mainly from tibialis anterior syndrome. Rarely the same clinical picture is presented by osteomyelitis, osteoid osteoma or other bone tumour.

Shin splints—shin soreness

This is a fairly common problem among athletes who complain of pain in the front of the leg on exercise.[57–59] It may be due to stress fracture, to tibialis anterior syndrome or to tendoperiostosis or tibialis posterior syndrome. Differentiation may be made from the site of the pain, and the fact that the mode of onset varies. Stress fractures exhibit the typical features described in Chapter 14.

Tibialis anterior syndrome
This is characterized by pain in the anterolateral muscular compartment of the leg on exercise. Various theories have been put forward to explain its aetio-

logy,[60-62] but all are based on the antomical peculiarity of the tibialis anterior
in that it lies enclosed between two bones, a fibrous septum and a well-developed
fascial layer. One view is that pain is due to ischaemia, the arterial supply being
jeopardized by the tight fascial layer;[63] the more likely explanation is that
symptoms are due to raised intramuscular tension, since symptoms persist even
when exercise is stopped. All muscles, particularly untrained muscles, swell after
exercise (see Chapter 17). In most muscle groups this swelling is encompassed
with no increase in intramuscular tension, but where expansion is restricted by
the surrounding tissues (as in the case of the tibialis anterior), engorgement
of the muscle and increase of interstitial fluid must result in the raising of intramuscular tension. This explanation receives support from Lloyd's observations
of the incidence of tibialis anterior syndrome in marathon runners at the
Cardiff Commonwealth Games.[6]

Treatment of this syndrome is difficult; various methods have been advocated,
of which elevation, massage and short wave diathermy appear to be the most
effective. In severe cases, operative decompression may be necessary. Even with
vigorous physiotherapy, symptoms may persist for a considerable time, so that
it becomes most important to recognize this condition as early as possible, and
to institute preventive measures. Chief of these are gradual and progressive build-
up of training with particular reference to the distance run at each session, and
avoidance of racing over distances greater than those covered in training sessions.
During each session the pace may be increased a little. On the first day of each
week the pace is dropped to compensate for an increased distance, being worked
up again to racing pace by the end of the week. This schedule may be regarded
as a form of controlled interval training—Fartlek may be included provided that
its length and severity is geared to the formal schedule. If symptoms recur the
patient goes back one week in his schedule and if they still persist he must rest
for a week and then start again.

Tendoperiostosis

This occurs typically on the medial side of the leg at the medial tibial border.
Pain occurs during exercise (not at rest or in bed at night in contradistinction
to stress fracture or osteoid osteoma), and may be quite severe although normally
well localized. There is no hint of direct trauma. On examination, a well-limited
tender area, sometimes slightly thickened, is palpable. This condition is due to
microtraumatic elevation of the periosteum by the jerk of the attached muscle
fascia during exercise. Treatment is injection with a local anaesthetic and hydrocortisone.

Widespread tendoperiostosis with scarring is a feature of posterior tibial compartment syndrome.

Posterior tibial compartment syndrome

When the tibialis posterior becomes hypertrophic it is trapped within its fascial
compartment in much the same way as the tibialis anterior[65] save that the fascial
attachments are less rigid. This allows for some stripping from the bony ridges
giving localized tendeoperiostosis.

In chronic cases or where the damage is widespread, considerable scarring with secondary tethering and adhesions will occur. Treatment is by operative decompression followed by intensive post-operative rehabilitation.

Intermittent claudication

True ischaemic leg pain is rare in athletes.[66] It may be due to early atherosclerosis, Buerger's disease or localized arterial thrombosis of indeterminate origin. The examination is directed towards eliciting absence of peripheral pulses, and any cases of suspected arterial insufficiency should be referred to a vascular surgeon for further investigation.

Muscle strains

The most common muscle strain in the lower leg is that of the gastrocnemius, frequently but erroneously described as 'ruptured plantaris tendon'. Onset is generally sudden, but may be drawn out over a period of minutes. Symptoms, signs and treatment are described in Chapters 16 and 17.

Bruises

Bruises of the lower leg are exceedingly common, and may cause considerable disability. Shin bruises may involve the tibial periosteum with production of subperiosteal haematomas.

Treatment is symptomatic with ice or lotio plumbi. The wearing of shin pads or leg guards will prevent many of these minor but uncomfortable injuries.

The possibility of underlying bone damage should always be considered.

Achilles tendon lesions

Pain around the Achilles tendon is a common cause of disability in sportsmen particularly in middle and long distance runners.[52, 67–69] The main features of the pathological conditions giving rise to Achillodynia have been set out in Chapter 16.

Table 25.1 Clinical fractures of Achillodynia

Achilles tendon	Onset	Appearance	Palpitation	Calf pinch test
Rupture: Complete	Sudden	Defect	Tendon tender±	Positive
Partial	Sudden	Swelling+	Tendon tender	±
Focal degeneration	Gradual	Swelling	Tendon tender++ Tender arc+	Negative
Tendonitis	Insidious	Swelling+	Tendon tender+	Negative
Peritendonitis: Acute	Rapid	Swelling+	Tendon not tender crepitus±	Negative
Chronic	Gradual	Swelling±	Tendon not tender paratenon thickened and tender±	Negative

Effective treatment depends upon an accurate differential diagnosis coupled with a clear understanding of the underlying pathology. The cardinal features of the main conditions involved are set out in Table 25.1.

Treatment of Achilles tendon pain

The choice of treatment will depend not only on the lesion under consideration but also the individual circumstances of the patient, the nature of his sport, and the facilities available for his clinical management.

Complete rupture

Complete rupture of the Achilles tendon (Fig. 25.40) may be treated conservatively or by operative repair.[70, 71] While conservative management is becoming increasingly popular, there seems little doubt that formal repair and satisfactory rehabilitation following a suitable period of immobilization in plaster of Paris

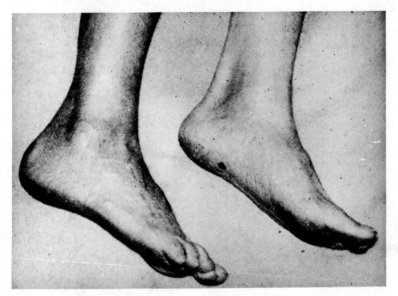

Fig. 25.40 Complete rupture of the Achilles tendon showing typical 'hollow' behind the right heel.

is the treatment of choice. This offers the earliest return to full sporting activity, and most athletes would regard the risks of complications of surgery (for example, infection and recurrent tear) as acceptable in the face of the somewhat variable outcome of conservative management.

Partial rupture

For many years a diagnosis of partial rupture was unacceptable in more conservative orthopaedic circles, but recent work has confirmed the existence of this condition.[67] When diagnosed, treatment should be surgical with exploration of the damaged tendon. Where only a few fibres are involved, debridement without any attempt at formal repair is acceptable (Fig. 25.41), and such a procedure

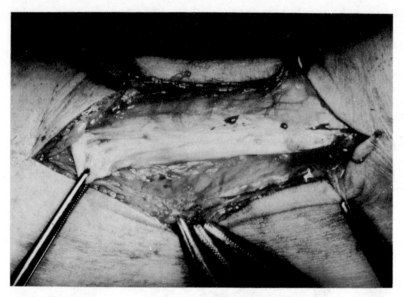

Fig. 25.41 Achilles tendon; partial rupture in a cross-country runner. The proximal part of the tear is held in artery forceps.

must be followed by intensive post-operative rehabilitation. Immobilization in plaster of Paris in such cases is not only unnecessary, but probably militates against a good long-term result. Where a partial rupture is more extensive, involving more than one third of the tendon's cross-sectional area, formal repair will have to be carried out, after which the post-operative management is similar

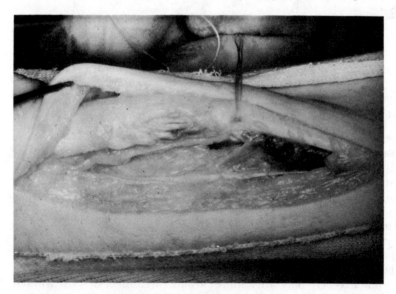

Fig. 25.42 Achilles tendon; focal degeneration in the superficial fibres in the deep surface.

to that of repair of a complete rupture of the tendon. In carrying out surgical repair of partial or complete rupture of the tendon, the problem of a paratenon must be considered. There are some authors who regard partial or complete rupture as following earlier degeneration in the tendon, but the evidence is equivocal.[72–75] Normal tendons showing no degenerative change whatever may be found after a post-mortem in even the most elderly subjects, and yet changes of degeneration have been seen at the margins of tendon ruptures even in the young. The association between inflammatory change in the paratenon and underlying focal degeneration (the 'central degeneration' of Burry and Pool,[76] although it is by no means always central in the tendon; Fig. 25.42) seems to be clearly established and indeed adhesions between the paratenon and foci of degeneration in the tendon can be demonstrated at operation (Fig. 25.43). In general, it seems appropriate to suggest that where a formal repair is carried out, the paratenon should be left *in situ* unless obviously diseased. Where debridement only is carried out, it is suggested that the paratenon should be stripped at the same time.

Focal degeneration
Focal degeneration of the tendon may be treated conservatively or by surgical intervention (Fig. 25.44). Various forms of conservative management have been tried in the past. Of these, rest together with padding of the heel and ultrasonic therapy appear to offer the best results.[77] Even so, there is very often considerable delay in returning to full normal training, and recurrences occur with monotonous regularity. Where facilities for early surgery and appropriate post-operative rehabilitation are *not* available, conservative management is the treatment of choice.

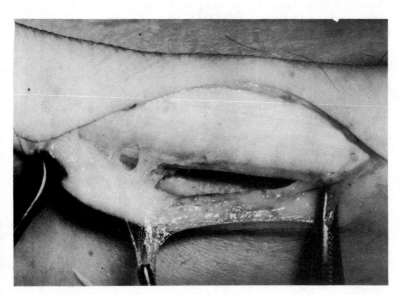

Fig. 25.43 Achilles tendon: peritendonitis showing adhesions between paratenon and tendon.

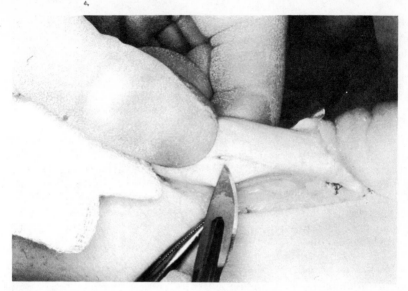

Fig. 25.44 Achilles tendon; focal degeneration showing nidus of granulation tissue deep in the tendon.

There is some argument as to whether or not the tendon itself should be injected, and most authorities agree that this is a dangerous procedure[78] [80] but the evidence is by no means unanimous and there are some authors who challenge the role of hydrocortisone injections in the production of complete rupture of the Achilles tendon, suggesting that it is the pre-existing focal degeneration that causes the rupture and not the hydrocortisone injection.[81] In the face of the available evidence, however, it seems at the present time unwise to inject lesions in the Achilles tendon.

If surgical treatment is selected, the method is simple. The tendon is exposed and the paratenon removed over 80 per cent of its circumference. The tendon lesion itself is identified and the tendon divided in its long axis down and through the lesion. The lesion itself and any granulation tissue is curetted and the wound is then closed in layers. An appropriate technique is to use interrupted catgut for the subcutaneous tissues and adhesive strips for the skin itself (Fig. 25.45). The patient remains in bed for the first four post-operative days, but during this time active dorsiflexion and plantar flexion are encouraged, particularly the former.[82] On the fifth post-operative day, the patient gets up and begins weight bearing, if necessary (when there is much muscle spasm in equinus) using a suitably built up but soft slipper. Progress with weight bearing is as rapid as the patient can tolerate and intensive rehabilitation is instituted before the end of the second post-operative week.

The objects of rehabilitation are to restore ankle mobility as rapidly as possible, and to build up both the power of the triceps surae and the general endurance of the limb. It is found that after a period of three weeks' intensive rehabilitation, the majority of patients are able to return to normal training; thus

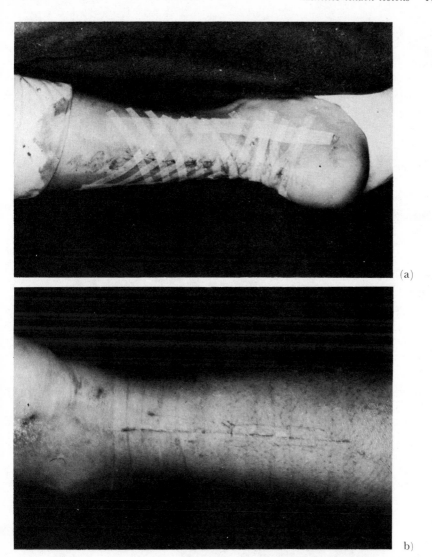

(a)

b)

Fig. 25.45 Achilles tendon decompression; skin closure using strips instead of sutures reduces the risk of wound margin necrosis. (a) At operation. (b) Twelve days later after removal of strips.

the post-operative morbidity of this procedure has been reduced to between four and five weeks which compares satisfactorily with the morbidity when the condition is managed conservatively.

Tendonitis

In some instances the change in the Achilles tendon is more widespread, the whole thickness of the tendon being involved over a length of 2 or 3 cm, occasionally with chondrification, although this is unusual in younger subjects (Fig. 25.46).

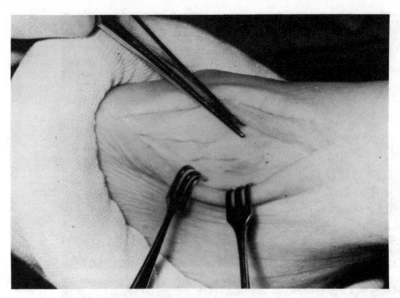

Fig. 25.46 Chronic Achilles tendonitis; the lesion in the tendon is widespread with punctate haemorrhage and areas of discoloration.

Results with conservative management are disappointing in that a very long period of rest and inactivity is required before the condition settles down satisfactorily. Response to surgical decompression is, however, good, and the post-operative disability period as a rule is not longer than six weeks.

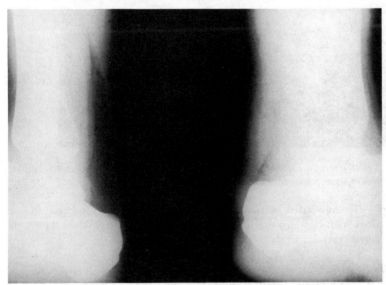

Fig. 25.47 Achilles tendon. Partial rupture with extensive peritendonitis. Lateral soft tissue radiograph showing obliteration of Kager's triangle on the right side.

Peritendonitis

Acute peritendonitis is best treated conservatively, and response to massive infiltration of the paratenon with a mixture of local anaesthetic, hydrocortisone, and hyaluronidase is usually satisfactory. This injection may need to be repeated on a number of occasions. In some cases, progress may be assessed radiologically when clearing of Kager's triangle is seen (Fig. 25.47).[83–85] It must, however,

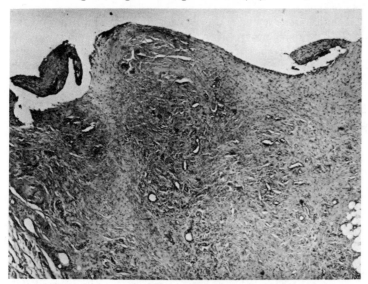

Fig. 25.48 Chronic peritendonitis; low power histological appearances showing haemosiderin deposits and pallisades of fibroblasts.

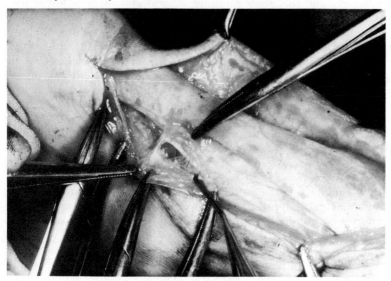

Fig. 25.49 Chronic Achilles peritendonitis showing constricting bands of adhesions.

be remembered that acute peritendonitis may be associated with an underlying lesion of the tendon itself. This is even more common in chronic peritendonitis. In such cases, the results of conservative management are generally poor, probably due to the fibrosis in the paratenon (Fig. 25.48) that causes permanent constriction around the moving tendon (Fig. 25.49). In such cases, exploration and stripping of the paratenon gives excellent results with a return to full training within four weeks of operation.[86, 87]

In all cases of Achillodynia treated conservatively, return to full training and competition must be cautiously progressive,[69] in contrast with post-operative rehabilitation which must be as energetic as the patient can tolerate. Indeed operation is *not* advised for patients with these tendon lesions if for any reason really energetic rehabilitation is not possible.

The paratenon

The role of the paratenon in the chronic Achillodynia is somewhat uncertain. A number of patients have come to surgery following recurrence of chronic Achilles tendon pain after one or more previous operations. In all cases it has been found that the paratenon was left *in situ* and not excised when the tendon was previously explored. While there have been other factors in the recurrence of chronic Achilles tendon pain after surgery, for example, post-operative immobilization, the one common factor has been the leaving of the paratenon. Furthermore, no cases of recurrence have so far been found in patients where the paratenon was formally excised at the first operation.

The long term post-operative results in cases of Achilles tendon pain in sport submitted to surgery are uniformly good, but patients have to be warned that healing of the skin and underlying tissues tends to be somewhat slower in this site than elsewhere, and that some morning stiffness and slight tightness may be felt for several months until the scar in the skin 'goes white'. Hypertrophic scarring is occasionally a minor problem and can be readily ameliorated by the application of bland emollient creams. In general, it now appears that the surgical management of most causes of chronic Achilles tendon pain as well as of acute partial rupture and focal degeneration, give excellent long-term results, provided that the paratenon is removed at the time of surgery and that early and vigorous post-operative rehabilitation is instituted. The mean post-operative disability time in such cases can be reduced to five weeks at the end of which the athlete is back to full training. This compares very satisfactorily with results of more conservative treatment.

Achilles tendon insertions

Lesions of the Achilles tendon insertion cause pain out of all proportion to their size. They are, however, happily less common than lesions of the tendon itself and the surrounding structures.[88] The most common cause of pain at the insertion is a chronic Achilles bursitis and this readily responds to infiltration with local anaesthetic and hydrocortisone. In recalcitrant cases, ultrasonics and/or short wave diathermy may also be helpful. In the most resistant cases of chronic Achilles tendon bursitis, and when there is either a spur of bone associated with the insertion or an erosion (Fig. 25.50), surgical exploration and a debridement is the

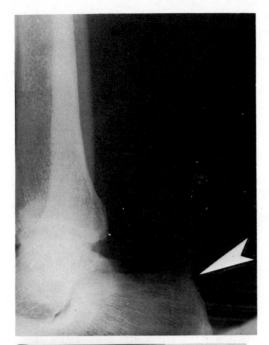

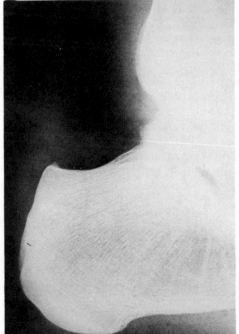

Fig. 25.50 Achilles tendon insertion; lesion of tendon attachment. (a) Erosion and (b) exostosis in runners. (Compare with olecranon: Chapter 24.)

treatment of choice. Post-operative management is as for surgery of the Achilles tendon and the long-term results are excellent.

The ankle

The ankle joint is the site of sprains, ligament rupture, and fractures.[89] In addition there are a few rare lesions involving surrounding structures and various types of degenerative changes.

Sprains

Acute capsular sprains of the ankle joint are probably the commonest single type of sports injury. The classical injury is that produced by inversion and internal rotation, which results in sprain of the lateral ligament of the ankle joint. Clinically there appear to be two main types.

In the first, pain is severe and soft tissue swelling is very pronounced, with obvious discoloration appearing early. So gross may be the swelling, so marked the limitation of movement (due to muscular spasm), and so severe the pain, that the presence of a fracture is suspected. This type of sprain is nearly always properly treated from the first.

The second, and less common, type of sprain has a far less well marked clinical picture. Pain varies in severity, there is little swelling and local tenderness may not be very acute. The only gross physical sign is limitation of movement, though careful inspection from behind will show filling of the sulci at the side of the Achilles tendon due to backward bulging of the effusion in the ankle joint. In simple ligament sprain or bruising only one sulcus is filled. This type of case tends to be overlooked in the absence of a very striking clinical picture, but if the ankle joint is needled, bloodstained synovial fluid is aspirated. Furthermore, follow up of cases of sprained ankle indicates that it is this second type which, if inadequately treated in the first place, tends to progress to 'chronic sprained ankle'.

The treatment of all cases of sprained ankle, once bony injury and complete ligament tear have been excluded (by X-rays including stress films if necessary), is as follows.

The leg is elevated and firm cold compresses are applied. Alternatively, Quigley's method[90] of immersing the ankle (to which a foam rubber pad and pressure bandage have been applied) in cold water for thirty minutes, following which the pressure bandage is reapplied dry and the leg is elevated, may be used. Swelling should have subsided in 24 to 48 hours, after which it possible to decide whether immobilization in a plaster of Paris cast is necessary. The vast majority of sprains do not require such immobilization, and should be treated by the application of a non-stretch adhesive strapping stirrup to prevent inversion or eversion (whichever is applicable), after which the leg and ankle are strapped from the toes to below the knee (Fig. 25.51). Prior to the application of any strapping, the leg is shaved and or treated with Friar's Balsam.

The patient is encouraged to walk normally from the first, and various exercises are prescribed to be carried out on a flat surface (for example a concrete playground, not a cambered road or grass playing field). After about one week, more vigorous exercises including tiptoeing are introduced, and full-range ankle exer-

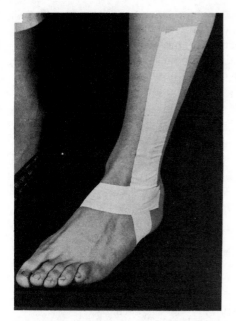

Fig. 25.51 Non-stretch adhesive strapping stirrup applied to the ankle to prevent inversion. An Elastoplast bandage is applied over this from the toes to below the knee.

cises (with strapping off) against steadily increasing resistance are added as soon as they can be carried out without pain.

Prior to resumption of competitive sport the ankle must be put through a severe 'fitness test' which should include walking twenty yards full-out with the ankle held first in inversion and then in eversion. Provided rehabilitation has been adequate these tests are carried out with no discomfort.

When a patient's skin is sensitive to adhesive strapping, Viscopaste can be used, or the strapping may be applied sticky side out, clothes and socks being protected by an outer layer of Stockinette or Tubegauz, or a cotton bandage.

Chronic sprained ankle

Not infrequently, and generally due to faulty treatment in the first instance, ankle sprains proceed to chronicity, but some caution must be observed in making this diagnosis, and other possible causes of symptoms eliminated. The differential diagnosis is from:

(1) 'Footballer's ankle'.
(2) Undiagnosed fracture.
(3) Undiagnosed complete ligament tear.
(4) Spastic flat foot—peroneo-extensor spasm.
(5) Peroneal tenosynovitis/tendovaginitis.

All these conditions apart from true peroneo-extensor spasm and the tendon sheath lesions can be diagnosed radiologically, if necessary with the help of stress films or special views. True chronic sprained ankle is more common in cases of 'undemonstrative' sprain described above. Various methods of treatment are available. Supportive exercises should always be prescribed, and localized tender spots respond to hydrocortisone by injection, or massage. If pain is felt even on quiet walking, the addition of a 'raise and float' to the heel of the shoe will help—$\frac{1}{4}$ in (6·35 mm) is about right for the average adult (Fig. 25.52).

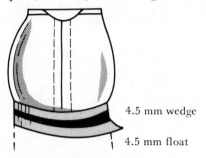

4.5 mm wedge

4.5 mm float

Fig. 25.52 Rear view of the heel of the shoe showing how the 'raise and float' is applied.

Really stubborn cases will often respond to manipulation (with or without general anaesthesia) followed by vigorous exercises. In all cases of chronic ankle sprain the possibility of a tubercular or rheumatoid aetiology should be borne in mind, and excluded by blood tests and serology.

Prevention of ankle sprains

The dictum 'once a sprain—always a sprain' should be regarded as an admission of defeat. In the previously uninjured subject ankle injuries may be very largely prevented by the development of an adequate supporting musculature, and the attention to the suitability of footwear for the ground conditions. Spikes or studs on boots or shoes that give excessive grip on track or field predispose to ankle injuries, as do overlong spikes which, because they do not penetrate to allow weight to be borne through the sole of the shoe or boot, render the foot unstable (Fig. 25.53).[91]

The correct use of release bindings by skiers contributes largely to prevention of ankle injury, but even without these such injuries may be prevented by adequate pre-season training.

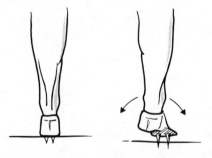

Fig. 25.53 Overlong spikes or studs render the foot unstable and the ankle liable to sprain because they do not permit weight to be carried through the flat of the sole.

Provided the initial diagnosis was correct and the treatment thorough, there is absolutely no necessity for ankle sprains to recur on the patient's return to sport. The Americans use involved systems of protective strapping for the ankles of their footballers,[92] and even in Britain it is common for footballers and others to festoon themselves with yards of bandage or elasticized stockings as ankle supports. There are two grave objections to this practice.[93, 94] Firstly, by as much as the joint receives extrinsic support, by just so much will the supporting muscles tend to atrophy, since they are no longer required to fulfil their supporting role. Secondly, when a stress is applied to an unsupported ankle it is able to give way when the stress reaches a dangerous level. If the ankle is firmly supported it is unable to give until the supports give way, generally to a far higher degree of stress, which being thrown on the now unsupported ankle, produces far more damage. Any athlete or gamesplayer who cannot get through a game without twisting his ankle should look to his exercises, not to his strappings!

Ligament tears and fractures

Complete tears of the deltoid, calcaneofibular or inferior tibiofibular ligaments are uncommon in isolation, being usually associated with fractures of the tibia and/or fibula.[95] Usually it is the fracture that is diagnosed, while the associated

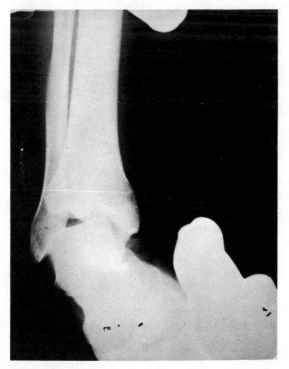

Fig. 25.54 X-ray photograph of ankle joint on anteroposterior projection to show 'talar tilt' due to rupture of lateral ligament demonstrated by applying inversion stress. (Photo: Middlesex Hospital.)

soft tissue injury is missed. In such cases the nature and site of the fracture may serve to indicate the presence of an accompanying ligament tear.

As a rule, however, it is possible to deduce the likely site of damage from analysis of the mechanics of injury, and in this respect it is as well for the surgeon to appreciate the mechanics of the sport. Unless there is obvious instability of the ankle joint in one plane it is usually impossible to diagnose complete tears with certainty without the help of stress X-rays; when stress X-rays are being taken the mechanism of injury should be reproduced (Fig. 25.54). When complete tear is discovered operative repair followed by immobilization in plaster of Paris must be undertaken. Subsequently rehabilitation must be gradual, with the accent on protective exercises.

The presence of associated fracture does not preclude repair of the ligament tear—indeed, it is more important in such cases that the ligament should be repaired. The practice of placing and internally fixing the bone fragment while leaving the ligament to take care of itself must be condemned. Provided that adequate and accurate repair of the ligament tear is carried out, the bone fragments will almost invariably reduce correctly and unite soundly without any internal fixation.

Sometimes X-rays of a severely sprained ankle show 'flake fractures' of the malleolar tips. These should be regarded as avulsion injuries and stress films should be taken to investigate the integrity of the joint. Demonstrable instability argues associated ligament tears which require repair.

Fractures without instability

Fractures without demonstrable instability are treated according to basic ortho-paedic principles. After initial immobilization, rehabilitation must be thorough, being directed to restoration of full movements on the one hand, and development of a strong supportive musculature on the other. *Controlled* training should be started as early as possible, but return to competition must be delayed as long as any symptoms persist.

Stable instability

From time to time patients present following ligament sprain, with a history of repeated 'giving way' of the ankle, in whom clinical instability cannot be demonstrated.[96, 97] In such cases it is postulated that there has been damage to the joint's proprioceptive feedback mechanism without solution of anatomical continuity of the capsule itself. Treatment is by appropriate neuromuscular re-education using the 'wobble board'.

Footballer's ankle

This condition may be regarded as a type of traumatic osteitis: it is not an osteoar-throsis as the joint surfaces are not involved. The patient complains of pain in the ankle on kicking the ball, and some general soreness at the end of the game.[98, 99] On examination, there may be a little swelling around the ankle joint together with diffuse tenderness. The condition is frequently regarded as a 'chronic sprain' but the diagnosis is easily established if X-rays are taken. The

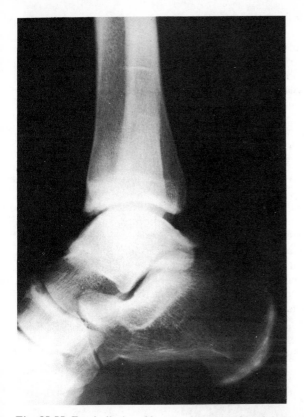

Fig. 25.55 Footballer's ankle; note hypertrophy of the anterior joint margin of the tibia.

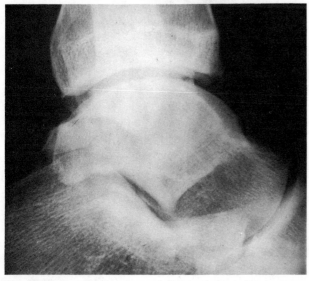

Fig. 25.56 Os trigonum in a triple/long jumper impinging on posterior margin of tibia during forced plantar flexion of ankle on take-off.

picture is typical, showing more or less well-developed outcrops of bone from the margins of the inferior articular surface of the tibia (Fig. 25.55).

Treatment consists of abstention from provoking activity together with ankle exercises (full range). Stubborn cases may require operative removal of the bony spurs, and if symptoms are severe a marked improvement may be expected after this procedure.

A somewhat similar condition involves fracture or degenerative change in the posterior part of the talus.[100] This may impinge on the 'third malleolus' (the posterior margin of the inferior articular surface of the tibia), which can develop a spur, or it may be represented by a separate os trigonum which is subject to repetitive trauma during forced plantar flexion of the ankle joint (Fig. 25.56). This condition is also seen in fast bowlers, particularly those who 'drag'.

Treatment is difficult, various forms of exercise, diathermy, and injection have been tried with inconstant results. Stubborn cases may require surgical exploration with removal of the bony outgrowths, and this is perhaps justified when symptoms are severe. The alternative is temporary or even permanent abandonment of the provoking form of activity. Many cases present with loose bodies or 'joint mice' which may require surgical removal if they interfere with joint function (Fig. 25.57). Progression is to frank osteoarthrosis.

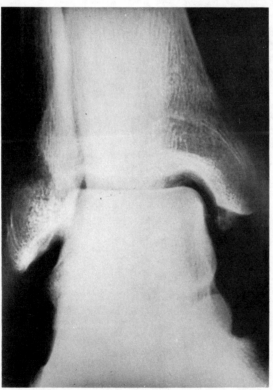

Fig. 25.57 Loose body: a tiny fragment may be seen nestling between the talus and the medial malleolus.

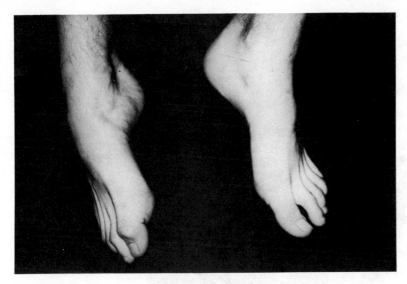

Fig. 25.58 Spastic flat foot; typical appearance.

Peroneo-extensor spasm

This is one form of 'spastic flat foot' and may be diagnosed in a patient who complains of pain in the outer aspect of the ankle and lower part of the leg after exercise, particularly running over hard or uneven ground. On examination there is painful limitation of inversion and dorsiflexion but no capsular tenderness at the ankle joint. After exclusion of bony abnormality (see below) treatment is directed to mobilization of the ankle by exercise, peroneal stretching and even manipulation under anaesthesia. An alternative is infiltration of the tarsal tunnel with local anaesthetic. Some severe cases respond to manipulation and immobilization in plaster of Paris in full inversion for a period of three to four weeks, but unfortunately recurrence must be expected. In long-standing cases spasm in eversion is marked, and proves particularly difficult to overcome. A similar spastic condition may affect the posterior tibial muscles (Fig. 25.58).

Peroneal tenosynovitis/tendovaginitis[101]

The symptoms and signs of these conditions are the same as those for similar lesions elsewhere, namely pain, limitation of movement and tenderness and crepitus, though the latter sign is rare.

Tenosynovitis may be treated by injection of hydrocortisone or supportive strapping. Limited exercise for a period of ten days to a fortnight and gradual resumption of full training complete the treatment.

Tendovaginitis is treated by the operation of tendovaginotomy with excellent results.

Posterior Tibial tenosynovitis/tendovaginitis[102]

A similar series of lesions may be found behind the medial malleolus. Treatment is the same.

Extensor retinaculum entrapment

An unusual form of over-use state is extensor retinaculum entrapment in which the hypertrophied inferior fibres of (particularly) tibialis anterior may be trapped beneath the extensor retinaculum. Treatment is division of the retinaculum.

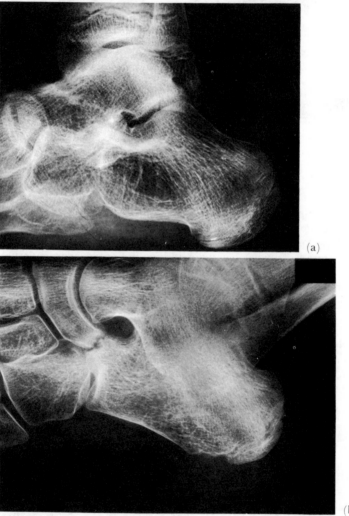

(a)

(b)

Fig. 25.59 Bony abnormalities of the tarsus. (a) Talocalcaneal bridge demonstrated on the oblique axial view. (b) Calcaneonavicular bridge demonstrated on the oblique lateral view. (Photo: courtesy *J. Bone Jt Surg.*)

Tarsal abnormalities—congenital 'bars'

Two types of congenital bony anomalies may produce the picture of 'spastic flat foot'. They are talocalaneal and calcaneonavicular bars.[103] [105] They may be complete, forming a bony fusion between the appropriate bones, or may be separated by a false joint. Their presence is demonstrated radiologically by the medial oblique axial or oblique lateral projections (Fig. 25.59).

Treatment consists of conservative measures in the first instance with rest, physiotherapy and heel wedges. Long-standing cases with severe deformity may be successfully treated by operative ablation of the bony bars, but more usually triple fusion is required.

The foot

Bruised heel

This is a common complaint among hurdlers and long or triple jumpers. Repeated heavy landings on the heel cause rupture of the fibrous septa between the under surface of the calcaneum and the skin so that the protective fat is 'milked out' from the point of contact allowing crushing of the skin by the bone (Fig. 25.60).

In early cases signs are minimal, the only positive finding being localized ten-

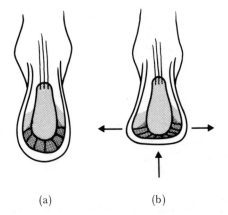

(a)   (b)

Fig. 25.60 Heel bruising. At rest (a) the skin of the heel is separated from the under-surface of the calcaneum by a fibro-fatty pad. This may be dispersed when the fibrous septa rupture under the stress of repeated heavy landings on the heel, allowing the skin to be compressed against the bone (b).

derness, but in chronic cases it is possible to feel a boggy softening of the subcuticular tissues under the heel. In veterans there may be a palpable nodule of scar tissue.

Bruised heel, once established, is difficult to treat. Prevention consists of training the jumper to 'give' as he lands rather than to ground the heel with the leg held rigid.

Early cases may be treated by the provision of a thick soft sponge rubber or Plastazote heel pad to be worn when jumping. At the same time the jumping schedule is eased off to allow the condition to settle down. Established cases require a heel pad with the centre cut out so that weight-bearing is distributed over the periphery. Alternatively, a moulded cup may be worn which 'reconstitutes' the natural heel pad by compressing the lateral aspects of the calcaneum and preventing lateral displacement of the soft tissue under the heel.

Occasionally heel bruising may be associated with the presence of a calcaneal spur demonstrated on X-ray. In a proportion of such cases, when conservative treatment has failed, recourse to surgical excision of the spur may lead to satisfactory results, but whether *per se* or because of the enforced period of rest which follows, it is difficult to determine.

Plantar fasciitis

This complaint is uncommon in athletes and may be confused with spring ligament sprain (Fig. 25.61).

There is pain under the foot on exercise and tenderness may be felt anterior to the calcaneal tubercles. It is thought to follow tearing of the plantar fascia,

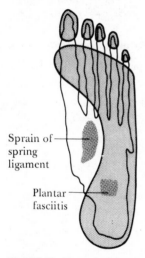

Sprain of
spring
ligament

Plantar
fasciitis

Fig. 25.61 Sites of tenderness in plantar fasciitis and spring ligament sprain superimposed on bony 'shadow' of foot to show how the former is under the weight-bearing aspect of the sole while the latter is under the arch.

though some cases may be due to stress fracture of the calcaneum. A relationship has been established between plantar fasciitis and rheumatoid arthritis; this last disease should be excluded by estimation of erythrocyte sedimentation rate and the Rose-Waaler test.

Treatment consists of local injections of hycrocortisone into the tender spot together with massage (deep friction) or a course of ultrasonics. When pain is felt even on gentle exercise a moulded high arch insole should be provided temporarily.

Sprain of the spring ligament

Sprain of the plantar calcaneonavicular ligament (the 'spring ligament') may follow unaccustomed running over uneven surfaces in soft shoes. The clinical picture is similar to plantar fasciitis but the pain is more aching in quality and tenderness is localized more deeply and medially.

Treatment consists of vigorous foot exercises including intrinsic exercises. When pain is severe, a moulded felt insole is applied to the sole of the foot and strapping is applied over it from the toes to just below the knee. This support is removed as soon as the patient can walk quietly in comfort. Chronic cases respond well to manipulation of the foot followed by exercise.

Chronic foot strain

This rather amorphous title is given to a condition quite frequently met among all kinds of track athletes and gamesplayers.[106] The story is one of gradually increasing ache in the rear half of the foot, at first intermittent during or just after exercise, but slowly becoming more constant. No precise localization of the pain is made, nor are there any very positive physical signs, though some limitation of subtalar and mid-tarsal movements may be elicited. It is thought that the condition may be due to chronic low-grade synovitis in the small joints of the tarsus. It is usual to find that the patient will admit to wearing unsuitable footwear for the ground conditions in the recent past. Many athletes have the habit of wearing one pair of spikes for training and reserving a special pair for competition. However economically desirable this practice may seem, it must be condemned. The athlete should always wear shoes of the same degree of resilience and length of spike for competition and training (if he wears spikes for training and not 'training shoes'). A common cause of foot strain is the wearing of light shoes for competition (to which the athlete is not accustomed and which

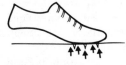 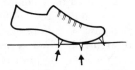

Fig. 25.62 This illustrates how overlong spikes which do not penetrate fully will prevent uniform weight-bearing through the sole of the show.

do not provide the same degree of support, however small this may be) with overlong spikes (which result either in too great a degree of adhesion in a 'sticky' track or in running on the spikes because they do not penetrate deeply enough for the weight to be taken through the sole of the shoe (Fig. 25.62).

Ideally, the athlete should buy two identical pairs of spikes at a time and use them turn and turn about so that should one pair become damaged he has a similar pair in reserve.

Foot strain is also common among footballers, particularly at the beginning and end of the season when grounds are hard. Under those conditions, strains may be prevented by the wearing of hockey boots rather than studded football boots. They are as comfortable for kicking, and more comfortable for being kicked!

Treatment for chronic foot strain consists of vigorous exercises, particularly of the intrinsic musculature of the foot (backed up if necessary by Faradic baths), and the avoidance of uneven surfaces for training. Contrast foot baths are valuable in dispelling any swelling and may produce marked amelioration of symptoms. They may be carried out in the patient's own home as follows. Two baths are filled, the first with water as hot as the patient can tolerate, the other with water as cold as possible. The patient places his foot in one bath keeping it there until he is no longer conscious of the temperature, then he transfers it to the other, and so on for about ten minutes. Contrast baths are of the utmost value in promoting circulatory activity.

Stubborn cases generally respond to manipulation followed by exercise, but occasionally even this fails. Only then should rest be advised, initially for three weeks, followed by very gradual controlled resumption of training.

Metatarsalgia—forefoot strain

There are four causes of pain in the anterior half of the foot. These are:

(1) Postural strains.
(2) Tendon insertion strains.
(3) March fracture—stress fracture.
(4) Morton's metatarsalgia—interdigital neuroma.

Of these, postural strains are the most common.

Postural strains

The patient complains of an ache in the front of the foot, generally under the second and third metatarsal heads. On examination it is usual to find a mild degree of pes planus with tenderness under the second and third metatarsal heads.

Treatment is by intrinsic exercises, and the patient must be greatly encouraged in their performance as they are somewhat tedious to carry out and improvement is usually far from dramatic, though none the less progressive.

Other forms of postural defect, for example pes cavus, dropped forefoot, and metatarsus primus varus do not, as a rule, provoke symptoms if mild. Their treatment is according to standard orthopaedic practice and requires no modification for athletes.

Tendon insertion strain

Pain may be felt over the fifth metatarsal styloid after a severe inversion or eversion strain, and the styloid may be acutely tender. After exclusion of fracture, typically of the *avulsion* type (Fig. 25.63), strain of the insertion of tibialis posterior may be diagnosed. In the early stages treatment is with support, ultrasonics and exercises. Chronic cases respond well to local steroid injection.

March fracture—stress fracture

This has already been discussed in Chapter 14. Onset of symptoms may be gradual or rapid. Tenderness is well localized and the callus may be palpable.

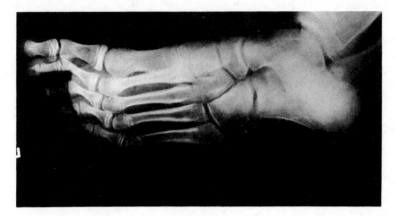

Fig. 25.63 Avulsion fracture of the 5th metatarsal styloid from the pull of posterior tibial tendon.

Rest from sporting activity and support with a felt undersole and strapping is the treatment of choice. After two to three weeks, training may be resumed and recurrence seldom occurs. When it does, the lay-off must be extended to six weeks.

Morton's metatarsalgia

Interdigital neuroma is not common in athletes but should be considered in the differential diagnosis of forefoot pain. The patient complains that the pain is 'like a knife' and is relieved by the removal of the footwear. Tenderness is localized between the metatarsal heads (usually 1/2 to 2/3) and the neuroma may be palpable. Treatment is by operative removal if local steroid injection fails.

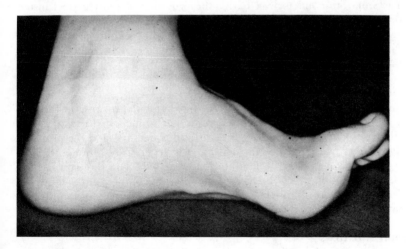

Fig. 25.64 Middle distance runner; inclusion dermoid in sole of foot. A cause of disability when running.

Fractures

The management of fractures of the foot in athletes in no way differs from the management of similar fractures in 'civilians', in so far as definitive treatment is concerned. If the period of immobilization is likely to be short-lived, vigorous supporting exercises should be organized. Subsequent rehabilitation is geared to the demands of the patient's sport or game.

Osteochondritides

These are discussed in Chapter 14.

Other complaints

Other unusual causes of foot-pain present from time to time (Fig. 25.64).

The toes

Apart from various skin conditions (see Chapter 7) the only significant lesions are:

(1) Hallux rigidus.
(2) Sesamoiditis.
(3) Subungual exostosis.
(4) Fractures.

Hallux rigidus
In this condition the patient complains of pain and stiffness in the first metatarso-phalangeal joint. There is marked limitation of movement on examination and frequently the joint is tender. Two main types are described— in adolescents it is more common in females, in adults it is more common in males.

Mild cases may respond to wax baths, the provision of a fitted steel insole, or hydrocortisone injections with or without manipulation under anaesthetic. Where limitation of movement is marked, phalangeal osteotomy provides good results with a remarkable increase in range of movement. In adults, Keller's operation is more likely to be successful.

Sesamoiditis
This is uncommon. It seems to be due to a form of avascular necrosis of the sesamoids in the tendon of flexor hallucis where they lie under the first metatarsal head. Mild cases may be treated by hydrocortisone injections and the provision of a sponge rubber pad. If this regime fails, and in severe cases, immobilization in plaster of Paris is necessary. Rehabilitation is started when the pain has disappeared, and attention should be paid to the internal contours of the footwear. Sesamoiditis may be precipitated by pressure of a stud forming a boss under the first metatarsal head (Fig. 25.65).

Subungual exostosis
This lesion is particularly disabling for footballers. Treatment is excision; terminal hemi-phalangectomy is a satisfactory method but should not be used if the

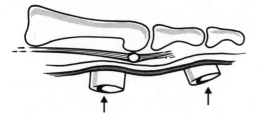

Fig. 25.65 Upward pressure on badly sited boot studs may cause 'bossing' inside the boot. Such an elevation under the 1st metatarsal head may provoke sesamoiditis.

patient has a long second toe. In such cases removal of the nail and curettage is to be preferred. Ingrowing toenail should always be treated energetically along orthodox lines as it may be the cause of considerable disability.

Care of the feet

It is remarkable how many otherwise healthy young men and women have demonstrable pathology in the feet. Many of the cases are attributable to the wearing of unsuitable footwear either for sport or in everyday life.[107]

Tight footwear is often dictated by fashion, but it gives rise to corns and callosities, blisters,[108] and minor postural defects, all of which can cause disproportionate amounts of trouble in the athlete.

Worn-out boots or shoes which are 'trodden over' or whose soles have given way to allow uneven upward pressure from studs or spikes are also a frequent source of trouble.

General care of the feet and the proper selection of footwear will do much to minimize injury and disability.

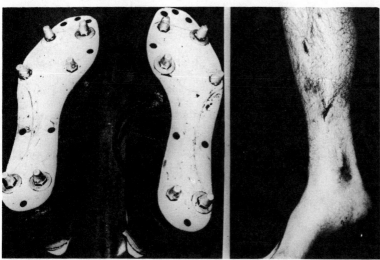

Fig. 25.66 Lacerations of the leg (Rugby football) and the boots that caused them. Note the sharp-edged metal discs under the studs, and the damaged surfaces of the stud ends.

Footwear for sport

In general, the design and manufacture of footwear for sport is atrocious. Although some research is being carried out, design is too often a matter of fashion as is manufacture one of business economics.[91]

Good footwear is light, supple and a good fit. Extra support is provided by the careful siting of suitable reinforcement. Too often, uppers are 'reinforced' by trade flashes and the like, often in unsuitable positions, which can cause rubbing or blistering. The design of the sole of all shoes needs care to ensure that cushioning is progressive, that the sole plate moulds to the contours of the moving foot and that any studs, spikes or other aids to grip are well placed. Nylon, though popular, is a most unsuitable material as it is unyielding, frequently bends in the wrong place (i.e. half way along the sole *not* under the metatarsophalangeal joints) and tends to sustain sharp edged lacerations from stones in the ground which makes it particularly unsuitable for football boots (Fig. 25.66). For heavy ground where long studs are needed, for example for football, uppers extending over the ankle make for safety and protect against the effects of excessive adhesion. Suitable footwear is an essential basis for sound and safe sports performance.

J.G.P.W.

References

1. Sperryn, P. N. and Williams, J. G. P. (1975) Why sports injuries clinics? *Br. med. J.*, **3**, 364.
2. Williams, J. G. P. (1973) Sports Injuries. *Folia Traumatologica*. Basle: CIBA-Geigy.
3. Williams, J. G. P. (1964) Knee injuries on the field of sport. *Rheumatism*, **20**, 76.
4. Carnevale, V. (1954) So called traumatic inguino-crural pain of football players. *Prensa med. argent.*, **41**, 355.
5. Howse, A. J. G. (1964) Osteitis pubis in an Olympic road walker. *Proc. R. Soc. Med.*, **57**, 88.
6. Adams, R. J. and Chandler, F. A. (1953) Osteitis pubis of traumatic aetiology. *J. Bone Jt Surg.*, **35A**, 685.
7. Klinefelter, E. W. (1950) Osteitis pubis: review of the literature and report of a case. *Am. J. Roentg.*, **63**, 368.
8. Williams, J. G. P. (In press) Limitation of hip joint movement as a factor in traumatic 'osteitis pubis'. *Br. J. sports Med.*
9. Cochrane, G. M. (1971) Osteitis pubis in athletes. *Br. J. sports Med.*, **5**, 233.
10. Reno, J. H. (1971) In *Encyclopedia of Sports Sciences and Medicine*, ed. Larson, L. A., London: Collier-Macmillan.
11. O'Donoghue, D. H. (1970) *Treatment of Injuries to Athletes*, 2nd edn. Philadelphia: W. B. Saunders.
12. Blazina. M. E. (1971) In *Encyclopaedia of Sport Sciences and Medicine*, ed. Larson, L. A., London: Collier-Macmillan.
13. Ryan, A. J. (1969) Quadriceps strain, rupture and Charlie horse. *Med. Sci. Sports*, **1**, 106.
14. Williams, J. G. P. (1971) Diagnostic pitfalls in the sportsman's knee. *Proc. R. Soc. Med.*, **64**, 640.
15. Blazina, M. E. (1969) Classification of injuries to articular cartilages of knee in athletics. In *Symposium on Sports Medicine*. St. Louis: C. V. Mosby.
16. O'Donoghue, D. H. (1959) Injuries to the knee. *Am. J. Surg.*, **98**, 463.

17. Klein, K. K. and Allman, F. (Jr.) (1969) *The Knee in Sports.* New York: The Pemberton Press.
18. Goldfuss, A. J., Morehouse, C. A. and Le Veau, B. F. (1973) Effect of muscular tension on knee stability. *Med. Sci. Sports,* **5,** 267.
19. Williams, J. G. P. (1975) Vastus medialis re-education in the management of chondromalacia patellae. In *Medical Aspects of Sports: 16.* Chicago: American Medical Association.
20. Nilsson, B. E. and Westlin, N. E. (1970) Muscle dysfunction following injury to the semilunar cartilage. *Ann. phys. Med.,* **10,** 281.
21. Reynolds, F. C. (1969) Diagnosis of Ligamentous Injuries of the Knee. In *Symposium on sports medicine.* Saint Louis: C. V. Mosby.
22. Pollacco, A. (1971) In *Encyclopaedia of Sports Sciences and Medicine,* ed. Larson, L. A., London: Collier-Macmillan.
23. Trickey, E. L. (1975) Personal communication.
24. Gollnick, P. D., Erickson, E., Hägmark, T. and Saltin, B. (1974) Recvery with a movable or standard cast following intra-articular reconstruction of the anterior cruciate ligament. In *Medical Aspects of Sports: 15.* Chicago: American Medical Association.
25. Tucker, W. E. (1969) Pellegrini-Stieda or post-traumatic para-articular ossification of the medical collateral ligament of the knee. *Br. J. sports Med.,* **4,** 212.
26. Slocum, D. B. (1969) Rotary Instability of the knee. In *Symposium on Sports Medicine.* St. Louis: C. V. Mosby.
27. Slocum, D. B., Larson, R. L. and James, S. L., (1974) Pes anserinus transplant: impressions after a decade of experience. *J. sports Med.,* **2,** 123.
28. Helfet, A. J. (1959) Mechanism of derangements of the medial semilunar cartilage and their management. *J. Bone Jt Surg.,* **41B,** 319.
29. Green, G. P. (1966) Osteochondritis dissecans of the knee. *J. Bone Jt Surg.,* **48B,** 82.
30. Lichtor, J. (1972) The loose-jointed young athlete. *J. sports Med.,* **1,** 22.
31. Hughston, J. C. (1969) Subluxation of the patella in athletes. In *Symposium on Sports Medicine.* St. Louis: C. V. Mosby.
32. Larson, R. L. and Osternig, L. R. (1974) Traumatic bursitis and artificial turf. *J. sports Med.,* **2,** 183.
33. Øwre, A. (1936) Chrondromalacia patellae. *Acta clin. scand.,* **77,** Supp. 41.
34. Wiles, P., Andrews, P. S. and Devas, M. B. (1956) Chondromalacia of the Patella. *J. Bone Jt Surg.,* **38B,** 95.
35. Bentley, G. (1970) Chondromalacia patellae. *J. Bone Jt Surg.,* **52A,** 221.
36. Fulford, P. (1969) Chondromalacia of the patella. *Br. J. sports Med.,* **4,** 198.
37. Robinson, A. R. and Darracott, J. (1970) Chondromalacia patellae. *Ann. phys. Med.,* **10,** 286.
38. French, P. R. (1969) The patello-femoral Joint. *Communication to British Orthopaedic Association.*
39. Bos, R. R. and Blosser, T. G. (1970) An electromyographic study of vastus medialis and vastus lateralis during selected isometric exercises. *Med. Sci. Sports,* **2,** 218.
40. Kearney, E. W. (1976) High riding patella as a factor predisposing to chronic dislocating patella in athletes—recognition and treatment. In *Proceedings XX World Congress of Sports Medicine,* Melbourne.
41. Hughston, J. C. (1964) Recurrent subluxation and dislocation of the patella. *J. Bone Jt Surg.,* **46B,** 787.
42. Cross, M. J. and Hughston, J. C. (1976) Instability of the patellofemoral joint in athletes. In *Proceedings XX World Congress of Sports Medicine,* Melbourne.
43. Harrison, M. H. M., Schajowicz, F. and Trueta, J. (1953) Osteoarthritis of the hip: a study of the nature and evolution of the disease. *J. Bone Jt Surg.,* **35B,** 598.

44. Williams, J. G. P. and Street, M. (In press) Sequential Faradism in vastus medialis re-education. *Physiotherapy*.
45. Hughston, J. C. (1972) Reconstruction of the extensor mechanism for patella subluxation. *J. sports Med.*, **1,** 1, 6.
46. Golski, A. and Devas, M. B. (1973) Treatment of chondromalacia patellae by transposition of tibal tubercle. *Br. med. J.*, **i,** 591.
47. Devas, M. B. (1960) Stress fracture of the patella. *J. Bone Jt Surg.*, **42B,** 71.
48. Devas, M. B. (1969) Stress fractures in athletes. *Proc. R. Soc. Med.*, **62,** 932.
49. Newman, P. H. (1969) Athletic injuries to the extensor mechanism. *Br. J. sports Med.*, **4,** 209.
50. Blazina, M. E., Fox, J. M. and Carlson, G. J. (1974) Basketball Injuries. In *Medical Aspects of Sport: 15.* Chicago: American Medical Association.
51. Williams, J. G. P. (1976) Surgical management of chronic patellar tendon strain. *Proceedings XX World Congress of Sports Medicine*, Melbourne.
52. Sperryn, P. N. (1971) Leg injuries in runners. *Ulmeanu Jubilee Symposium*, Bucharest.
53. Williams, J. G. P. (1971) Aetiological classification of injuries in sport. *Br. J. sports Med.*, **5,** 228.
54. Williams, J. G. P. and Sperryn, P. N. (1972) Overuse injury in sport and work. *Br. J. sports Med.*, **6,** 50.
55. Muckle, D. S. (1973) Dislocation of the superior tibiofibular joint—an unusual soccer injury. *Br. J. sports Med.*, **7,** 365.
56. Devas, M. B. (1958) Stress fractures of the tibia in athletes or 'shin soreness'. *J. Bone Jt Surg.*, **40B,** 227.
57. Slocum, D. B. (1967) The shin splints syndrome: medical aspects and differential diagnosis. In *Proceedings of 8th National Conference on Medical Aspects of Sport.* Chicago: American Medical Association.
58. Paul, W. D. and Sodenberg, G. L. (1967) The Shin splints confusion. In *Proceedings of 8th National Conference on Medical Aspects of Sports.* Chicago: American Medical Association.
59. Rasmussen, W. (1974) Shin splints. *J. sports Med.*, **2,** 111.
60. Maver, G. E. (1956) The anterior tibial syndrome. *J. Bone Jt Surg.*, **38B,** 513.
61. French, E. B. and Price, W. H. (1962) Anterior tibial pain. *Br. med. J.*, **ii,** 1290.
62. Clement, D. B. (1974) Tibial stress syndrome in athletes. *J. sports Med.*, **2,** 81.
63. Hughes, J. R. (1948) Ischaemic necrosis of the anterior tibial muscles due to fatigue. *J. Bone Jt Surg.*, **30B,** 581.
64. Lloyd, K. (1959) Some hazards of athletic exercise. *Proc. R. Soc. Med.*, **52,** 151.
65. Critchley, J. E. (1972) The posterior tibial syndrome. *Aust. N. Z. J. Surg.*, **43,** 31.
66. Harris, J. D. and Jepson, R. P. (1971) Entrapment of the popliteal artery. *Surgery*, **69,** 246.
67. Ljungqvist, R. (1968) Subcutaneous partial rupture of Achilles tendon. *Acta orthop. scand.*, Suppl. 113.
68. Stanescu, N. (1971) *Hyperfunctional Disorders of the Locomotor System.* Bucharest: Sports Medicine Centre.
69. Williams, J. G. P. (1967) Cause and prevention of Achilles peritendonitis in middle and long distance runners. *Br. Ass. Sport med. Bull.*, **3,** 16.
70. Lea, E. B. and Smith, L. (1972) Non-surgical treatment of tendo Achilles rupture. *J. Bone Jt Surg.*, **54A,** 1398.
71. Di Stefano, V. J. and Nixon, J. E. (1973) Ruptures of the Achilles tendon. *J. sports Med.*, **1,** 2, 34.
72. Burry, H. C. (1971) The pathology of the painful heel. *Br. J. sports Med.*, **6,** 9.
73. Arner, O., Lindholm, A. and Orell, S. R. (1958) Histological changes in subcutaneous rupture of the Achilles tendon. *Acta. chir. scand.*, **116,** 484.

74. Ippolito, E., Postacchini, F. and Puddu, G. (1973) Le alterazioni strutturali del tendine di Achille in rapporto all'età. *Med. del. Sport.*, **26**, 258.

75. Sønnischsen, H. V. (1966) Tendinitis Chronica. *Nord. Vet. Möte X.*

76. Burry, H. C. and Pool, C. J. (1973) Central degeneration of the Achilles Tendon. *Rheum. Rehabil.*, **12**, 177.

77. Sperryn, P. N. (1971) Runner's heel. *Br. J. sports Med.*, **5**, 228.

78. Lee, H. B. (1957) Avulsion and rupture of the tendo calcaneus after injection of hydrocrotisone. *Br. med. J.*, **i**, 395.

79. Unverferth, L. J. and Olix, M. L. (1973) The effect of local steroid injections on tendon. *J. sports Med.*, **1**, 4, 31.

80. Ismail, A. M., Balakrichnan, R., Rajakumar, M. K. and Lumpur, K. (1969) Rupture of patellar ligament after steroid infiltration. *J. Bone Jt Surg.*, **51B**, 503.

81 Matthews, L. S., Sonstegond, D. A. and Philps, D. B. (1974) A biomechanical study of rabbit patellar tendon: effects of steroid injection. *J. sports Med.*, **2**, 349.

82. Williams, J. G. P., Sperryn, P. N., Boardman, S., Street, M., Mellett, S. and Parsons, C. (In press) Postoperative management of chronic Achilles tendon pain in sportsmen. *Physiotherapy*.

83. Kager, H. (1939) Zur klinik und diagnostic des Achillessehnenrisses, *Chirurg.*, **2**, 691.

84 Arner, O., Lindholm, A. and Lindvall, N. (1958) Roentgen changes in subcutaneous rupture of the Achilles tendon. *Acta chir. scand.*. **116**, 496.

85. Sperryn, P. N. (1976) Diagnostic radiology in Achilles tendon pain. In *Proceedings XX World Congress of Sports Medicine*, Melbourne.

86. Williams, J. G. P. (1969) Treatment of chronic Achilles peritendonitis by stripping of the paratenon. *Br. J. sports Med.*, **4**, 223.

87. Snook, G. A. (1972) Achilles tendon tenosynovitis in long distance runners. *Med. Sci. Sports*, **4**, 166.

88. Williams, J. G. P. (1973) Lesions of tendon attachments. *Rheum. Rehabil.*, **12**, 82.

89. Lettin, A. W. F. (1971) In *Encyclopedia of Sports Sciences and Medicine*, ed. Larson, L. A., London: Collier-Macmillan.

90. Quigley, T. B. (1959) Management of ankle injuries sustained in sports. *J. Am. med. Ass.*, **169**, 1431.

91. Williams, J. G. P. (1976) The problem of football boots. In *Proceedings Centenary Medical Congress*, Dublin: Irish Rugby Football Union.

92. Garrick, J. G. and Requa, R. (1973) Role of external support in the prevention of ankle sprains. *Med. Sci. Sports*, **5**, 200.

93. Ferguson, A. B. (1973) The case against ankle taping. *J. sports. Med.*, **1**, 2, 46.

94. Williams, J. G. P. (1965) *Medical Aspects of Sport and Physical Fitness*. London and Oxford: Pergamon Press.

95. Freeman, M. A. R. (1965) Treatment of ruptures of the lateral ligament of the ankle. *J. Bone Jt Surg.*, **47B**, 661.

96. Freeman, M. A. R. (1965) Instability of the foot after injuries to the lateral ligament of the ankle. *J. Bone Jt Surg.*, **47B**, 669.

97. Freeman, M. A. R., Dean, M. R. E. and Hanham, I. W. F. (1965) The etiology and prevention of functional instability of the foot. *J. Bone Jt Surg.*, **47B**, 678.

98. McDougall, A., (1955) Footballer's ankle. *Lancet*, **ii**, 1219.

99. McMurray, T. P. (1950) Footballer's ankle. *J. Bone Jt Surg.*, **32B**, 68.

100. Borsay, J. and Kardos, G. (1952) Isolated fracture of the posterior process of the talus in footballers. *Z. Orthop.*, **82**, 430.

101. Parvin, R. W. and Ford, L. T. (1956) Stenosing tenovaginitis of the common peroneal tendon sheath. *J. Bone Jt Surg.*, **38A**, 1352.

102. Williams, R. (1963) Chronic non-specific tendovaginitis of tibialis posterior. *J. Bone Jt Surg.*, **45B**, 542.

103. Isherwood, I. (1961) A radiological approach to the subtalar joint. *J. Bone Jt Surg.*, **43B,** 566.
104. Webster, F. S. and Roberts, W. M. (1951) Tarsal anomalies and peroneal spastic flat foot. *J. Am. med. Ass.*, **146,** 1099.
105. Jack, E. A. (1954) Bone anomalies of the tarsus in relation to 'peroneal spastic flat foot'. *J. Bone Jt Surg.*, **36B,** 530.
106. Savastano, A. A. (1971) In *Encyclopedia of Sports Sciences and Medicine*, ed. Larson, L. A., London: Collier-Macmillan.
107. Sperryn, P. N. (1971) Heels of athletes' shoes. *Br. J. sports Med.*, **5,** 188.
108. Spence, W. R. and Shields, M. N. (1968) New insole for prevention of athletic blisters. *J. sports Med phys. Fitness*, **8,** 177.

26

First aid

It is desirable that a significant proportion of all members of a sports club, including officials and ground staff, have an elementary knowledge of the principles and practice of first aid, such as that given in England by the St John Ambulance Association.[1] In addition, they should have extra training for any hazards that are specific to the sport concerned. It is also necessary that they should take refresher courses from time to time, to learn new techniques and to revise knowledge and skills that may not have been used frequently.

Physiotherapists, nurses, and scientifically trained physical educationalists should possess all the knowledge of the lay first aid worker, and in addition should be able to carry out certain special jobs for which they have been trained—postural drainage and aspiration of the airway, supervision of a transfusion, and application of plaster of Paris splints and back-slabs. They should be able to instruct first aid workers in some of their training.

The club or team doctor should have all the first aid knowledge and practical skill of trained first aid and paramedical workers. He must take responsibility for treatment, direct his assistants, and perform certain duties outside the scope of those without medical qualification, including, if necessary, the pronouncement of death, the prescription of Controlled Drugs, and the performance of emergency operations, e.g. tracheotomy or pleural tap. It is also desirable that he be able to train others in first aid, and assess their competence.

Unfortunately, in many medical schools there is little if any first aid taught to students. The doctor must be able to make independent decisions, even under pressure from team manager, coaches, ambulance personnel or police, whilst accepting that there are limitations to his privileges; for example, he has no right on the football field or in the boxing ring unless invited by the referee.[2] He also has responsibilities to colleagues, to the law (whether national or just to the rules of the sport involved), and above all to his patient.

Principles of first aid

(1) The preservation of life.
(2) The prevention of further injury to the patient and to others.
(3) The relief of pain and anxiety.
(4) The first stage in the rehabilitation of the injured sportsman.

The scope of first aid in sports medicine is very wide. The range of sporting activities, each with its special hazards, for which provision should be made is great and almost any emergency can occur without warning in any sporting venue, either to participants or spectators (Fig. 26.1). Asphyxia, cardiac arrest,

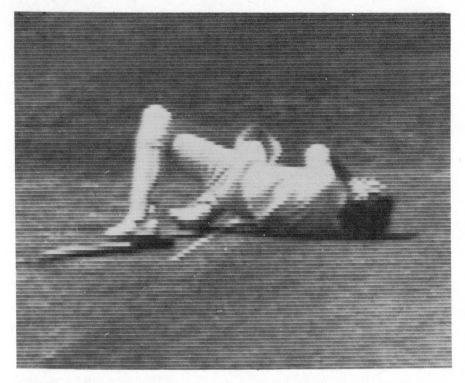

Fig. 26.1 'Almost any emergency can occur without warning'; batsman laid out by a fast ball at cricket. (Photo: Central Press Photos.)

severe trauma and thermal stresses can occur in any sport, anywhere. First aid treatment must be concentrated first upon those conditions in which life is endangered, and afterwards other procedures can be carried out to reduce pain. Nobody will be grateful for an expertly splinted corpse! Asphyxia, cardiac arrest and severe haemorrhage must be treated first.

Asphyxia

Even in sports, asphyxia may occur (see also Chapter 23). Causes include:

(a) breathing irrespirable mixtures, for example swimming pool water, gases;
(b) inspiration of foreign bodies into the respiratory passages, for example inhalation of dentures or chewing-gum;[3]
(c) tissue damage, for example laryngeal oedema following a 'short arm tackle'; and
(d) external obstruction such as strangulation by parachute harness.

Signs of asphyxia

(1) Cessation of respiration. Some respiratory muscles, such as the muscles of the nostrils, mouth, and pharynx may continue to work for some time, but both the diaphragm and intercostals are inactive.

(2) Colour. The skin is pale in cardiac asphyxia, but cyanosed when the asphyxia is limited to the respiratory system.

(3) Partial asphyxia is often much more difficult to diagnose and may progress insidiously to complete asphyxia. The gradual progression of such a condition as haemopneumothorax can be characterized by a slow increase in respiration rate, with progressively more shallow breathing. A gradual onset of cyanosis may be present, but often this useful sign is absent.

Treatment of Asphyxia

Oxygen must be supplied to the lungs as soon as any mechanical obstruction is cleared, so the first essential is urgently to establish an adequate airway.[4] Foreign matter such as leaves or dentures should be removed with the finger. Fluid should be aspirated as soon as improvised or correct equipment is available. A foreign body impacted in the airway may be expelled by the firm sudden com-

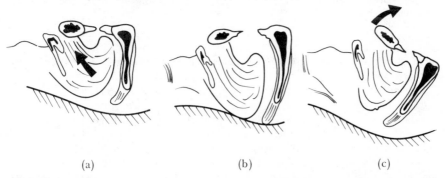

(a)	(b)	(c)

Fig. 26.2 Obstruction of the airway by the tongue in the unconscious patient. (a) Normal tone in the muscles of the tongue leaves the airway patent. (b) In unconsciousness the muscles lose tone and the tongue falls back causing obstruction. (c) Pulling the chin forwards restores the airway.

pression of the thoracic cage. Because of the attachment of the tongue musculature to the mandible, lack of tone in this muscle mass in deep unconsciousness allows the tongue to fall against the vertebral column and causes mechanical obstruction of the pharynx (Fig. 26.2). Extension of the neck combined with support of the jaw in a forward position, will allow adequate air flow above and behind the tongue.

Resuscitation[5, 6] can now be started by the expired air method (mouth-to-mouth or mouth-to-nose) or by use of properly applied breathing apparatus such as an airway or mechanically operated equipment such as the 'minute man', Ambu, or similar bag (Fig. 26.3). This permits simultaneous closed chest cardiac massage[7] if it is indicated. Great care must be taken to prevent inhalation of

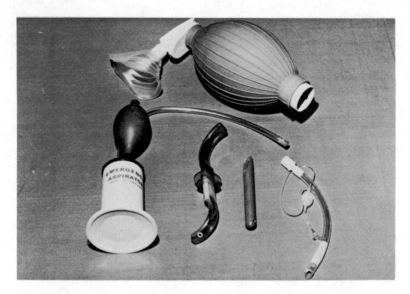

Fig. 26.3 The contents of a simple resuscitation kit (by Vitalograph) includes hand-operated ventilating equipment, hand-operated aspiration sucker pump, two-way airway (different sizes and suitable for expired air resuscitation), wedge for opening jaws, and endotracheal tube.

regurgitated gastric contents, and immediate aspiration or gravity draining by turning the patient three-quarters on to his face must be carried out, with resumption of resuscitation as soon as possible (Fig. 26.4).

Particular care must be taken with artificial airways to ensure that they are inserted into the correct place, are fully patent, and are not curled up inside the mouth or blocked by mud or packing material. It is also essential that the lips be closed firmly round the airway and that the nose be clipped or the nostrils held together to prevent the escape of the air or gases being supplied.

It must also be ensured that the air administered actually enters the lungs and not the oesophagus. A stomach inflated with air effectively prevents inflation of the bases of the lungs, and hinders diastolic filling of the ventricles. The only really reliable artificial airway is an inflatable endotracheal tube, which is easier to pass in the deeply unconscious patient who is not breathing than in one whose cough reflex is still active.

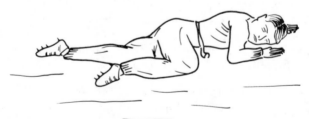

Fig. 26.4 The coma position; this may not look very tidy on a stretcher but is much safer for the patient.

The rescuer's expired air is a most efficient breathing mixture, and its 2 per cent or so of carbon dioxide is a respiratory stimulant.

There are problems of ventilating patients with facial injuries, but the modified Silvester method of arm extension alternating with thoracic compression can be successful, provided that the neck is hyperextended.

Once respiration has been established, the patient should be placed in the three-quarter prone coma position. Frequent observations must be made to ensure that breathing continues, the airway is clear, and that there is no constriction to the neck, chest or abdomen by tight clothing.

Other emergency measures may be needed to deal with specific complications.

Tension pneumothorax

This is common after penetrating wounds to the chest. It is necessary to make the wound as airtight as possible by an occlusive dressing, such as a piece of polythene sheet, tulle gras or wet cloth. If there is increasing respiratory distress, the dressing can be removed, the wound edges opened, and the lungs reinflated by mechanical means or expired air resuscitation. Much more of the rescuer's expired air is needed than in normal mouth-to-mouth respiration.

Pulmonary oedema

Following head injury, respiration may sometimes become more difficult, with froth expelled from the mouth or nose, and diminished percussion note in the chest.

Pulmonary oedema can occur insidiously at any time from half an hour to a day after brain injury. Respiration must be maintained, with frequent aspiration of the frothy fluid, and as soon as possible a diuretic such as frusemide (Lasix) should be injected (20 mg intravenously initially, and repeated if there is little response).

Laryngeal oedema

If due to anaphylaxis, immediate injection of adrenaline should be given, and this can be followed by antihistamines such as chlorpheniramine maleate (Piriton) (10 mg intramuscularly, repeated half an hour later if necessary). Intubation should be carried out, and if unsuccessful, a tracheostomy may be needed, but this step is indicated only very rarely.

Cardiac arrest

Cardiac resuscitation must always be accompanied by an effective form of artificial respiration, performed either by a machine, a second rescuer, or single-handed by alternating cardiac with respiratory measures. Closed chest cardiac massage should not be attempted if there is a proper heart beat present. Great care must be taken when practising cardiac massage on the healthy volunteer during training or on any conscious person. The signs of cardiac arrest are:

(1) Unconsciousness.
(2) No palpable pulse at the carotid arteries.
(3) No respiration.

(4) No heart sounds or palpable apex beat.
(5) Fixed dilated pupils.

It is not possible to differentiate between asystole and fibrillation by palpation and auscultation—this requires use of the ECG. Defibrillation is best performed by the electric defibrillator carried by specialist cardiac resuscitation teams, but in an emergency a firm blow on the precordium may stop fibrillation, and this should be followed immediately by intermittent pressure over the sternum at approximately the normal pulse rate. Five or six cardiac compressions should be interspersed by inflation of the lungs. The carotid pulse must be checked frequently, and as soon as systoles recur, cardiac compression must be suspended. Unfortunately, the chances of restarting a heart in complete asystole are not good, but it is always worth attempting.

Cardiac tamponade

This may follow penetrating wounds of the thorax or upper abdomen, or even closed fractures of the ribs. The jugular venous pressure is raised, but a carotid pulse differentiates tamponade from arrest. It may be possible to aspirate blood from the pericardium, if a syringe and wide-bore needle are available, and so enable ventricular filling to take place pending operation and closure of the myocardial wound.

Inevitably biochemical changes occur during cardiac and respiratory arrest, with at least a change of blood pH. Proper laboratory investigations are needed to rectify these changes, so hospital admission is essential. Following drowning, there are risks of chemical or bacteriological contamination, for which precautions have to be taken, and a sample of the water from which the victim was recovered should be made available to the laboratory if it is needed. It is not necessary to remove a drowning victim from the water before commencing resuscitation. Mouth-to-mouth respiration can be performed as soon as the victim is brought to the surface, and even a couple of lung inflations at this stage can increase the chances of survival. Occasional inflations can be carried out while towing towards shallow water; they are done more efficiently when the rescuer can touch bottom or the bank.

In resuscitation after asphyxia time is of the essence and seconds count.

Hypothermia

Acute hypothermia can be a severe problem for those engaged in winter sports, and in aquatic and mountaineering activities at any time of the year (see also Chapter 5).

Signs of acute hypothermia

The onset of hypothermia is usually marked by cortical changes and the patient becomes talkative, slightly inco-ordinated and excitable. His judgement increasingly becomes impaired, and he may complain of feeling cold. Heat loss can be reduced by waterproof clothing, and even a thin plastic clothes bag with a hole cut for the head can be a life-saving measure.

If any member of an expedition shows even the earliest signs of hypothermia, the expedition should be abandoned immediately, and the patient returned to roadhead or shelter where he can be warmed as soon as possible. Unless treated, the patient becomes progressively inco-ordinated, slurred in speech, and incapable of making any rational decision. Intense weakness, then paralysis follows, so it is best to seek warmth long before the patient becomes a stretcher case, always assuming that a stretcher can reach him in time.

Treatment of hypothermia—acute

There has been some controversy over whether reheating should be carried out slowly or rapidly. In acute exposure in young healthy people, rapid warming is essential, and the sooner it is instituted, the better the prognosis. There is no need to wait until the patient is brought to roadhead or hospital before starting reheating.

(1) Prevention of further heat loss can be assisted by wrapping the patient in waterproof material—groundsheet, anorak, plastic bag, or the special heavy duty rubber survival bags recently developed for cave rescue. Much heat can be lost through the skin of the hands and face, so as much of the surface should be covered consistent with the patient's ability to breathe. The minimum interference should be made in the examination and treatment of injuries, to avoid further exposure. If rescue is delayed, for example, through clearing rock or other debris, or awaiting a stretcher, the patient can be warmed by close contact with his colleagues, who can also help to screen him from the wind.

(2) Application of external heat. Cave rescue teams now bring hot water tanks to the cavemouth for filling the survival bags as soon as they can reach the victim. Hot water bottles, any other container with hot liquid, or cooling stones from a camp fire, well wrapped to prevent burning, can all supply external heat during transport. Unless unconscious, the patient should be immersed in a hot bath as soon as he reaches a house or hospital. Mouth or axillary temperature give little indication of core temperature, so rectal temperature must be recorded; the temperature of recently voided urine is a good guide to core temperature.

(3) Oxygen can be administered when available, and is best given warm. Apparatus for supplying warmed oxygen has been developed for cave rescue, and will prevent the considerable heat loss that occurs during expiration.

(4) Warm drinks can be given to the conscious patient and glucose or other sugar will assist in increasing metabolism and heat production. Under no circumstances should alcohol be given until reheating is complete, because of its vasodilating effect upon the skin vessels with consequent increase in heat loss.

Shock

When tissue is damaged through injury, crush, or burns it liberates a histamine-like substance that acts as a peripheral vasodilator, leading to capillary stagnation in the muscles and splanchnic area. This results in a progressive diminution of the circulation to the brain, heart and lungs, and the classical signs of shock are due to the body's attempts to compensate for this anoxia.

Signs of shock

(1) Cold sweating skin.
(2) Pallor, and perhaps slight cyanosis.
(3) Rapid faint pulse.
(4) Hypotension.
(5) Rapid breathing—air hunger.
(6) Cerebral excitement, later leading to confusion then coma.
(7) Oliguria.

The cold damp pale skin is due to attempts to produce cutaneous vasoconstriction, hence the pallor. The worst treatment that can be given is overheating, which increases the vascularity of the surfaces and therefore deprives the essential circulation to the brain, heart and lungs of yet more blood. Tachycardia and rapid respiration are compensation for cerebral anoxia, but as blood loss or stagnation increases, the blood pressure eventually falls despite these compensatory mechanisms. Cerebral anoxia is characterized by excitement at first—the patient often asking the same, usually irrelevant, question over and over again.

Treatment of shock

Because of the circulatory stagnation, the only really effective treatment of severe shock is the *transfusion of whole blood*, whether there has been any significant haemorrhage or not. If this is not available immediately, some of the capillary stagnation can be partly overcome by a saline or glucose drip, or preferably plasma or dextran.

The use of warm sweet drinks can be justified where transfusion has to be delayed for many hours—on a mountain, or at sea—but not when hospital services are a few hours away.

The failing circulation can be helped by lying the patient flat (in the semi-prone coma position if unconscious). The limbs can be raised to assist gravity in venous drainage, but tilting the body head down can embarrass respiration as the weight of the viscera keeps the diaphragm elevated. Tight clothing at the neck and waist must be loosened, and an adequate airway ensured.

Further blood loss must be prevented by securing haemostasis, and elevation of the bleeding limb. Fractures must be immobilized very carefully to prevent crepitus, which will increase the state of shock. Pain must be relieved. Although some authorities use pentazocine hydrochloride (Fortral) (30 or 60 mg intramuscularly) as the drug of choice, others do not find it very effective, and prefer morphia (10–15 mg by slow intravenous injection). If pain is severe, but the peripheral circulation adequate, the injection can be given intramuscularly or subcutaneously. Morphia must *not* be given in head, chest or abdominal injuries.

Oxygen should be given to the severely shocked, but the use of adrenaline is contraindicated. Cortisone is sometimes given, but is of doubtful value in hypovolaemic shock.

Haemorrhage

Blood loss is variable in effects but the patient is at risk to life if the effective loss reaches 25 per cent. Concealed bleeding is difficult to estimate. A litre of blood may be lost into the tissues in a closed fracture of the tibia and far greater volumes may be lost through haemorrhage into pleural or peritoneal cavities.

Treatment of haemorrhage

(1) External arterial haemorrhage can usually be controlled by grasping the wound edges together with the fingers and thumb, and maintaining that grasp for at least ten minutes. The grasp is then re-applied if there is further bleeding. When dressings are available, a large absorbent pad should be applied and outside this a firm bandage. More padding and another firm bandage should then be applied and nothing more done to the wound until the patient is in the operating theatre.

(2) External venous haemorrhage. In an athlete during competition the large blood flow to active limbs can lead to profuse haemorrhage if a leg vein is spiked or caught on a thorn in cross-country running. Bleeding is easily controlled with a pad and firm bandage, and elevation of the injured limb. The dressing should be left alone for 24 hours, unless surgical cleansing or suture are needed.

(3) External capillary haemorrhage. Small wounds are often deep and contaminated, and as the best material for washing out a wound is fresh blood, haemostatic measures can be left until the wound has bled enough to clean itself. If there is little bleeding, it can be encouraged by the application of a light venous tourniquet such as a handkerchief wrapped round proximal to the lesion, and/or swinging the limb to encourage bleeding by centrifugal force. Brief immersion in warm water can also increase bleeding.

Once the wound is clean, and anaerobic bacteria have been well oxygenated in its depths, a dressing is applied and the limb is elevated (and sutured if necessary).

(4) Epistaxis. Facial contusions associated with epistaxis are common in sports. Epistaxis can usually be controlled by application of:

(a) ice (or other source of cold);
(b) compression (by compressing the nostrils together);
(c) elevation (by sitting the patient upright).

Nasal fractures with displacement will need reduction soon after injury. If haemorrhage cannot be controlled by simple means, packing of the nose with several metres of adrenaline-soaked ribbon gauze may be necessary.

(5) Internal bleeding. Intra-abdominal haemorrhage may be from a ruptured solid viscus, or from the tearing of a branch of the aorta, almost invariably an anterior branch, the coeliac or a mesenteric artery. Curling the patient up with his knees near his chin compresses the abdominal wall and tends to compress the tear and reduce the leakage of blood (Fig. 26.5). Lying the patient supine at attention may make him look tidy on a stretcher, but stretches the torn vessel and encourages bleeding. The curled-up position

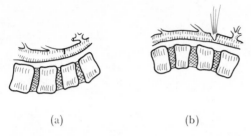

(a)   (b)

Fig. 26.5 Trunk flexion usually reduces aortic haemorrhage. (a) Flexion. (b) Extension.

should be maintained until a transfusion is running and the surgeon is ready to perform a laparotomy.

'Pattern bruising', where the pattern of clothing is imprinted on the skin, indicates severe compression with the possibility of visceral rupture. The possibility of ruptured ectopic pregnancy must be remembered as a cause of emergency in the sportswoman.

(6) Haemorrhage into tissue. Because of the increased vascularity of 'fit' muscles, particularly during exercise, interstitial haemorrhage following tear, sprain or fracture tends to be profuse. Treatment is application of cold packs together with compression and elevation.

Fractures

All suspected fractures and dislocations should be treated by immobilization using suitable splints, followed by evacuation to hospital. The pneumatic inflatable splint is particularly useful since it not only immobilizes the limb but its compression minimizes haemorrhage (Fig. 26.6).

Head injuries and suspected spinal fractures require particular care. The patient should be moved as far as possible 'in one piece' and this can best be done by six lifters (three each side) co-ordinated by a seventh who controls the patient's head.

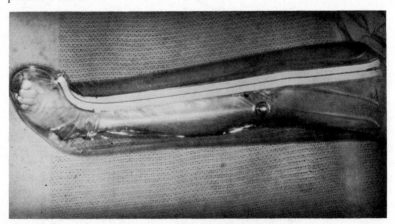

Fig. 26.6. Inflatable pneumatic splint; a 'must' for the first aid bag.

Fractured pelvis also requires special care. The patient may feel 'flattened out', so the first aim is to restore the body to its usual cylindrical state, by firm supporting bandages round the pelvis, and by holding the legs together by a figure-of-eight bandage round the feet and ankles, and a bandage around the thighs. There is usually an urgent desire to micturate, but this must be prohibited to prevent possible extravasation from a ruptured urethra and consequent perineal cellulitis.

Burns

Burns other than sunburn, are uncommon in sport but may follow accidents in motor-car, motor-cycle or motor-boat racing. First aid involves removal from the cause of the burn, protection of the lesion from infection, and treatment of pain or shock along usually accepted lines. The immediate application of cold water for 20 minutes or so usually reduces blistering and relieves pain.

Other conditions

Various other less traumatic but frequently disabling conditions may occur in sport, the morbidity of which may be much reduced by prompt and efficient first aid.

Insect stings and bites

Mosquito, gnat and flea bites rarely need treatment, other than the application of a commercial sting-relief lotion.

Temporary relief can be given immediately by spraying with a topical freezing anaesthetic such as ethyl chloride or Skefron. Antihistamine tablets and creams are not very effective, and the former can induce drowsiness.

Wasps usually retract the sting, but bees leave it *in situ* after stinging. If the sting has been left in, it should be removed with fine forceps or a sterilized needle. Stings in the mouth may lead to oedema, with possible respiratory obstruction in patients with an allergy to the insect's sting. A mouthwash with sodium bicarbonate should be given immediately, the sting removed, and an antihistamine injection given as soon as possible. It may be necessary to administer corticosteroids as well.

Snake bites

These are a hazard to cross-country runners, even in Britain, in adder-infested areas. There is usually a severe degree of shock, both neurogenic and hypovolaemic, and fatalities are due to the former. A constrictive bandage should be applied proximal to the lesion and released for a short time at twenty-minute intervals.

Urgent evacuation to hospital or to a centre where the appropriate antivenom is available must be carried out.

Dog bites

A runner's or cyclist's legs can prove a temptation to excited canine spectators. As these wounds are usually contaminated, and there is bruising to the skin edges, wound cleansing by the encouragement of fresh bleeding, and closure by strapping rather than suture is the safest course. Antitetanus vaccine should be given unless the patient has been immunized (see Chapter 7).

Foreign bodies

An insect buzzing in the ear is a frightening occurrence; it can be floated out if warm vegetable oil is instilled into the external auditory meatus, the patient lying on his side with the affected ear uppermost. If oil is not available, warm water may suffice. Syringing is rarely necessary.

Stitch

This occurs usually in distance running, especially when running downhill, and often when the stomach is fairly full. There are probably several aetiological factors concerned, but one of the most important is tension on the ligament of Trietz, supporting the pylorus from the diaphragm, and containing skeletal muscle and cerebrospinal nerve endings. Cessation of abdominal movement relieves the condition, and it may be possible to continue running but with the trunk flexed, a difficult and inefficient technique, but one that should enable a competitor at least to complete the course.

Winding

Winding is due to a blow on the abdomen, causing temporary delay in venous return in the inferior vena cava, and overstimulation to the autonomic (especially parasympathetic) fibres in the coeliac plexus. There is temporary bradycardia and bronchospasm, which will recover with rest. Forceful spinal flexion is contraindicated as symptoms could be due to vertebral injury caused by the sudden flexion from the abdominal blow.

Cramp

Cramp can be due to several causes; muscle anoxia, cold, imbalance of salts (as in heat cramp following sodium chloride loss), or hormonal factors (especially the tendency to cramp during the menstrual period). The attack can usually be relieved by relaxation of the affected muscles, assisted by massage towards the periphery. Female swimmers are advised to train in the outside lanes during menstruation, and to float, relaxed, if affected by cramp while in the water. There is danger of cramp in anyone swimming too soon after a meal (while much of the circulation is devoted to absorption and digestion and is not readily available to the active skeletal musculature).

Distance-runner's heat collapse

During prolonged muscular effort in a hot humid environment, the heat production of the active muscles can exceed heat loss by sweating and evaporation, so that the body core temperature rises, and there is loss of cerebral function. If the patient is allowed to lie flat and rest, and cooling is accelerated by removal of clothing, fanning, and tepid sponging, he will recover rapidly. The use of very cold water causes cutaneous vasoconstriction, therefore heat retention. Pulling the patient to his feet and walking him around is the worst way to overcome cerebral anoxia. Crowding round him keeps a cooling breeze away. The wrong treatment and delay in correcting cerebral anoxia has been known to leave permanent brain damage.

Conclusion

Most first aid is the application of common sense, based upon the knowledge of elementary principles. The priorities of treatment must be observed; preservation of life, prevention of further injury, relief of pain and suffering, and avoidance of any action that might make the condition of the patient worse, or cause unnecessary distress to his family and colleagues.

Certain essential equipment should be available in places where it is likely to be needed,[8] but the doctor or first aid worker in attendance must be able to improvise, and to use his initiative to carry out treatment even under the most difficult conditions.

The best way to learn first aid is to teach it.

H.E.R.

References

1. Anonymous (1975) *First Aid Manual*, 3rd edn revised. St. John Ambulance, St. Andrew Ambulance Association and British Red Cross Society, London: St. John Ambulance.
2. Kelleher, K. D. (1976) The referee and injuries on the field. *Proceedings Centenary Medical Congress*. Dublin: Irish Rugby Football Union.
3. Moncur, J. A. (1973) Inhalation of chewing-gum: fatality during rugby. Proceedings XVIII World Congress of Sports Medicine. *Br. J. Sports Med.*, **71**, 162.
4. Combs, L. W. (1965) Establishing the proper airway in athletic emergencies. *J. NATA*, **1**, 18.
5. Haid, B. C. (1971) In *Encyclopedia of Sports Sciences and Medicine*, ed. Larson, L. A., London: Collier-Macmillan.
6. Gordon, A. (1961) The principles and practice of heart-lung resuscitation. *Acta anaesth. scand.*, Supp. **9**, 134.
7. Kouwenhoven, W., Jude, J. R. and Knickerbocker, G. (1960) Closed chest cardiac massage. *J. Am. Med. Ass.*, **173**, 1064.
8. Straub, W. F. (1971) In *Encyclopedia of Sport Sciences and Medicine*, ed. Larson, L. A., London: Collier-Macmillan.

27

Sport and age

Introduction

Physical activity is necessary throughout life if the human organism is to remain healthy and independent. The term 'play' is often used to describe the physical activities which are indulged in by adults and children, and confusion has arisen in an attempt to equate what are two entirely different things. The play of the child is an exploration of the environment without which normal development is not possible and which may or may not be physically demanding, while the play of the adult is a pastime and generally has no other aim than the pleasurable occupation of spare time. Too often this 'play' in the adult is replaced by non-physical activities to the detriment of physical health. Consequently it is frequently found that simple physical activity must be prescribed as a therapeutic measure in later years. Sport in some sense can be used as a tool in both these types of play by parents, teachers, doctors, and by politicians to further aims which have nothing to do with 'sport' as such. As long as these aims are directed towards the benefit of the individual in terms of educational, psychological, social, or medical advantage this use of sport is legitimate. Indeed, as far as health is concerned, sport must be the most palatable dose of social medicine yet devised!

'Better to hunt in fields, for health unbought,
Than fee the doctor for a nauseous draught.'
(John Dryden)

What can be claimed for sport? Claims have been made of the value of games in the inculcation of courage, leadership, character building, etc., but evidence for such claims is lacking and few would still argue 'The Battle of Waterloo was won on the playing fields of Eton'!

Firm claims can be made only on the basis that sporting activities are physical and can be shown to improve cardiovascular function, joint mobility, muscle strength, certain neuromuscular skills, and can be used as an occupational therapy to a limited extent in psychological disorders. It must, however, also be recognized that it is possible to overdo physical activity,[1] and that the very nature of sport lays the participant open to a greater or less risk of injury with some long-term effects in the shape of joint damage.[2,3]

The purpose of this chapter is to examine briefly the line which sporting activities should take at various ages so that maximum benefit and minimum damage may accrue, and to suggest that Childhood and Youth should be a preparation for a vigorous Old Age. The idea that a man's progress through life is an inevitable decline from childhood to senility is no longer valid, and sporting activities can undoubtedly play a part in promoting the interest, companionship, activity, and altertness which influence the quality of life, whether or not contributing to longevity.

The physical activity required for the various age groups, i.e. the pre-school child, the school child, the adult, and the elderly will now be considered. Apart from the arbitrary selection of 5 years (when in Great Britain a child begins school), and the onset of puberty, the borderlines between the schoolboy and the adult, and between the adult and the elderly are becoming increasingly difficult to define. Any advice given to an individual on the sporting activity in which he should indulge must therefore be given with regard to his individual needs and potential, and not because he falls into an arbitrarily defined group.

The pre-school child

Since the maintenance of activity throughout life depends upon the progress of the degenerative diseases, it follows that anything which can be done to slow the progress of degeneration will be valuable. It is generally accepted that minor

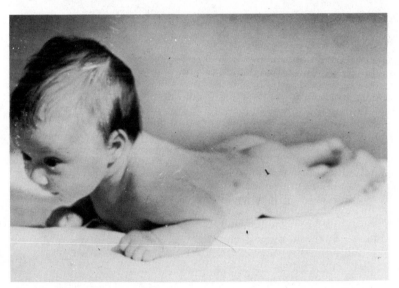

Fig. 27.1 An eight-week-old baby that as learnt to raise his head—and enjoy it.

disturbances of joint function will contribute to an earlier onset of degenerative joint disease,[4] and anything which can be done to promote and maintain the mobility, strength, and sound mechanics of those joints where degeneration is commonest, should play some part in ensuring a longer active and symptom-free life for those joints. From the earliest days infants can indulge in gymnastics to strengthen their muscles and a mother naturally plays with her baby whether or not she knows that she is preparing his limbs for future activity. What is less well known is that babies can raise their heads from the first weeks of life. If a baby is made to lie in the prone position he will raise his head and quickly learn to control it with nothing but benefit for his vertebral muscles, and a flying start for his next activity of crawling (Fig. 27.1). At the standing and walking stage babies should be given the opportunity to walk barefoot on rough surfaces, e.g. shingle, to promote development of the intrinsic musculature of the feet. Any footwear should be non-constricting. Even at this stage babies may take part in sport with their parents (Fig. 27.2)!

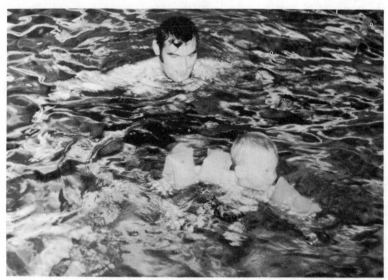

Fig. 27.2 This young man is 14-months-old and has been participating in bathing from the age of eight months.

The school child

Until a child begins to participate in major sports, particular attention should be given to the maintenance of mobility in joints, and to the use of these joints in non-injurious ways. Much has been written about the importance of footwear for the developing foot, and there is no doubt that foot disability is to a great extent due to badly fitting shoes and socks. It has been suggested[5] that while this is undoubtedly true, the strong active foot is more likely to be able to resist the insults of faulty footwear. Physical educationalists in the schools should be aware of this and plan their programmes accordingly. Similarly, mobility and sound posture of the vertebral column should attract as much attention as the feet, and any physical activity which promotes these is to be commended. The well-trained teacher of physical education has an unequalled chance to observe children undressed in the gymnasium and swimming pool, and should be the first to recognize poor posture. It is likely that adequate provision of sporting activities will ensure healthy physical development in the majority of children, but there will always be some who will require special attention, and appropriate exercises should be instituted at the earliest suggestion of deviation from 'normal'. This is not to say that there is a norm to which every child should conform, but there is an optimum posture for each particular build, subjective though this assessment may be, and the skilled physical educationalist should be aware of this. It is tragic

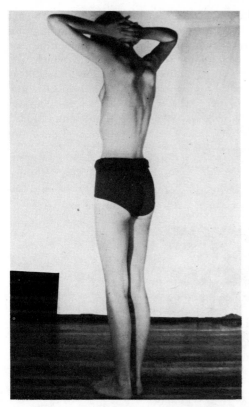

Fig. 27.3 Stiff deformed back in a 12-year-old girl.

that children should be allowed to pass through school without for example a matured spinal deformity (Fig. 27.3) being discovered.[5]

The adult

Further up the school, children are young adults and will indulge in the sporting activities preferred by their social group whether their physique is suitable or not. It is not desirable to prevent this even were it possible, but at least guidance should be given as to suitable activities for different physiques, and some attempt made to reduce, as far as possible, the accidents to which healthy active young adults are prone (for example by the provision of suitable facilities). The question arises as to whether those sports which produce a great many accidents also have some value commensurate with the risks involved in playing them. It may be heresy to suggest that there might be better activities for the young than, for example Rugby football, but is there not something particularly to be said in favour of those activities such as hill-walking, sailing or camping which have potentially a value other than that of a pure pastime and which can be continued to a more advanced age than the more vigorous team games? There is no easy answer to this since activities are chosen according to temperament and social pressures, and no one would wish to deny to the young the vigour and adventure which they seek. It is, however, unwise to demand that all young men be cast in the same mould, and to make claims for the traditional games, which are, to say the least, questionable. Since it is only a matter of time before major team games must be abandoned, it would seem wise to introduce young people to those games which are less physically demanding, so that when the time came it would be possible to transfer to a suitable physical activity rather than to be reduced to developing a paunch at the Club bar!

The later years

To what age should people indulge in vigorous physical activity? The answer would appear to be 'as long as they feel like it, without becoming too distressed'.

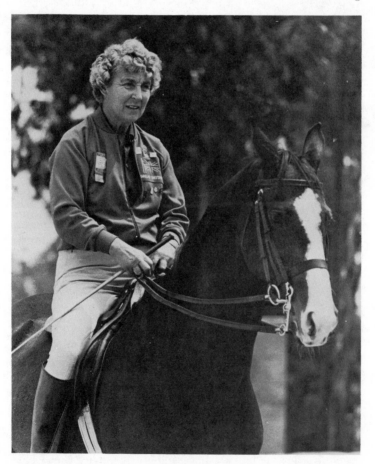

Fig. 27.4 Mrs. Lorna Johnstone (G.B.), an Olympic Competitor at the age of 70. (Photo: E. D. Lacey.)

Borotra played tennis at Wimbledon at the age of 73; Mrs Lorna Johnstone competed in Olympic dressage at the age of 70, and most people will know less famous people who are looked upon as being 'remarkable for their age' (Fig. 27.4). It is likely that many more could emulate these older athletes if they could be reassured that they would not put themselves in imminent danger of death by so doing. Such reassurance (modified by a measure of common sense) can in most cases be given. The evidence for increased longevity in the physically active, is however, equivocal. There have been studies which suggest that exercise plays a protective role in the development of coronary atherosclerosis,[6-8] but other studies deny that the connection between activity and decreased coronary disease has been adequately shown.[8-10] A post-mortem study has, however, shown less coronary artery disease in the physically active,[11] and is encouraging. Unfortunately, prediction of coronary efficiency is not possible, and more recent examinations of the problem[12,13] have not improved on previously held views[14] that the only guide to the effect of exercise is close observation of the subject. If this is undertaken it would seem to be unjustified to restrict the activity of the elderly unless there is a clear reason for so doing.

It is, however, suggested that sport for the elderly should be selected so that skill, patience, and equanimity are at a premium as opposed to the vigour, immediacy and excitement required by the younger participant. But to lay down a specific age at which this transfer should be made would be a mistake since it is in fact impossible. Advice from a medical attendant who himself takes part in the sport concerned could be sought, but many continue in sport to an advanced age relying on their own feelings and their own common sense to tell them when to ease up. Indeed, it is likely that the older sportsman who feels it is necessary to consult his doctor about this problem has probably already answered his own question!

The elderly beginner in sporting activities and the former sportsman wishing to resume sport after many years absence present similar problems which are in turn different from those of the continuously active. The overweight executive who suddenly decides he wishes to participate in a 'jogging' programme because it is fashionable, should be discouraged until he has gradually worked himself up under close supervision to the level of energy output required. This will mean supervised, progressive activity, with monitoring of pulse rate and pulse recovery time until better methods are available. (Ballistocardiography[15] or displacement cardiography[16] may possibly have a predictive value but these techniques are at present not generally available.) The return to exercise should not be taken in isolation. Attention to obesity, smoking, and drinking habits is mandatory, but if all these precautions are taken there is no doubt that 'training' of the elderly unfit in the absence of cardiac decompensation and pulmonary disorders (such as emphysema) is both possible and beneficial.

It will frequently be found that participation in sport by the elderly has become restricted because of pain in degenerated joints. In most cases this will be because of muscle insufficiency and early limitation of movement, but rather than reduce his activities the sportsman should be advised to train for his selected sport by indulging in exercises which will increase the mobility of his damaged joints and strengthen his weakening muscles. These exercises may have to be artificial because joints are not normally carried to their full range of movement, and movement in the little-used range of a joint will become uncomfortable, encouraging the subject to restrict his movement still further, and so on. It has been known for some time that sufferers from degenerative joint disease who are physically active complain less than the sedentary worker.[17]

The opportunities for participation in sporting activities are increasing rapidly and with the advent of an increasing number of Community Sports Centres it is becoming ever more possible for sport to be a family concern. The advantages which this brings to both the young and the old cannot be overemphasized and, apart from the obvious social advantages in the shape of bridges between the generations, there is a vast untapped area of active therapeutics in the psychological[18] as well as the physical field which those concerned with Health should exploit.

J.A.M.

References

1. Williams, J. G. P. and Sperryn, P. N. (1972) Overuse injuries in sport and work. *Br. J. sports Med.*, **6,** 50.
2. Murray, R. O. (1965) The aetiology of primary osteoarthritis of the hip. *Br. J. Radiol.*, **38,** 810.
3. Tucker, W. E. and Armstrong, J. R. (1964) *Injury in Sport.* London: Staples Press.
4. Hollander, J. L. (Ed.) (1960) *Arthritis and Allied Conditions.* Philadelphia: Lea and Febiger.
5. Moncur, J. A. (1958) An investigation into minor orthopaedic deformities in first year secondary schoolchildren. *Br. J. sports Med.*, **3,** 204.
6. Morris, J. N., Heady, J. A., Raffle, P. A. B., Roberts, C. G. and Parks, J. W. (1953) Coronary heart disease and physical activity of work. *Lancet* **ii,** 1053, 1111.
7. Morris, J. N. and Crawford, M. D. (1958) Coronary heart disease and physical activity of work—evidence of a national necropsy survey. *Br. med. J.*, **ii,** 1485.
8. Spain, D. M. and Bradess, V. A. (1960) Occupational physical activity and the degree of coronary atherosclerosis in 'normal' men. *Circulation*, **XXII,** 239.
9. Brunner, D. and Jokl, E. (1970) *Physical Activity and Aging.* Basel: Karger.
10. Shapiro, S., Weinblatt, E., Frank, C. W. and Sager, R. V. (1969) Incidence of coronary heart disease in a population insured for medical care, *Am. J. publ. Hlth,* **59,** 1 (Suppl.).
11. Morris, J. N. and Gardner, M. J. (1969) Epidemiology of ischaemic heart disease. *Am. J. Med.*, **46,** 674.
12. Anonymous (1972) Life pattern for coronary arteries. *Br. med. J.*, **iv,** 63.
13. Short, D. and Stowers, M. (1972) Earliest symptoms of coronary heart disease and their recognition. *Br. med. J.*, **ii,** 387.
14. Williams, J. G. P. (1965) Exercise and the diseased heart. *Research Reviews* 1964–5. London: Trafford Press.
15. Holloszy, J. O., Skinner, J. S., Toro, G. and Cureton, T. K. (1964) Effects of a six-month program of endurance exercise on the serum lipids of middle-aged men. *Am. J. Cardiol.*, **14,** 753.
16. Vas, R. (1972) Changes in heart movements during controlled physical activity. *Br. J. sports Med.*, **6,** 147.
17. Lawrence, J. S. (1955) Rheumatism in coal miners. *Br. J. ind. Med.*, **12,** 249.
18. Platt, R. and Parkes, A. S. (1967) *Social and Genetic Influences on Life and Death.* Edinburgh: Oliver and Boyd.

28

Sport and disability

Sport has much to offer the injured and disabled. It provides not merely a vehicle for therapeutic exercise under particular conditions of competition[1] and physical enjoyment, but offers opportunities for interest and fulfilment in individuals permanently disabled who, by virtue of their disability, might not have other satisfactory outlets. In this context therefore, sport has that quality of liberality defined by Newman in his *Idea of a University* which takes it beyond the more mundane concept of a mere method of carrying out physical activity.[2]

The purely therapeutic aspects of sport require little elaboration.[3] Exercise in the treatment of locomotor disease is clearly established and its role in the treatment of other illnesses, for example cardiac and mental illness, is becoming more clearly defined.[4, 5] It is, however, in its role as a means to fulfilment for disabled people that sport has a very special medical and social value.

Historical

Many examples have been recorded of certain types of sport which have been successfully promoted amongst disabled adults and children, both for rehabilitation and for continuing physical recreation. Early instances of organized activities are the provision for amputees and blind ex-servicemen in Germany after the First World War. Later came an organization in the U.S.A. providing golf for leg and arm amputees, while in Britain the Society of One-Armed Golfers was formed in 1932. During and after the Second World War there was a great increase in sporting provision, particularly in rehabilitation. In several European countries and the U.S.A., skiing became popular for amputees and those with visual handicaps. National voluntary organizations for disabled ex-servicemen used various sports, both competitive and non-competitive, for rehabilitation and recreation. Notable for the subsequent world-wide effect were the International Stoke Mandeville Games, which did much to establish competitive segregated games for people in wheelchairs (Fig. 28.1). Table-tennis, basketball, fencing, shot, discus, javelin, archery, bowling, wheelchair dashes and swimming have become associated with disabled people in the minds of the public. The International Sports Organization for the Disabled was founded under the aegis of the World Veteran's Federation and later became independent. There are member organizations in Japan, Italy, Indonesia, Germany, Iceland, Denmark, U.K., U.S.A., Czechoslovakia, New Zealand, Spain, Yugoslavia and several other countries. In recent times there have been established the European Basketball Championships, international volleyball competitions for amputees, athletic competitions organized the International Cerebral Palsy Society, World Skiing Championships for blind people and amputees, and the World Games for the

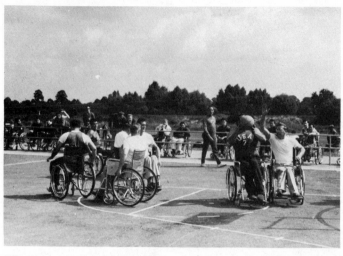

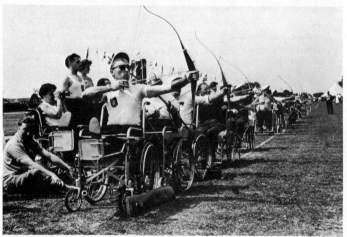

Fig. 28.1 Basketball and archery from a wheelchair; sports in the Stoke Mandeville Games.

Deaf which have been held annually for more than a dozen years. The Special Olympics Programme for mentally handicapped young people began with an event for a thousand children in Chicago in 1968. Two years later there were 1400 meetings in 49 States of the U.S.A. as well as in Canada and France. In 1972 a quarter of a million children and young adults took part in local and regional games, and Puerto Rico is now included in the scheme. The organizers estimated that two million young mentally handicapped people did not have an opportunity to join in sports in the U.S.A.

There is room for both integrated and segregated provision; total integration within the community, however desirable this may be, is not always possible nor even appropriate in sport. It is not surprising that disabled athletes seek situations in which they can compete as nearly as possible on equal terms, and that restricts them in some sports to taking part with people who have 'similar' handicaps (similar in name, but often not in degree). There seems no case against segregated groups which teach, for instance, swimming or riding; if a man is integrated in normal social and working life, does it matter if for an hour or two a week he likes to go to a riding or swimming club where his limitations may be understood better than in the usual club? So that experienced instruction and willing helpers may be readily available, it seems sensible and natural to have some specialist provision (Fig. 28.2). However, it does seem preferable to lean as much as possible towards integration wherever this is realistic.

The frequently repeated statement that competitive sport helps to instil or restore self-confidence and self-respect must be questioned. Is it not inherent in

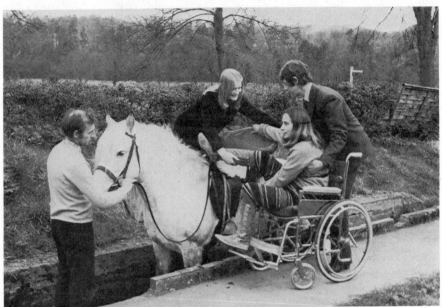

Fig. 28.2 For some activities specialist provision may be necessary; note the special 'pit' for the pony, and the special saddle. Normally a hard hat would be worn. (Photo: Disabled Living Foundation and Town and Country Productions Ltd.)

a situation where the winner's self-confidence and self-respect may be increased that for the loser the opposite effect may result? The question is particularly relevant for a newly disabled person. In a letter to the *British Journal of Sports Medicine*,[7] the following opinion was expressed: 'To those of us familiar with the consequences of failure in highly competitive non-handicapped sport, there appears to be no reason why "normal" competitive attitudes in the disabled should not lead to a similar problem of failure and thus provide for the majority of competitive disabled sportsmen the bitterness of sporting failure as well as of the underlying handicap.'

It must be remembered that sporting failure is not confined to competitive events; it can be very disappointing for some paraplegics or people with cerebral palsy to find that canoeing, for instance, is not safe or possible for them. False expectations should not be raised, but neither should people be discouraged from trying, in safe situations, sports which may well suit them.

Flemming and Melamed[8] write, 'At this point it is sufficient to say that there is a psychological difference between team-competitive games and adventure sports, and that people who are attracted to one are often not attracted to the other. Thus, granted that sports have a rehabilitative value, adventure sports reach a new section of the disabled population.'

This applies also, of course, to non-competitive sports outside the adventure bracket. It is not unreasonable to assume that for many individuals, whether disabled or not, there may be only one sport that becomes significant in their lives, and that will often be the activity in which they perform best. People will judge their own best performances in different ways: one may be delighted to be placed fifteenth out of forty competitors in a table tennis competition with able-bodied opponents, while another may prefer to be first out of five in a competition for physically-handicapped people. Another may choose to sail without ever joining in competitions, and someone else may like playing golf alone. Variety in human sporting aspirations should be respected to ensure the maximum range of opportunities for sporting fulfilment. The message of the words which Wheeler and Hooley applied[9] to a school situation could be used of the whole field of sport for disabled people: '... the teacher must know his field so thoroughly that adapted physical education becomes a matter of choosing from a wide range of possible activities. He cannot be versed solely in aquatics or team games.'

But Lancaster-Gaye, chairman of the Sport and Leisure Group of the International Cerebral Palsy Society asks,[10] 'What about the non-competitive sports? Horse-riding, sailing, canoeing, swimming, climbing, camping—these are not new activities, yet lack of finance and lack of opportunity still seem to limit their popularity.'

Developments outside competitive games

During the first few decades of this century there were isolated instances of disabled people following a great variety of sports including cycling, angling, canoeing, camping, sailing and hiking. There is, however, a lack of information on the numbers involved, and it is impossible to establish the extent of this 'hidden' participation. Organized provision received much publicity and this has had an influence on the development of competitive, segregated games: in consequence it is not always appreciated how many other forms of sporting activity are possible for disabled people. A number of examples below help to illustrate the range of what has been taking place. It will be noticed that in many of these sporting activities targets of achievement are not vital; anyone who enjoys camping or angling is a 'winner'. Several of the cases cited involve activities which *may* lead participants, once they have gained in confidence and proficiency, to practise them in clubs or other groups with able-bodied members. It need hardly be pointed out that there are a great many medical and safety considerations to be taken into account in deciding which sports are suitable, and each person must be assessed individually.

(1) The Blind Outdoor Leisure Division, based at Aspen, Colorado, U.S.A., has a summer programme of hiking, climbing, camping, riding, fishing, swimming and ice skating. The winter programme includes skiing, ice skating and swimming.

(2) Groups where riding is taught exist in Australia, Malta, the U.S.A., Bermuda, Rhodesia, Eire, New Zealand, Lesotho, and the United Kingdom. Some of the organizations are quite large: the riders in one association in New Zealand number six hundred, and in a similar association in the U.K. and Eire there are more than four thousand five hundred. Disabilities involved include cerebral palsy, spina bifida, mental handicaps, muscular dystrophy, blindness, and limblessness.

(3) Six members of the Israel Defence Forces wounded soldiers rehabilitation programme attended a course to assess certain physiological and rehabilitative factors of sub-aqua (SCUBA) diving. Four were paraplegics (T4, T6, T12, L3), and two were double leg amputees. Although several paraplegics and leg or arm amputees had dived before, until this course there had been 'little formal attempt to define standards of diving instruction and diving qualifications so that disabled people may acquire safe diving training.'[8] The subjects also used snorkels, as have many severely handicapped individuals: choice of reliable equipment is essential in both sub-aqua diving and snorkelling.

(4) An army surgeon, Major Clark, reported on a group of single leg amputee soldiers who took part in a skiing rehabilitation programme in the U.S.A.: 'Physically, every one of the eleven patients demonstrated definitive, objec-

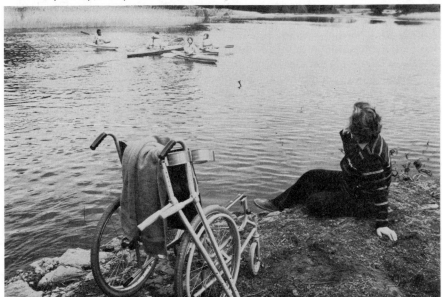

Fig. 28.3 Canoeing. Suitably supervised (as for the able-bodied) canoeing is an excellent physical recreation for the disabled with full control of their upper limbs. (Photo: Disabled Living Foundation and Town and Country Productions Ltd.)

tive improvement in strength, range of motion and/or decreased pain ...
all within two half days of this training. Mentally there was a singular and
very obvious change noted in every individual ... changes in deportment,
carriage and general attitude.'[11] The group who organized the programme,
the National Inconvenienced Sportsmen's Association, are concerned with
blind, deaf and neurologically damaged people as well as amputees. Trampolining, shooting, water skiing and snowmobile (motorized sledge) driving
are some of the sports of the association.

Ski courses for certain types of disabled men and women have been held
in Norway, Switzerland, Austria, Poland, France, Canada and Germany.

(5) There are many factors to be taken into account before it can be decided
for whom canoeing is suitable (Fig. 28.3). Participants have included men-
tally-handicapped children, paraplegics, leg amputees, people with quite
serious paralysis following poliomyelitis, and blind individuals who have
used double canoes with sighted companions. The physical education
adviser of the Spastics Society in Britain estimates that approximately five
hundred cerebrally palsied children and adults canoe regularly.

(6) Competitive and non-competitive rowing has suited those with visual
handicaps (accompanied by one or more sighted persons to row or cox),
cerebral palsy, and amputation of a leg—one rowing club had three one-
legged coxswains, one of whom took part in the Olympic Games.

(7) As an example of large scale provision for mentally handicapped young
people, the National Federation of Gateway Clubs in Britain provides
opportunities for table tennis, football, rounders, swimming, trampolining,
canoeing, riding and mountain walking. The Federation has over three
hundred affiliated clubs and twelve thousand members.

(8) Sailing has been widely practised in many countries, and one paraplegic
(T9/10 complete) has recently qualified as a sailing instructor. Blindness,
amputation of both legs or an arm or both hands have not prevented some
people from sailing in certain circumstances. A sailing catamaran which
will embark wheelchairs has proved popular in the United Kingdom and
other countries have been keen to copy it (Fig. 28.4). Motor boating has
obvious potential too.

(9) Levels of independence in tent camping vary from those who camp alone
to the organized camps where each handicapped person has at least one
helper, and medical staff are in attendance. Camps accommodated in permanent buildings include those of the Muscular Dystrophy Association of
America, at which professional staff make regular rounds in the night to
turn people in bed. Prescribed treatment and therapy are administered by
medical teams supervized by physicians. More than two thousand campers
with muscular dystrophy attend each year and undertake sports such as
swimming and riding.[12]

Through the Scouts, groups of boys with many different, and in many
cases severe, physical and/or mental handicaps are introduced to camping
throughout the world. In Canada and the U.S.A., the National Camps for
Blind Children organization runs about ten camps a year with an average
of eighty boys and girls at each site. The range of activities at the camps
is wide, including baseball (with a special ball), archery (with balloons as

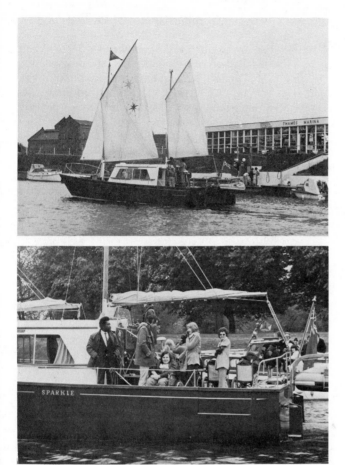

Fig. 28.4 (a) and (b) 'Sparkle', a catamaran which can embark wheelchairs. (Photo: Wey Studio, courtesy 'SPARKS'.)

targets), sailing, canoeing, gymnastics, riding, swimming and trampolining, as well as nature trail walks.

(10) It may at first seem surprising that one of the successful pursuits at the camps for blind children in (9) above is water skiing. Hundreds of blind boys and girls have been able to water ski and many get up on their first or second attempt. Obviously, boat handling takes on a special significance when the skier is blind or partially sighted, and instructors usually ski alongside to give signals to the boat. Reports have been received of one-legged water skiers in South Africa, Australia, Britain, Canada and the U.S.A., and people with leg handicaps through poliomyelitis have managed this sport.

A minimum requirement for water skiing is the ability to stand, but some non-ambulant individuals have used an aquaplane—a board towed behind a boat.

(11) One blind, handless man uses a rod mounted on a chest harness for sea

angling. Large numbers of severely handicapped men, women, and children fish with ordinary rods.

(12) Rambling and hill and mountain walking are growing in popularity both for individuals who go with able-bodied companions, and for groups of disabled people. The Colorado Mountain Club and Denver Association of the Blind join in a project called 'White Cane Hiking', in which blind people enjoy the sounds, smells, and touches of the mountains while taking healthy exercise. A group of blind people have successfully undertaken the long hike up Kilimanjaro, 19 565 ft (5963 m). A blind, one-legged man, and groups of cerebrally palsied people find hill walking possible. In Britain there is a thriving club for deaf mountaineers, and as well as walking, members of the club climb serious mountain and rock routes. A blind French woman, Colette Richard, rock climbed, mountaineered and caved, once reaching over 13 000 ft (3962 m) in the French Alps.[13] Geoffrey Yung, who had one leg amputated above the knee, climbed the Matterhorn before the Second World War.* One man who had one foot of shoe size 4 (European continental size 37), four sizes smaller than the other through poliomyelitis, walked over fifty miles in a day in rough country and was an active member of a Himalayan expedition. One of his friends took size 16 boots, and when walking side-by-side in the snow they left a very interesting set of tracks!

For those who use wheelchairs, wild country is rarely accessible except where motor transport can be taken over tracks and roads. Some special nature trails have been laid out in a few parts of the world, and the use of modern powered wheelchairs increases the opportunities of access.

(13) Leg handicaps as a result of poliomyelitis, amputation, etc. are common amongst cyclists and there have also been several one-armed cyclists. Tricycles are suitable for many, and are much used by cerebrally palsied people for races, slalom event and casual transport (Fig. 28.5). Blind people, with sighted 'pilots', ride tandems.

(14) Shooting does not provide the same amount of useful physical exercise as archery, but it must be remembered that there are more considerations than just what is physically beneficial. In shooting, as in archery, some disabled people have an opportunity to take part with able-bodied competitors. Generally the archer needs two reasonably strong arms and two hands (there are exceptions, including one-handed archers who use mechanical devices for holding the bow). Arm strength is not so critical in shooting, and a person with the use of one arm only can shoot a pistol; indeed the Hungarian pistol shot, Karoly Takacs, won Olympic Gold Medals in 1948 and 1952 shooting with his left hand after losing the other (with which he had previously been a National Champion).[14]

With a rifle mounted on a swivel stand and constrained to shoot within a limited area, blind people are able to aim by means of oscillators emitting sounds which change in pitch as the rifle is trained on different areas of the target.[15]

(15) Amongst glider pilots are single and double leg amputees, and people affected quite badly by poliomyelitis and cerebral palsy. One deaf and blind man wears a helmet with a cable by means of which his companion in a

*As in 1974 did Norman Croucher, a bilateral leg amputee: Ed.

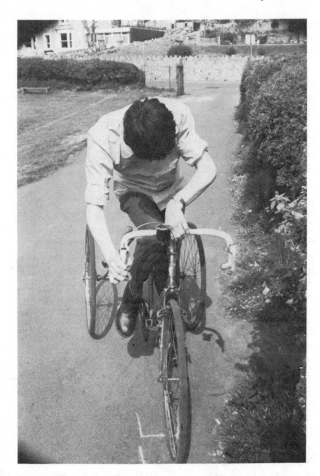

Fig. 28.5 The tricycle can be a most suitable vehicle for victims of cerebral palsy. (Photo: Disabled Living Foundation and Town and Country Productions Ltd.)

two-seater glider can operate plungers to tap the deaf/blind man's head. The taps signal how the controls should be moved at any time, and through this greatly modified form of sport the disabled man enjoys many of the sensations of gliding, particularly in a cockpit with no canopy.

Powered flying has suited single and double leg amputees and at least one paraplegic (T10, incomplete).

(16) Many instances are known of handicapped people taking a less physically active part in sport as passengers, and spectators and in administrative or coaching/instructing roles. Particularly bearing in mind the large numbers of elderly people who become physically handicapped, these aspects of sport are very significant. Unfortunately, access to and within spectator facilities, club houses, etc. is all too often poor or impossible. Gliders, boats, sand yachts, powered aircraft, sledges, and horse-drawn vehicles have all been used for joy-rides by disabled passengers. Danny Hearn (quadriplegic, C4)

since an accident while playing rugby for England, coaches rugby teams from a wheelchair.[16] A paraplegic sailing instructor has already been mentioned above, and there have been ski instructors with single and double leg amputations.

Thus a great many possible areas of participation have been explored. However, in several sports there has been little or no organized provision for disabled people in general. Many need at least a special introductory course at which they can try a sport on their own rather than join in with able-bodied people from the start. Of the illustrations given above, many are isolated examples. Disabled people with initiative have pursued opportunities on their own, but overall development has been uneven, with a bias towards competitive, segregated games. One reason for the unevenness of opportunity stems from the fact that organizers and doctors sometimes make decisions about the suitability of a sport based on a thorough knowledge of the handicap involved, but a lack of knowledge of the sport in question. They are rightly cautious, but may fail to take the next step of consulting experts in that sport.

The time is now ripe for expansion, for the gaps to be filled. It is not a partisan issue, not a question of non-competitive sport in place of competitive sport: there is room for both. Similarly, it is not a case of integrated sport versus segregated sport, although moves towards integration are welcome. New developments should not take place instead of competitive games, but as well as those games. More needs to be done in the area of competitive games and *much* more needs to be done about other sports for disabled people. The aim should be the provision of all sports for all disabled people, as long as the sport does not aggravate the disability or expose the participant to great risk. In some sports the risks must be weighed up and the handicapped participant may have to take part only in certain carefully chosen and restricted situations. Decades of experience have led to the adoption of commonly accepted (albeit sometimes hotly debated) standards of safety for the able-bodied. Similar but often modified guidelines need to be established for disabled people, and these may vary from person to person depending on the handicap.

The advantages of absorbing handicapped people within the social and sporting framework of ordinary centres or clubs for anglers, bowlers, archers, pistol-shooters or darts players are many. It is often the grouping together of disabled people which produces problems of access, transport, accommodation, etc., whereas the disabled sportsman with his problems may be more easily absorbed when spread thinly throughout the community. Further, a positive attitude towards the solving of individual problems is very necessary if people are not to be denied sports which are suitable for them.

Problems and solutions

Progress has depended to some extent on the solving of practical problems, and several notable solutions have been found. Mention has already been made in (15) of a deaf/blind glider pilot, in (11) of a handless angler, and in (14) of one-handed archers and blind rifle shooters. The rifle described was adapted for a handless man so the trigger could be pulled by means of a foot pedal. For a deaf and blind man the rifle was fitted with a tactile stimulator to replace the sound oscillators. One man with poor co-ordination who could not balance a canoe found the answer to his problem was a simple outrigger. Outrigger ski sticks help one-legged and other leg-disabled skiers. In water sports such as sub-aqua diving, canoeing and sailing, there is a danger of damage to areas of skin without sensation; protective clothing and padding of pool edges and parts of craft have been the solutions. The list of devices and modifications continues to grow, and includes Braille maps and compasses, devices to enable handless people to hold a bowling wood, ramps to prevent wheelchairs from marking bowling greens, wet suits made to fit arm or leg stumps, swivelling footboards for an oarsman with limited ankle flexibility, purpose-built seats for boat anglers, tracks cut in the snow for the skis of blind ski-tourers and adjustable back-rests on tricycles.

Lack of experience in a sport prior to the occurrence of disability is not a great problem, as many congenitally handicapped people have proved. Of amputee skiers Major Clark reported that they '... demonstrated commendable proficiency and progress in the early techniques of downhill skiing, traversing and turning, regardless of prior pre and/or post amputation ski experience.'

Some limiting factors

Medical conditions often preclude forms of sport, and in particular people with hernia, any degree of detachment of the retina, bronchiectasis, or moderate or severe heart disease should not take part in strenuous activities. Allergies may dictate where sports should be followed as much as which sports are appropriate. It must always be borne in mind that for diabetics small blisters and cuts may be serious as they may not heal. The usual dietary and insulin considerations apply to diabetics, and before exercise extra sugar in slowly absorbed form should be taken. For haemophiliacs, any sport with a risk of cuts, falls or bodily collision, or which requires great physical effort, cannot be advocated. Epileptics pose a particular problem and many factors must be weighed; the likelihood of fits and degree of control by drugs, the presence or absence of warning of an impending fit, and the outcome of having a fit in any of the circumstances which may be encountered in the sport must all be taken into account.

Many handicaps do not preclude participation but make certain extra precautions essential. For instance, because of the increase of the likelihood of spasm, and partly also because they may become chilled in paralysed parts of the body without realizing it, many disabled people should take part in water sports only in warm water (and for some the risk of spasm may always prevent participation). Protection of paralysed limbs has already been mentioned.

Certain handicaps which vary from time to time in severity, such as multiple sclerosis and emphysema, can mean that an activity which is possible on one day may not be appropriate on another. Obviously in many cases continued medical review of a person's involvement in sport may be necessary.

Double or multiple physical handicaps and combined mental and physical handicaps are common and may greatly narrow choice. But even if an activity has to be restricted, such as sub-aqua diving confined to a swimming pool, the psychological benefits of limited participation should not be underestimated.

In deciding on suitable activities it is essential to remember how much one type of handicap can vary in degree from person to person. Amongst paraplegics the range of ability, depending much on the site of the lesion, is very great. The same applies to leg amputees, and particularly evident is the difference between an above-knee and a below-knee amputation. The extremes of handicap grouped under the title of cerebral palsy are perhaps the most noticeable. It is impossible to say generally that all people with the handicaps mentioned can or cannot join in some sports; each individual's circumstances must be considered in detail. The medical adviser who has little knowledge of a specific activity may welcome the advice of experts in that sport. The merging of expert medical and coaching knowledge, and a certain amount of very careful experimentation in safe situations will establish what can and cannot be done. The temperament of the disabled person, as well as physique, will set the limits, and the availability of medical personnel, coaches, instructors, and helpers can be of paramount importance.

Calipers and prostheses create obvious hazards in water sports as they may cause wearers to sink. Even buoyant artifical legs cause problems because they may hinder swimming and affect the proper functioning of a lifejacket: an unconscious person lying face down in the water may not be turned on to his back by the action of the lifejacket if a buoyant leg is worn. A false sense of security may result from the fact that an artificial limb or caliper wearer is a very good swimmer when not wearing the appliance. It is usual in many water sports to remove calipers and artificial legs, but artificial hands and arms are frequently retained. However, no absolute recommendation can be made on this matter as there are several exceptions, such as experienced single below-knee amputee water-skiers and sailors who wear their lower limb prostheses. Intelligent, well-informed assessment of the hazards is vital in every individual case. For the doctor or coach the alternatives are on the one hand to deny a sport unnecessarily and on the other to sanction participation unwisely. The difference between being justifiably opposed to someone taking part or being prejudiced is not always easy to judge. Just as it cannot be said that cycling or hockey are *absolutely* safe for able-bodied people, neither can complete guarantees be given about the safety of some sports for disabled individuals. But certainly participation should not be sanctioned if there remains any unease about safety aspects after the medical considerations and the potential hazards of the activity have been taken into account.

Several sports are rendered possible for those with visual handicaps only by the presence of sighted companions: tandem cycling and rowing are examples.

Mentally handicapped people do not face the usual access barriers (unless they are physically handicapped too), but lack of supervisory personnel can cause them to be barred from facilities. For people with physical handicaps access to sports centres, spectator facilities, club houses, water spaces and the like can impose limits, firstly by preventing entry altogether (especially to wheelchair users), and secondly by restricting independent movement. Some people do not object to being lifted over rough ground or up and down stairs, but for reasons of dignity and safety adults, particularly, may dislike being carried. Even in buildings where access is possible, design often prevents ingress to certain areas like sports halls, toilets, changing rooms, spectator areas, bars and restaurants. For an occasional event people may prefer to be carried rather than be excluded, and unsuitable access is not always a valid reason for keeping them out. Several courses for disabled campers and sailors have been successful even though based in unsuitable centres.

Conclusion

Dialogue between the medical profession, coaches, instructors, administrators and the 'consumers' is much needed. In sports where participation by disabled people is not common, close medical supervision and a high standard of coaching is especially important. Well-meaning, enthusiastic leadership is not enough if leaders are insufficiently informed about the hazards.

While all suitable forms of sport should be encouraged as physically and psychologically beneficial, the encouragement should be done with sensitivity, for many disabled people feel that they are pressurized into doing what is expected of them. As Dr Roger Salbreux wrote,[17] 'If it is necessary to offer a wide choice of leisure activities to spastic children, one must try not to impose this on them.'

Unfortunately there is a possibility that the more diffident person will be frightened away by the real or apparent superiority of others, and while winners may be an encouraging example to many, the more some people are put on a pedestal the more others will be put off joining in. Naturally there will be champions, but the involvement of as many disabled people as possible in sport should be seen as more important than producing an élite group of winning competitors. Though the importance of medal winning should not be underestimated, more emphasis could be put on fun and exercise. For many, participation rather than perfection or excellence will be sufficient (Fig. 28.6). The attainment of difficult goals will be important for others, and while the goals should be within the bounds of possibility, not everyone can come first or achieve all that they set out to do. The success of a sporting programme must be judged not only by its best results

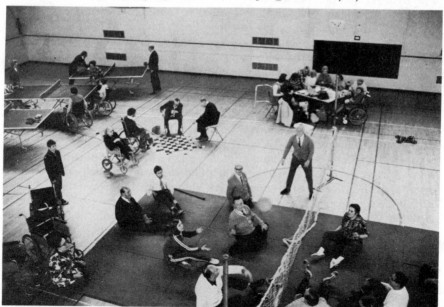

Fig. 28.6 'Participation rather than perfection'; with a wide range of choice. (Photo: Disabled Living Foundation and Town and Country Productions Ltd.)

in the shape of champions, but also by its physical and psychological effects on people of medium and low ability. However beneficial sport is believed to be, it is not imperative for any man, woman or child to *achieve* in sport. Indeed, while not detracting from the value of sporting achievement, it is important to steer clear of the prevalent feeling that the most worthy of disabled people must have a list of sporting successes or several medals to their credit. The picture must be kept in perspective: to hold down a job day after day, to run a home, to put up with pain, may call for far more courage and determination than to take part in games occasionally. Just like their able-bodied fellows, disabled people may not choose sport to express themselves and fill their leisure hours. Although they have less of an element of physical exercise, activities like chess, painting, music and crafts give opportunities for achievement and enjoyment equal to those of sport. Other leisure activities have in common with sport an element of physical exercise, e.g. music and movement, wheelchair dancing, field studies and gardening. These are already popular amongst disabled people and are likely to appeal to older men and women who may not be so attracted to sport. A large number of disabled people are active and receive quite a lot of exercise in their daily lives through walking on crutches, looking after children, using tools at work, and so on, but others have transport, sedentary jobs and a way of life which involves very little exercise. In consequence the need for sporting exercise will vary from individual to individual.

Disabled people are not a race apart, but members of the public are frequently accused of treating them as such. Yet how can members of the public be expected to react properly when within some games for disabled adults are seen organizers who treat the competitors like a separate, superior and different group?[18] It is *not* surprising when people with leg disabilities beat able-bodied competitors at archery; on the contrary, it is realistic to believe that they can. If they practise hard and become good then they are good archers, and their disabilities may have no effect at all on that particular sport. (It is another matter if they are handicapped in the arms.) While organizers make proud boasts such as, 'That man with one leg can beat able-bodied men at billiards, and we've got a paraplegic who won an award in archery which a lot of able-bodied archers couldn't get,' those organizers have no grounds for complaint when someone says, 'Isn't he marvellous' if a paraplegic buttons his own coat. The mistakes are of a different degree but of the same nature. Especially for the sake of the potential participant who may be nervous about joining in, difficulties and lack of difficulties should be portrayed as realistically as possible. The words of Wendell Johnson[19] are appropriate here: 'The astonishment with which many individuals regard a one-armed lawyer or a stuttering novelist recalls one of the more droll remarks of Artemus Ward: "I knew a man in Oregon one time who didn't have a tooth in his head, not a tooth in his head—and yet that man could play the bass drum better'n any man I ever saw"'

It is necessary to recognize that neither all able-bodied nor all disabled adults and children are suited to a system of segregated competitive sport for an élite group. The tendency towards the integration of disabled people in the community should be followed wherever possible, but voluntary segregation is not to be seen as necessarily undesirable. It needs to be questioned, however, particularly where no alternative provision exists. It must be remembered that to train a man in

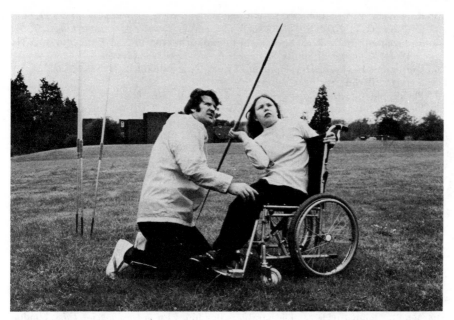

Fig. 28.7 Throwing the javelin from a wheelchair. 'A backwater where he competes only with a separate minority?' (Photo: Disabled Living Foundation and Town and Country Productions Ltd.)

a wheelchair to throw a javelin is to teach him a sport in which he can compete fairly against only a few other people in wheelchairs (Fig. 28.7). To train him to shoot or use a bow is to give him the opportunity of joining in with others whether they are disabled or not. The more he has a chance to measure his skill in fair competition against all-comers, the more he can feel that he is in the mainstream of life instead of in a backwater where he competes only with a separate minority.

It is not surprising that sport for disabled people should have grown in the twentieth century, for this is the century during which sport for the able-bodied has flourished.[20] The time has now come for further responsible development of sport for physically and mentally handicapped people. Decisions about risk will have to be faced. Anyone who has watched a game of wheelchair basketball will appreciate that there is some risk of injury; the idea that disabled people should never face any physical risk is unacceptable.

As much as their able-bodied fellows, and often more, disabled people can benefit from exercise, and what better form of exercise can there be than one which is enjoyed?

N.C.

References

1. Cochrane, G. M. (1967) Competitive sport in rehabilitation. *Br. Ass. Sport Med. Bull.*, **3**, 28.
2. Newman, J. H. (1852) *Idea of a University*. London: Longman Green and Co.

3. Karpovich, P. V. (1968) Exercise in medicine: a review. *Archs phys. Med.*, **49,** 66.
4. La Cava, G. (1967) The role of sport in therapy. *J. sports Med. phys. Fitness*, **7,** 57.
5. Strauzenburg, S. E. (1973) Sport in the therapy of internal disease, Proceedings XVIII World Congress of Sports Medicine, *Br. J. sports Med.*, **7,** 259.
6. Guttmann, L. (1973) Development of sport for the disabled. In *Sport in the Modern World*. Berlin: Springer-Verlag.
7. Pheidippides. (1973) Correspondence. *Br. J. sports Med.* **8,** 2.
8. Fleming, N. C. and Melamed, Y. (1974) Report of a SCUBA diving training course for paraplegics and double leg amputees with an assessment of physiological and rehabilitation factors. From British Sub-Aqua Club, London.
9. Wheeler, R. H. and Hooley, A. M. (1969) *Physical Education for the Handicapped*. Philadelphia: Lea and Febiger.
10. Lancaster-Gaye, D. (1973) In *Int. Rehabil. Rev.*, 2nd Issue, **XXIV,** No. 2.
11. Leaflet. (undated) National Inconvenienced Sportsmen's Association, 3738 Walnut Avenue, Carmichael, Calif. 95608.
12. Anonymous (1973). In *Performance*, the President's Committee on Employment of the Handicapped. Washington, D.C.
13. Richard, C. (1966) *Climbing Blind*. London: Hodder and Stoughton.
14. Jokl, E. (1958) *The Clinical Physiology of Physical Fitness and Rehabilitation*. Springfield, Ill.: Charles C. Thomas.
15. Anonymous. (1969) *Special Aids for War Blinded*. London: St. Dunstan's.
16. Hearn, D. (1972) *Crash Tackle*. London: Arthur Barker.
17. Salbreux, R. (1974) In *Int. Cerebral Palsy Soc. Bull.*, January.
18. Kipling, Rudyard (1923) The parable of Boy Jones. From *Land and Sea Tales*. London: Macmillan.
19. Johnson, W. (1946) *People in Quandaries*. London: Harper and Row.
20. Pollono, F. and Tessore, A. (1964) Physical disablement and sport. *J. sports Med. phys. Fitness*, **4,** 229.

Index